Vaccine Hesitancy in the Nordic Countries

Bringing together studies from across the Nordic region, this book examines the challenges brought by the COVID-19 pandemic, with a particular focus on vaccine hesitancy. Shedding light on the political tensions that emerged as a result of the pandemic and the debates that ensued both within and between the Nordic nations, it investigates the vociferous discussions surrounding the COVID-19 vaccines and their presumed negative side effects through the lens of trust; trust in and between the neighbouring countries, in healthcare systems, fellow citizens, and experts; in public authorities, politicians, researchers, journalists, and pharmaceutical companies. The first volume to explore vaccine hesitancy in the Scandinavian context, this ground-breaking volume offers fresh perspectives on vaccine scepticism not as a form of ignorance or lack of knowledge, but as a manifestation of a more fundamental lack of faith in modern government and science. As such, it will appeal to scholars of sociology, politics, anthropology, media studies, communication and cultural studies with interests in public health, popular and political discourse and questions of public trust.

Lars Borin is Professor of Natural Language Processing at the Department of Swedish, Multilingualism, Language Technology, University of Gothenburg, Sweden. He is the co-editor of *Approaches to Measuring Linguistic Differences* and *Constructicography: Constructicon Development across Languages*.

Mia-Marie Hammarlin is Reader in Ethnology and Senior Lecturer in Media and Communication Studies in the Department of Communication and Media at Lund University, Sweden. She is the author of *Exposed: Living with Scandal, Rumour and Gossip*.

Dimitrios Kokkinakis is Reader in Language Technology at the Department of Swedish, Multilingualism, Language Technology, University of Gothenburg, Sweden.

Fredrik Miegel is Reader and Senior Lecturer in Media and Communication Studies in the Department of Communication and Media at Lund University, Sweden.

Vaccine Hesitancy in the Nordic Countries

Trust and Distrust During the COVID-19 Pandemic

Edited by Lars Borin, Mia-Marie Hammarlin, Dimitrios Kokkinakis, and Fredrik Miegel

Routledge
Taylor & Francis Group
LONDON AND NEW YORK

First published 2024
by Routledge
4 Park Square, Milton Park, Abingdon, Oxon OX14 4RN

and by Routledge
605 Third Avenue, New York, NY 10158

Routledge is an imprint of the Taylor & Francis Group, an informa business

British Library Cataloguing-in-Publication Data
A catalogue record for this book is available from the British Library

ISBN: 978-1-032-30599-8 (hbk)
ISBN: 978-1-032-30600-1 (pbk)
ISBN: 978-1-003-30585-9 (ebk)

DOI: 10.4324/9781003305859

Typeset in Times New Roman
by SPi Technologies India Pvt Ltd (Straive)

Contents

Figures

Tables

Contributors

Sofie á Rogvi is a PhD student in medical science and technology studies at the Department of Public Health, University of Copenhagen. She has a background in public health and her research includes ethnographic studies of chronic disease care, reactions to the COVID-19 response, and transplantation medicine.

Lars Borin is Professor of Natural Language Processing at the University of Gothenburg. He is director of Språkbanken (the Swedish Language Bank), a national research infrastructure funded jointly by the Swedish Research Council and partner institutions, and the national coordinator of the Swedish activities in the European CLARIN ERIC research infrastructure. Borin is part of the Rumour Mining project team.

Bastiaan Bruinsma is a postdoctoral researcher at Chalmers University of Technology in Gothenburg, Sweden. His research topics and interests lie with voting advice applications, quantitative text analysis, and political methodology.

Joanna Doona is Associate Senior Lecturer in Media and Communication Studies at Lund University. Her research mainly concerns the intersection of the serious and the silly, through studies of popular and political culture, and civic engagement.

Tove Ingebjørg Fjell is Full Professor of Cultural Studies at the Department of Archaeology, History, Cultural and Religion at the University of Bergen.

Trine Krigsvoll Haagensen is Associate Professor of Technology and Society at Oslo Metropolitan University. Her background is in gender studies, media studies, and art history. Her main research interests include image theory and history, technology studies, visual culture, history of knowledge and surveillance studies.

Mia-Marie Hammarlin is PI for the research project Rumour Mining, a 4-year (2020–2023) mixed-methods collaboration with the goal to investigate rumours on- and offline surrounding vaccines as well as vaccine reluctance in a Swedish context. She is Associate Professor of Ethnology, and Senior Lecturer in Media and Communication Studies, Lund University.

Klaus Hoeyer is Professor of Medical Science and Technology Studies in the Department of Public Health, University of Copenhagen. He has his background in social anthropology and medical ethics. His research covers a range of topics relating to ethics, exchange systems for human biological material, and data politics.

Vetle Hove is a research assistant at the Department of Culture Studies and Oriental Languages, at the University of Oslo, as well as a master's student at Department of Culture Studies and Oriental Languages and Department of Philosophy, Classics, History of Art and Ideas.

Karine Aasgaard Jansen is a senior researcher at the Chr. Michelsen Institute. She has a PhD in cultural studies from the University of Bergen and was a post-doctoral fellow at Umeå University in the research project "Epidemics, Vaccination, and the Power of Narratives" funded by the Marcus and Amalia Wallenberg Foundation.

Katri-Maria Järvinen holds a PhD in social policy. She works as a postdoctoral researcher in the Data Literacy for Responsible Decision-Making (DataLit) project at the University of Eastern Finland. Her research spans from data use for public sector decision-making, construction of survey knowledge in research practices, working life, and vaccine hesitancy.

Mikael Klintman is Professor of Sociology, Lund University. His research interest is on the roles, values, and preconditions of people and organisations for making choices that reduce environmental and social harm. How people and organisations create, interpret, sort, and sometimes ignore/resist knowledge and insights in these areas is a central part of his research.

Dimitrios Kokkinakis is Associate Professor of Computational Linguistics at the Department of Swedish, Multilingualism, Language Technology, University of Gothenburg, Sweden. His research interests lie in the area of applied computational linguistics, natural language processing, and text mining. Kokkinakis is part of the Rumour Mining project team.

Aapo Kuusipalo is a researcher at Tampere University, Finland. He is a sociologist interested in contestations of health and well-being and is currently working in the VAX-TRUST research project, which studies vaccine hesitancy as a broad societal phenomenon across seven European countries.

Fredrik Miegel holds a PhD in sociology and is Associate Professor of Media and Communication Studies, Lund University. His main fields of research are youth culture and lifestyle, the sociology of culture, and civic culture and the media. Miegel is part of the Rumour Mining project team.

Johanna Nurmi is university lecturer in social sciences at the University of Turku, Finland. She holds a PhD in sociology and has focused on vaccine hesitancy and alternative health cultures. She has published multiple articles on these topics and edited the volume *Assembling Therapeutics* on alternative health practices.

John Ødemark is Professor of Cultural History with an emphasis on cultural encounters. His background is in cultural history, cultural theory, and the history of knowledge. He is the PI of the research project Bodies in Translation: Science, Knowledge and Sustainability in Cultural Translation.

Emma Ricknell has a PhD in political science and is a postdoctoral researcher in the interdisciplinary research group *A Questioned Democracy* (if-dem) at Linnaeus University. Her research focuses on social media, online communities, and disinformation.

Björn Rönnerstrand has a PhD in political science and is a researcher at the SOM Institute of the University of Gothenburg.

Tony Sandset is a research fellow at the Center for Sustainable Healthcare Education (SHE), Faculty of Medicine, at the University of Oslo. His research has focused on HIV/AIDS and the social and political aspects of prevention and the development of pre-exposure prophylaxis (PrEP) and its impact upon the HIV epidemic.

Jullietta Stoencheva is a PhD candidate in media and communication studies at Malmö University, Sweden. She is interested in the democratic backlash, proliferation, and transnationalisation of oppositional counter narratives across Europe. Her PhD project "Tracking, Attuning and Limiting the Spread of Extremist Narratives" explores the strategies for mainstreaming right-wing extremist narratives in Sweden and Bulgaria.

Jana Sverdljuk is a postdoctoral fellow at the Department of Media Studies, University of Agder, Norway. She has worked as research librarian and curator of migration archives at the National Library of Norway. She has a PhD from the Centre for Gender Research at the Norwegian University of Science and Technology (NTNU).

Pia Vuolanto has a PhD in sociology. She is an academy research fellow at Tampere University, Finland. She is PI of the *Addressing Vaccine Hesitancy in Europe* (VAX-TRUST) research project. Her research centers on complementary and alternative medicine, vaccine hesitancy, contestation of expertise, and controversies over health and the medical sciences.

Preface

The general background and scientific context in which the present volume is set is a research collaboration initiated a few years back, in 2018, between, on the one hand, an ethnologist (Hammarlin) and a sociologist (Miegel) interested in the phenomena of rumour and vaccine hesitancy; and, on the other hand, two computational linguists/language technologists (Borin and Kokkinakis), working in the general area of digital humanities, specifically in developing and applying language technological tools to large bodies of text in order to address research questions in the humanities and social sciences.

This collaboration resulted in a successful research project proposal – entitled *Rumour Mining* – receiving financial support under the Mixed Methods scheme of the Swedish funding agency *Riksbankens Jubileumsfond* (grant # MXM19-1161:1, 2020–2024). As the title of the project indicates, it is about rumour, notably about viewing the propagation of vaccination hesitancy encouragement on the internet as rumour-mongering. The second part of the title – *Mining* – is used in the special sense that this word has acquired in computing, where it appears in terms like *data mining*, *text mining*, etc. One central goal of the project is to develop methods based on language technology and artificial intelligence for reliably retrieving and classifying rumours and rumour threads on vaccination from very large text data sets (on the order of millions or even billions of words), primarily in Swedish and English. Our project thus mixes qualitative and quantitative methodology in order to investigate the form, propagation, and effects of anti-vaccine sentiment on the internet, primarily in various social media.

The topic of the present book emerged out of serendipity (although such a positively connoted term may not be the most appropriate under the circumstances): the Rumour Mining project proposal took shape in mid-2019, i.e., at the same time when WHO singled out the increase of vaccine hesitancy as one of the ten most important and urgent threats to global health. Thus, the project was conceived before the first cases of a new virus disease were attested in late 2019 in Wuhan in China.

Enter COVID-19, which understandably led to a partial realignment of the project goals: instead of studying vaccine hesitancy in general, we have focused on the rich material offered by the online COVID-19 vaccine discourse, as well as traditional media coverage of the same debate. In this volume, we have endeavoured to investigate specifically how this discourse has unfolded in the Nordic context, a distinct political and cultural entity from more than one point of view.

We extend our warmest thanks to Riksbankens Jubileumsfond, for the grant which has supported the research resulting in the present volume as well as enabled its open-access publication. Our thanks also go out to our respective departments (Department of Communication and Media at Lund University and the Språkbanken Text section in the Department of Swedish, Multilingualism, Language Technology at the University of Gothenburg), which generously have covered part of the overhead costs of our joint project as well as provided rich and stimulating academic environments for our research.

The members of our scientific advisory board – Fausto Colombo, Università Cattolica del Sacre Cuore; Elżbieta Drążkiewicz-Grodzicka, Lund University; Bernice Hausman, Penn State University; Lars-Eric Jönsson, Lund University; and Andrea Kitta, East Carolina University – have throughout our project given us their unfailing support and constant sage advice, for which we are more grateful than words can express. Last but not least, the volume editors would like to express their gratitude to our always helpful and unerringly professional editorial assistant at Routledge, Gemma Rogers.

Lund and Gothenburg, June 2023

Lars Borin
Mia-Marie Hammarlin
Dimitrios Kokkinakis
Fredrik Miegel

1 Introduction

Vaccine hesitancy and the COVID-19 crisis in the Nordic countries

Lars Borin, Mia-Marie Hammarlin, Dimitrios Kokkinakis, and Fredrik Miegel

Introduction

In 2019, the World Health Organization (WHO) singled out the increase of vaccine hesitancy as one of the ten most important and urgent threats to global health.[1] Infectious diseases like measles are returning in parts of the world, partly as a result of the activities of the anti-vaccination movements which have become more visible and vocal over the last decade, in no small part due to the new global community-building opportunities afforded by social media. Between 2016 and 2020 worldwide measles deaths climbed by 50%, a figure that might rise even more due to the recent coronavirus pandemic's negative effects on vaccination willingness in some countries.[2]

Truly global in scope and quite deadly,[3] the COVID-19 pandemic[4] changed the world as we knew it in a very short time. It largely paralysed international travel and even set some countries on something reminiscent of a war footing, with lockdowns, curfews, and other forms of tangible restrictions put in place and enforced – often in a quite heavy-handed manner – by governments. The pandemic's effects on the everyday lives of people are profound and long-lasting, spanning all dimensions of human existence: biological, political, economic, technological, cultural, and social.

In this anthology, we endeavour to address some of these effects and challenges by investigating the pandemic, despite its global reach, as a phenomenon that is handled, interpreted, and experienced at both a national and a regional level. We believe that this crisis cannot be fully understood without a thorough investigation of national, regional, and even local aspects of its consequences. Notably, surprising differences surfaced among the Nordic countries with regard to their official policies and communication strategies in the face of the COVID-19 pandemic.

For this reason, we have asked our contributors to investigate the reactions to the pandemic in different segments of the Nordic societies, ideally charting these in the context of the general notion of *trust*, a property often ascribed in the literature to all the modern Nordic societies, and with an emphasis on expressions of vaccine hesitancy.

DOI: 10.4324/9781003305859-1

The contributions that make up the present volume fall naturally under three general headings:

- *Nordic societal trust under stress*
- *COVID-19 in Nordic public discourses*
- *The growing chorus on the margin*

Even though the context in which the present volume was conceived is one of a mixed-methods research collaboration among its editors (see the preface to this volume), we have allowed the authors free rein with regard to their methodology, and we are happy to note that two of the chapters (Hammarlin et al., Chapter 10, this volume; Sverdljuk & Bruinsma, Chapter 11, this volume) indeed present studies where a mix of quantitative and qualitative methods is applied.

Nordic trust under stress

Background

There have long been many concrete grounds for thinking of the Nordic countries – Denmark (with the autonomous territories Faroe Islands and Greenland), Finland (with the autonomous territory Åland), Iceland, Norway, and Sweden – as constituting one community. Since the 1950s, they form a common labour market with completely free movement of its citizens over the whole Nordic area (the so-called "Nordic passport union"), established long before the EU's Schengen area. They have similar societies, which continually rank high in international surveys measuring values associated with modern liberal democracy, such as low levels of corruption, equality of the sexes, etc., and – significant in the present context – high levels of societal trust.

Despite this perceived unity, the Nordic countries chose to handle the crisis in conspicuously differing ways, causing heated debates both within and between the nations (see the contributions in Johansson et al. 2023b, in particular Blach-Ørsten et al. 2023). For example, distrust and political tensions between the Nordic countries came to the fore during 2020, explicitly addressed by the then Swedish Minister of Foreign Affairs Ann Linde, quoted in *Dagens Nyheter*, a major Swedish national daily, as saying: "I worry about how long these wounds will remain" (2020-06-14; our translation). What Linde among other things referred to was that the usually open borders between Sweden and its neighbouring countries Denmark, Finland, and Norway were abruptly shut down due to the pandemic, causing immediate negative effects for cross-border work commuters, and even disastrous effects for separated parents living geographically close to each other, but in neighbouring countries, who suddenly could not commute back and forth to maintain their families' everyday routines (Johansson et al. 2023a: 16).

Sandberg (2023: 46) notes that while there are clear recognised differences with historical roots between West (Denmark, Iceland, and Norway) and East (Finland and Sweden) Nordic administrative traditions, which are relevant in this context, at the present day the main dividing line in this respect runs between Sweden on the one hand and the other Nordic countries on the other. Consistent with this and notably, Sweden attracted global fame – or, perhaps, infamy – during the pandemic, by not locking down the country at any point, and instead putting trust into the Swedish people's willingness to observe, in international comparison, softer restrictions, with significantly higher mortality figures than other Nordic countries.[5] Sweden's strategies have been heavily criticised by both public authorities and politicians in the neighbouring countries, who chose to lock the nations down for many months.

The Scandinavians' willingness to follow their countries' established vaccination programmes can be related to a long-term historical development towards a social democratic, egalitarian welfare state model, which seems to have enabled the accumulation of an exceptionally strong social capital in this part of the world. Social capital can, in simple terms, be interpreted as a kind of societal lubricant comprising qualities and resources that facilitate collective actions and cooperation with ultimately beneficial effects on democracy and on civil morality, for instance generalised trust between people, social networks of different kinds, and an experience of reciprocity (Putnam 1993: 65–78; 2000). The Swedish political scientist Bo Rothstein has devoted a significant part of his professional life to the study of social capital, in particular social trust, which is an aspect of Putnam's original concept. The overarching question informing this body of work is this: *Which qualities in social relationships result in people's cooperation being based upon trust?* In several studies, Rothstein's point of departure is his own native country and Scandinavia more broadly (Rothstein & Stolle 2003), consistently found at the top of global statistics with respect to social capital and generalised trust among people (Rothstein 2007). In 2014, 64% of Swedish citizens answered in the affirmative to the assertion that "Most people can be trusted", a remarkably high figure, globally speaking, which has fluctuated only marginally over time. The same holds true also for Sweden's neighbours, expressed by the researchers behind the global survey in the following words:

> In one extreme, in countries such as Norway, Sweden and Finland, more than 60% of respondents in the World Value Survey think that people can be trusted. And in the other extreme, in countries such as Colombia, Brazil, Ecuador and Peru, less than 10% think that this is the case.[6]

Investigations show that the likelihood that people one does not know will behave honestly increases if public institutions function in the manner they are meant to. Expressed in terms of trust, one can say that if you trust the honesty of public officials, you probably also trust people in general (Rothstein 2013). In summary, Scandinavia is known for both its individualistic and its authorities-trusting culture, which makes the countries unique in many respects in a global comparison.

It has been claimed in the literature that the Nordic nations have developed an exceptionally strong connection between the state and the individual, at the expense of the relationship between the individual and the family. In this sense they are reminiscent of Germany, but the view of what constitutes the basic unit in society is different. In Scandinavia, the individual citizen is at the centre. It is towards him or her that measures and resources are directed, without going through the family or private organisations, protecting the individual from the risk of ending up in a position of dependency on spouses, parents, or charity organisations (Berggren & Trägårdh 2015: 82). As a consequence, Scandinavians have over time been able to develop an individualism which is exceptional in an international comparison, with independence and self-realisation as bywords, showing trust in authorities and public institutions by following rules and regulations, and at the same time creating room for the personal life project.

Arguably, the high level of trust purportedly characterising the Nordic societies described and discussed by scholars (see, e.g., Trägårdh 2013; Svedin 2017; Helkama & Portman 2019) is a defining characteristic of the *imagined communities* described by Anderson (1983/2006), defined by *acts of identity* as discussed by Le Page and Tabouret-Keller (1985). However, imagination gets increasingly strained as a result of globalisation and the changed conditions of public discourse. Similarly to the notion of a regimented *standard language* characterised by minimal internal variation (Milroy & Milroy 1985/2012; Joseph 1987), now increasingly showing cracks with hegemonic access by a small, privileged clique to the written word already long a thing of the past due to the internet, the very same communication medium also reveals unexpected diversity in the imagined communities that are our nations. In this context, we hypothesise that the high-trust community indicated earlier in actual reality encompasses far from all residents or discernible groupings of the Nordic countries.

In the literature discussing (societal) trust, a terminological distinction is sometimes made between *mistrust* and *distrust* (e.g., Kuusipalo et al., Chapter 7, this volume), although general language usage does not generally seem to make this distinction.[7] When attempts are made to enforce such a distinction in general language, *mistrust* is taken to mean 'suspicion or doubt based on feelings and instinct rather than direct experience', while *distrust* expresses 'lack of trust stemming from a specific experience or certain knowledge',[8] which approximately corresponds to the distinction suggested by Kuusipalo et al. (Chapter 7, this volume): *mistrust*, 'cautious, doubtful, questioning and sceptic mindset'; vs. *distrust*, 'established belief of untrustworthiness' (see also á Rogvi & Hoeyer, Chapter 6, this volume).

Nordic societal trust under stress: The studies in this volume

The chapters in this part of the present volume all make broader, more theoretical contributions to the general question of the relationship between (generalised) trust and the discourses and actions prompted by the COVID-19 pandemic in the different Nordic countries.

In Chapter 2, Klintman suggests that vaccination-related distrust/mistrust and trust are primarily adaptations to social environments rather than irrationality or lack of knowledge. He introduces the concepts of *Apollonian trust*, focusing on the issue-specific problem-solving potential of vaccination, and *Dionysian trust*, emphasising group identity and social cohesion, broadly similar to the *scientific–narrative rationality* dichotomy discussed by Engebretsen and Baker (2023) in the context of the COVID-19 pandemic. Klintman further argues on the basis of examples from Denmark and Sweden that organisations promoting vaccination have focused primarily on enhancing Apollonian trust, viewing vaccine hesitancy as irrational and often emotional. This may have worked against a reduction in vaccination hesitancy among groups whose hesitancy is rooted in cultural and ideological identity and hence amenable to argumentation invoking primarily Dionysian trust. Klintman further notes that experiments have revealed that merely providing additional scientific information – i.e., attempting to promote Apollonian trust – has been shown to have little effect on vaccination hesitancy. However, the solution cannot be to reject Apollonian strategies in favour of Dionysian ones, primarily because this is already done by unscientific and populist attempts aiming at increasing and spreading vaccination distrust, so that the public would be unable to distinguish between unscientific and science-based messages, and hence unable to make well-informed decisions about vaccination. Still, all is not lost: the image of science as an inherently self-correcting process – imperfect, but the best knowledge process we have – is relatively easy for people to translate into sound, social interaction, and Klintman consequently suggests that official accounts should strive to employ a combined Apollonian–Dionysian communication strategy, aiming at imbuing the public with a reflective trust in the process of science.

In his contribution, Miegel (Chapter 3) notes that while it is well-known and generally acknowledged that vaccines have potential negative medical side effects, researchers are equally generally in agreement that the benefits of vaccination far outweigh the negative effects, on the scale of populations. Drawing an analogy to the medical case, Miegel discusses *civic side effects* of public – in particular social-media – discourse on vaccination. His point of departure is that while potential medical side effects of vaccination are extensively discussed, and in particular stressed by vaccine sceptics, mass vaccination campaigns like the one related to the recent pandemic may also have considerable consequences for civic culture and democracy, brought about by an intense civic engagement on the internet. He describes and examines two notable

Swedish cases of such engagement – in both cases counter-campaigns waged primarily on the internet against the vaccines and against Sweden's vaccination strategy – and concludes that the ongoing public deliberation concerning vaccines and vaccination policies needs to be studied in a wider democratic context, examining the relation between knowledge, civic culture, and democracy. *Civic side effects* can be described as unintended outcomes of people's engagement in matters related to the vaccines and mass vaccination campaigns: formation of (online) communities of adherents to different beliefs regarding these matters; academic reactions to this engagement among researchers regarding the significance of such engagement for civic culture and democracy; and the dawning questioning of democracy as an adequate political system. Finally, Miegel identifies a basic social epistemic question common to these manifestations of civic side effects, viz. the relation between knowledge and democracy.

Rönnerstrand (Chapter 4) considers the COVID-19 pandemic as a problem that requires large-scale societal cooperation, which in turn relies on trust. Hence, Rönnerstrand explores the link between distrust and COVID-19 pandemic vaccine hesitancy. Drawing on two nationally representative Swedish surveys from 2021, two hypotheses are formulated and empirically tested.

Firstly, vaccine hesitancy is hypothesised to be linked to distrust. This hypothesis is relevant against the background that it is desirable to maximise immunisation uptake in the population in order to reduce overall morbidity and mortality.

Secondly, in order to achieve the public good of community protection against COVID-19, high immunisation coverage must be obtained also in groups with low risk of severe COVID-19 infection. Since trust is argued to stimulate cooperation for the common good, this kind of trust is theorised to be a particularly important driver of vaccination acceptance outside risk groups. Thus, hypothetically, distrust is particularly strongly linked to COVID-19 vaccine hesitancy among younger people and those who do not believe themselves vulnerable to the virus.

With regard to the first hypothesis, the results demonstrate that distrust is generally linked to vaccine hesitancy, also when controlling for potential confounders. However, the results are mixed when it comes to the second hypothesis, concerning risk factors as moderator of the link between distrust and vaccine hesitancy. In line with predictions, the association between social trust and vaccine hesitancy is stronger among people who do not (*subjectively*) perceive themselves to be vulnerable. But the association between distrust and vaccine hesitancy was not significantly stronger among younger people, as compared to people of average age in the sample, or older people, i.e., it is not sensitive to the *objective* risk factor age.

One way of interpreting this finding is that distrustful people who do not think they are subject to risk of a serious COVID-19 infection lack both personal and other-regarding motivations to vaccinate. They do not fear the disease, and they do not feel obliged to contribute to the collective goal of herd immunity.

The general methodological framework of investigating anti-vaccine rumour propagation using internet sources – in particular, social media – is broad enough to allow for many different investigative approaches. Looking at what we could call a genre-related aspect of this communication, Doona (Chapter 5) studies humorous vaccination and pandemic policy internet memes – which she refers to simply as "memes"[9] – to understand how memes as symbolic levelling construct trust or distrust.

Doona analyses humorous pandemic and vaccination memes in different meme-sharing communities on Reddit, in order to understand how memes and their associated processes of civic symbolic levelling construct institutional and interpersonal trust or distrust. Memes are polysemous, and their ambiguity is frequently used to create what Doona refers to as *ironic space*, where the uncertainty characterising the pandemic context – in particular that between trust and distrust and between analytical distance (characteristic of Klintman's Apollonian trust) and "myopia" (Klintman's Dionysian trust) – is expressed through humour.

COVID-19 in Nordic public discourses

Background

The contributions in this part of the volume look more concretely at public discourses on COVID-19, vaccination, and vaccine scepticism in the four Nordic societies covered in the book (Denmark, Finland, Norway, and Sweden). A common thread running through the chapters in this part is an ambition to contrast more "official" and more "private" public discourses.

COVID-19 in Nordic public discourses: The studies in this volume

Though vaccine hesitancy has long been associated with some form of assumed knowledge deficit on the part of the hesitant, not least in policy circles, recent research has suggested focusing instead on trust and trustworthiness in order to understand the choices people make. Inspired by this, á Rogvi and Hoeyer (Chapter 6) explore processes through which trust and mistrust in COVID-19 vaccines have emerged in Denmark. In their case study, they investigate how the official Danish narrative – referring to COVID-19 vaccines as a "super weapon" which would bring societal life back to normal, and refusal of which would be immoral – is reflected and countered in individual narratives collected through ethnographic fieldwork and interviews about the coronavirus pandemic and COVID-19 vaccination.

The picture of trust and mistrust which emerges out of their study is complex. Contrary to the frequently expressed view that vaccine mistrust grows out of a propensity to listen to conspiracy theories, á Rogvi and Hoeyer show that both supporters of vaccines and the vaccine hesitant share general doubts about the incentives and intentions driving pharmaceutical industry and global vaccine actors. The vaccine hesitant, however, also have more specific experiences informing their mistrust and how they make sense of the pandemic. They are unlikely to neglect these concrete experiences because of generalised appeals to "science": more and correct information will not diminish vaccine hesitancy by itself. When authorities or individuals shame people who hesitate to vaccinate, it will probably only make them gravitate towards those who accept them.

Kuusipalo et al. (Chapter 7) compare vaccine-hesitant and vaccine-critical discourses in Finnish mainstream media and alternative channels. In order to make this comparison, they introduce some theoretical terms: *confidence*, *trust*, *mistrust*, and *distrust*. Discourse characterised by *confidence* corresponds roughly to Klintman's (Chapter 2) Apollonian trust, mentioned earlier, while the other three terms all refer to his Dionysian trust. This fine-grained conceptual space allows Kuusipalo et al. to distinguish several different stances among these discourses, and to trace their fluctuations over time during the course of the pandemic.

Kuusipalo et al. identify confidence as the prevalent mode of trust-building in both mainstream and alternative channels. Thus, scientific references, statistics, and expert statements were utilised to build confidence in both sets of materials, although obviously with clear differences in the selection of publications, studies, and experts which were deemed valid and credible, as well as their interpretations (see, e.g., Santos et al. 2022: 162).

Trust-based argumentation also played a significant role, especially in the alternative discourse, where a distinct temporal shift in focus was noticeable from a predominantly mistrusting tone in the earlier materials to an increasingly distrusting orientation in the later ones. Vaccine hesitancy and criticism were generally not very visible themes in mainstream media discourse, and reports covering these phenomena often featured marginalising, mocking, and dismissive tones. These practices left little room for expression of critical views and pushed those wishing to express such views to form alternative channels of communication.

Chapter 8 by Jansen aims to increase our knowledge about vaccine hesitancy and trust in Norway during COVID-19, by comparing Norwegian public health communication during the earlier 2009–2010 swine flu A(H1N1) pandemic to that during the more recent coronavirus pandemic. She notes that in terms of Norwegian public health communication, there appears to have been a rhetorical shift from one pandemic to the next.

While public health has traditionally framed vaccine hesitancy as a problem to be overcome by persuasion instead of transparent communication and information, this can ultimately increase rather than decrease mistrust in health authorities and public vaccination programmes. Then again, transparency is not unproblematic and may in some cases weaken rather than strengthen trust in health care.

In contrast to the swine flu, the conditional transparency which characterised the Norwegian public health communication during COVID-19 proved to be successful. This time, Norwegian public health authorities appear to have recognised and reflected laypeople's concerns, rather than rejecting them. This rhetorical strategy may not have been possible unless trust in public institutions was not already as high as it is in Norway. In the case of COVID-19 communication in Norway, it appears thus as if the Norwegian public health authorities learned from previous shortcomings during the swine flu pandemic, a conclusion receiving further support from the study reported by Fiskvik et al. (2023).

Swedes are generally trusting of both government and each other, and are happy to count on government to provide the service and support needed to live a life where there is no need to rely on another person. Despite all the uncertainties coupled with the pandemic, and eventually the COVID-19 vaccine, Swedes remained trusting, and a vast majority accepted the vaccine. Ricknell (Chapter 9) has aimed to examine what happens when individuals interact with each other on a social media platform while under considerable pressure due to the coronavirus pandemic and in the context of an intense spread of both accurate and inaccurate information. The COVID-19 vaccine roll-out is treated as a critical test, and the online context is one far removed from the more extreme corners of the internet, namely Facebook conversations relating to the vaccine among local public radio listeners. Ricknell notes that individuals who were hesitant towards the vaccine, particularly those who felt apprehensive regarding potential side effects, were willing to make their sentiments public and engage in conversation about their views with others who had taken part of the same local public radio news story. After a period of such comments being relatively common while the vaccine was still being rolled out, they eventually declined in number, as did comments that were straightforward in their opposition to the vaccine. This highlights the importance of open and constructive communication between the public and professionals during a stressful time.

The growing chorus on the margin

Background

Societal trust is not a status-quo phenomenon, however, and a global pandemic is, among many other things, a political issue with implications for most citizens, which puts people's trust in authorities to the test. The various measures taken to restrict the spread of the disease have affected most people's private and professional lives. Hence, these issues have created a hotbed for intense and often heated debates and discussions about the strategies used to fight the pandemic not only among officials and experts, but also among the general public. The possibilities for people to engage civically in matters of importance to them are greater than ever; to give public voice to one's opinion is only a few clicks away on the phone, tablet, or laptop (Coleman & Blumler 2009; Dahlgren 2009, 2013). Social media like Facebook and Twitter[10] contain countless posts on the matter, inviting further comment, and on internet forums like Reddit and its Swedish counterpart Flashback, the threads dedicated to various aspects of COVID-19 vaccines are constantly growing. Generally regarded as something principally good and desirable in a democratic culture, the civic engagement regarding how the pandemic is dealt with by the governments, public health agencies, officials, and authorities raises important questions about the democratic implications of contemporary civic engagement. A significant number of the threads and forums dedicated to discussions about the pandemic are ruthlessly critical and impugning, which also in general is increasingly characteristic of civic discussions on the internet (Rosanvallon 2008). Rooted in a growing distrust in political institutions, experts, and authorities, it is possible to term this kind of engagement *counter-democratic*; negative judgemental and dismissive engagement is on the increase at the expense of a constructively critical civic debate. This culture of civic distrust, identified by Rosanvallon (2008), Coleman and Blumler (2009), and others, is particularly well demonstrated by the growing anti-vaccination movement's questioning of not only political decisions but also established scientific knowledge and research. It is clear that vaccine scepticism is not primarily a question of ignorance and lack of knowledge to be eliminated by information and education, but an expression of a much more fundamental matter, namely a decreasing "citizen faith in modern governments and medical science", as (Hausman 2019: 49) puts it (see also Klintman 2019).

The previously loosely organised protests in different parts of Europe against the various established national vaccine programmes, sometimes legally requiring people to take certain vaccines, were in 2020 and 2021 fuelled by pandemic restrictions and regulations, causing vast illegal manifestations and demonstrations of a more coordinated kind in many countries, e.g., France, Italy, Germany, and England, targeting COVID-19 vaccines and restrictions brought about by the pandemic. Clearly, antivax demonstrations are no longer a rare phenomenon in the public space, even in the Nordic countries; if they until recently were regarded as an American anomaly, they have now successively become increasingly spread over the globe, and to some extent normalised. The vaccination reluctance problem is as old as vaccines themselves; it comes and goes over time, depending on the general development in societies. The pandemic undoubtedly brought fuel to the debate, where the critical discussions concerning measles-mumps-rubella (MMR) vaccines seemed to be transferred and adjusted to the pandemic, making potential negative side effects of COVID-19 vaccines a topic on everyone's lips.

The growing chorus on the margin: The studies in this volume

Drawing on rumour theories and social cognitive perspectives, Hammarlin et al. (Chapter 10) aim to account for the purpose and spreading of medical rumours about mRNA COVID-19 vaccines. To this end, they study Swedish-language tweets spurred by the publication of a molecular biological journal article by a group of medical researchers at Lund University, Sweden. The Lund study has been widely interpreted as supporting an already-established rumour about mRNA vaccines, viz. that mRNA vaccines alter the human genome (something that the study's authors explicitly did not set out to investigate, and did not show). Hammarlin et al. (as also Sverdljuk & Bruinsma, Chapter 11, this volume) combine a quantitative distant-reading method – structural topic modelling of a large number of tweets – with traditional qualitative close reading and thematic analysis of the results of the quantitative investigation.

Their analysis indicates that scientific facts (such as those presented in the Lund study) are (selectively) used to strengthen the arguments for a vaccine-sceptic stance, and also that vaccine-sceptic rumours, including mRNA rumours, are based primarily not on ignorance, but rather on distrust regarding the officially sanctioned, positive narrative of new vaccine technologies, expressed through what Hammarlin et al. term *counter-scientific argumentation*. What is questioned is consequently not the science *per se*, but rather the official interpretation of the scientific results and the measures taken based on them.

In their contribution, and similarly to Hammarlin et al., Sverdljuk and Bruinsma (Chapter 11) apply a combination of (quantitative) structural topic modelling and (qualitative) thematic analysis, in order to analyse the COVID-19 vaccine discussion on Twitter during the pandemic based on a corpus of over 1 million tweets in English, and focusing in detail on the sub-corpus from Nordic countries (3,401 tweets), looking at the main discussion topics and the core arguments behind vaccine acceptance or scepticism, and whether the opponents and advocates of vaccination remained in the framework of social trust. They show that while vaccine supporters spoke of solidarity, sceptics were concerned with free choice.

Although the majority supported vaccination, the debate resulted in sharp political, philosophical, and value-based divisions between defenders and opponents of vaccination. The main problem, in many cases, was in the manner of communication and the inability to adhere to the basic rules of decency. There were instances of hate speech, disrespect, and othering. Especially problematic was the style of radical groups, which demonstrated mistrust at many levels towards others, medical institutions, and the whole of society. At the same time, representatives of the majority, instead of trying to include these groups in a meaningful conversation, made them objects of public ridicule. Thus, there was a noticeable acute lack of mutual respect and the ability to conduct a constructive dialogue between the two groups. Sverdljuk and Bruinsma conclude that for Nordic societies to maintain a basic level of trust, it is necessary to include various groups in decision-making and public deliberation processes based on respect.

Fjell (Chapter 12) notes that vaccine hesitancy is not a new phenomenon in Norway, but has a history going all the way back to the early days of vaccination in the 19th century. While trust in authorities is normally high in Norway, vaccine hesitancy does exist and is communicated by a heterogenous mix – right-wing groups, alternative health groups, and Christians, as in Protestant charismatic movements – uniting in the face of perceived authoritarian repression.

Based on material collected from traditional media (newspaper articles) and social media items (Facebook pages and YouTube videos), Fjell analyses COVID-19 vaccine hesitancy in Norwegian Christian charismatic movements. In addition to the familiar widespread vaccine hesitancy counter narratives, this community also presents counter narratives with Bible references – notably the Revelation of St. John – in an ostentatious demonstration of belief and trust in the Bible, rather than in some health advice presented by authorities. In part, Fjell attributes this to these movements' marginalised position in society, with a certain distrust of, and disagreement with, liberal values and authorities' scientific medical know-how.

Many of the cases of COVID-19 in Norway (as well as in Finland and Sweden; see Backholm & Nordberg 2023) have been in migrant and minority populations, prompting a debate about cultural factors in the spread of the virus. While it was regularly claimed that the Norwegian success in disease control was due to a high level of trust in the authorities, the spread of COVID-19 in some migrant and minority communities was moralised and interpreted as a lack of social responsibility on the part of immigrants by anti-immigration politicians. Liberal voices contested this interpretation and pointed to social and economic factors behind the spread of COVID-19 among migrants and minorities.

Ødemark et al. (Chapter 13) examine how concepts of "culture" were deployed in the debate about COVID and minorities in Norway in mainstream newspapers, notably that "culture" is what "others" (like ethnic minorities) have. Members of the majority were mostly held individually responsible for (not) complying with rules for social distancing. Moreover, Norwegian customs like Christmas celebrations and Easter holidays were seldom framed as cultural dangers for public health.

In this discourse, immigrants and their risk of COVID-19 infection are not only framed as marked by culture and cultural "properties" but are, also discursively marked through what they lack: lack of language skills; lack of health literacy; and lack of trust. Language barriers, low health literacy, and low levels of trust are all well-documented barriers to health care and can be seen as determinants of health, and also as promoting vaccine hesitancy. However, what is particular in this case is how "lack" is regularly framed asymmetrically as something that only immigrants have.

Summing up: Unity in diversity

The studies in the present volume together provide a kind of mosaic: rich in variegated detail when seen up close, but also with some more general patterns discernible if we take a step back and view it from a little distance away.

In particular, complementing and sometimes cross-cutting the three main themes of this volume, we find some additional common threads among some of the chapters.

The Apollonian–Dionysian dichotomy introduced by Klintman is also found (although not named as such) at least in Doona's, á Rogvi and Hoeyer's, and Kuusipalo et al.'s chapters (Chapters 5–7), as well as to some extent in Jansen's chapter (Chapter 8).

The importance of transparent communication and information on the part of public authorities for maintaining societal trust is stressed by both Jansen and Ricknell, and shaming and confrontational and exclusionary language are pointed out as unfortunately occurring and (obviously) inimical to trust-building, e.g., by á Rogvi and Hoeyer, Kuusipalo et al., and Sverdljuk & Bruinsma.

The authors of several chapters point out that vaccine hesitancy is due not primarily to lack of knowledge, but rather to lack of trust, inclining the mistrusting to reject, not scientific facts *per se*, but official interpretations of and conclusions from these facts (e.g., the chapters by Klintman, Kuusipalo et al., and Hammarlin et al.).

Related to the preceding, e.g., Kuusipalo et al. and Hammarlin et al. note that not only vaccine proponents, but also vaccine sceptics frequently cite scientific findings, statistics, and expert statements in order to build trust in their viewpoint.

All in all, the contributions in this volume paint a many-faceted picture of vaccine hesitancy in the Nordic countries during the COVID-19 crisis. They pose and answer a fair number of research questions, but the topic is enormous, and they also consequently point out many exciting future research directions.

Notes

1 https://www.who.int/emergencies/ten-threats-to-global-health-in-2019
2 https://www.who.int/news/item/12-11-2020-worldwide-measles-deaths-climb-50-from-2016-to-2019-claiming-over-207-500-lives-in-2019
3 Professor Azra Ghani of Imperial College London, as cited by O'Hare (2020), notes that "[a]lthough the case fatality ratio [of COVID-19] is significantly lower than SARS [severe acute respiratory syndrome], the spread has been much, much greater".

4 In the nomenclature used by the WHO, the COVID-19 outbreak is a *public health emergency of international concern* (PHEIC).
5 This narrative took an unexpected turn at the time of writing of this Introduction in early 2023, when Statistics Sweden on their website published commented statistics – widely noted in Swedish media – on excess mortality in Sweden during the coronavirus pandemic:

> Our summary shows an excess mortality in Sweden during 2020–2022 in the range from upwards of four to seven percent, depending on which of several measuring methods was used. Regardless of measure, Sweden and the other Nordic countries are among the European countries with the lowest excess mortality.
>
> (Statistics Sweden 2023; our translation)

6 https://ourworldindata.org/trust
7 "In their noun forms, distrust and mistrust are essentially interchangeable [in everyday usage]" (https://www.dictionary.com/e/mistrust-vs-distrust/; accessed on 2023-05-03).
8 https://www.dictionary.com/e/mistrust-vs-distrust/ (accessed on 2023-05-03)
9 As Doona (Chapter 5, this volume) mentions, the main sense of meme has drifted since the term was invented by Dawkins (1976), who defined it as

> a unit of cultural transmission, or a unit of *imitation*.... Examples of memes are tunes, ideas, catch-phrases, clothes fashions, ways of making pots or of building arches. Just as genes propagate themselves in the gene pool by leaping from body to body via sperms or eggs, so memes propagate themselves in the meme pool by leaping from brain to brain via a process which, in the broad sense, can be called imitation.
>
> (Dawkins 1976: 192, emphasis in original)

For her "internet memes", Doona cites a definition by Shifman (2014) which is narrower in at least two respects than the original sense; first, since it concerns only the internet, and second, because of a "created with awareness of each other" component, lacking from Dawkins's original notion of meme: imitation of an idea, etc., can certainly occur unbeknownst to its originator.
10 Since July 2023, Twitter is known as X. The chapters in this volume were essentially finished well before this date, and for this reason, references to "Twitter" and "tweets" have not been changed in the book.

References

á Rogvi, Sofie & Klaus Hoeyer. 2024. Trust, mistrust and data narratives about COVID-19 vaccines in Denmark: How people reflect on the past, present and future when navigating the pandemic. In Lars Borin, Mia-Marie Hammarlin, Dimitrios Kokkinakis & Fredrik Miegel (eds.), *Vaccine hesitancy in the Nordic countries: Trust and distrust during the COVID-19 pandemic* (Chapter 6, this volume). London: Routledge.

Anderson, Benedict. 1983/2006. *Imagined communities*. 2nd edn. London: Verso.

Backholm, Klas & Camilla Nordberg. 2023. Efficient authority communication in times of crisis: Examining how vulnerable language minorities experienced Covid-19 communication strategies in Finland, Norway, and Sweden. In Bengt Johansson, Ihlen Øyvind, Jenny Lindholm & Mark Blach-Ørsten (eds.), *Communicating a pandemic: Crisis management and Covid-19 in the Nordic countries*, 325–346. Gothenburg: Nordicom, University of Gothenburg. DOI: 10.48335/9789188855688-15

Berggren, Henrik & Lars Trägårdh. 2015. *Är svensken människa: Gemenskap och oberoende i det moderna Sverige* [Is the Swede human: Community and independence in modern Sweden]. Stockholm: Norstedts.

Blach-Ørsten, Mark, Anna Maria Jönsson, Valgerður Jóhannsdóttir & Birgir Guðmundsson. 2023. The role of journalism in a time of national crisis: Examining criticism and consensus in Denmark, Iceland, and Sweden during the Covid-19 pandemic. In Bengt Johansson, Ihlen Øyvind, Jenny Lindholm & Mark Blach-Ørsten (eds.), *Communicating a pandemic: Crisis management and Covid-19 in the Nordic countries*, 261–282. Gothenburg: Nordicom, University of Gothenburg. DOI: 10.48335/9789188855688-12

Coleman, Stephen & Jay G. Blumler. 2009. *The internet and democratic citizenship: Theory, practice and policy*. Cambridge: Cambridge University Press.

Dahlgren, Peter. 2009. *Media and political engagement: Citizens, communication and democracy*. Cambridge: Cambridge University Press.

Dahlgren, Peter. 2013. *The political web: Media, participation and alternative democracy*. Palgrave Macmillan: New York.

Dawkins, Richard. 1976. *The selfish gene*. Oxford: Oxford University Press.

Doona, Joanna. 2024. "Read the room Sweden": Memes, trust and vulnerability in pandemic engagement. In Lars Borin, Mia-Marie Hammarlin, Dimitrios Kokkinakis & Fredrik Miegel (eds.), *Vaccine hesitancy in the Nordic countries: Trust and distrust during the COVID-19 pandemic*. London: Routledge.

Engebretsen, Eivind & Mona Baker. 2023. *Rethinking evidence in the time of pandemics: Scientific vs narrative rationality and medical knowledge practices*. Cambridge: Cambridge University Press.

Fiskvik, Jannicke, Andrea Vik Bjarkø & Tor Olav Grøtan. 2023. Vaccine rhetoric, social media, and dissensus: an analysis of civic discourse between Norwegian health authorities and citizens on Facebook and Twitter during crisis. In Bengt Johansson, Ihlen Øyvind, Jenny Lindholm & Mark Blach-Ørsten (eds.), *Communicating a pandemic: Crisis management and Covid-19 in the Nordic countries*, 241–260. Gothenburg: Nordicom, University of Gothenburg. DOI: 10.48335/9789188855688-11

Fjell, Tove Ingebjørg. 2024. COVID-19, the mark of the beast, and the Last Days: A study on vaccine hesitancy in Norwegian Christian charismatic movements. In Lars Borin, Mia-Marie Hammarlin, Dimitrios Kokkinakis & Fredrik Miegel (eds.), *Vaccine hesitancy in the Nordic countries: Trust and distrust during the COVID-19 pandemic*. London: Routledge.

Hammarlin, Mia-Marie, Dimitrios Kokkinakis, Fredrik Miegel & Jullietta Stoencheva. 2024. Fearing mRNA: A mixed methods study of vaccine rumours. In Lars Borin, Mia-Marie Hammarlin, Dimitrios Kokkinakis & Fredrik Miegel (eds.), *Vaccine hesitancy in the Nordic countries: Trust and distrust during the COVID-19 pandemic*. London: Routledge.

Hausman, Bernice L. 2019. *Anti/vax: Reframing the vaccination controversy*. Ithaca: Cornell University Press.

Helkama, Klaus & Anneli Portman. 2019. Protestant roots of honesty and other Finnish values. In Kaius Sinnemäki, Anneli Portman, Jouni Tilli & Robert H. Nelson (eds.), *On the legacy of Lutheranism in Finland: Societal perspectives*, 81–98. Helsinki: Finnish Literature Society • SKS. DOI: 10.21435/sfh.25

Jansen, Karine Aasgaard. 2024. Uncertainty at the needle point: Vaccine hesitancy, trust and public health communication in Norway during swine flu and COVID-19. In Lars Borin, Mia-Marie Hammarlin, Dimitrios Kokkinakis & Fredrik Miegel (eds.), *Vaccine hesitancy in the Nordic countries: Trust and distrust during the COVID-19 pandemic*. London: Routledge.

Johansson, Bengt, Ihlen Øyvind, Jenny Lindholm & Mark Blach-Ørsten. 2023a. Introduction: Communicating a pandemic in the Nordic countries. In Bengt Johansson,

Ihlen Øyvind, Jenny Lindholm & Mark Blach-Ørsten (eds.), *Communicating a pandemic: Crisis management and Covid-19 in the Nordic countries*, 11–30. Gothenburg: Nordicom, University of Gothenburg. DOI: 10.48335/9789188855688-1

Johansson, Bengt, Ihlen Øyvind, Jenny Lindholm & Mark Blach-Ørsten (eds.). 2023b. *Communicating a pandemic: Crisis management and Covid-19 in the Nordic countries*. Gothenburg: Nordicom, University of Gothenburg. DOI: 10.48335/9789188855688

Joseph, John Earl. 1987. *Eloquence and power: The rise of language standards and standard languages*. London: Frances Pinter.

Klintman, Mikael. 2019. *Knowledge resistance: How we avoid insight from others*. Manchester: Manchester University Press.

Klintman, Mikael. 2024. Apollonian & Dionysian trust in vaccination. In Lars Borin, Mia-Marie Hammarlin, Dimitrios Kokkinakis & Fredrik Miegel (eds.), *Vaccine hesitancy in the Nordic countries: Trust and distrust during the COVID-19 pandemic*. London: Routledge.

Kuusipalo, Aapo, Johanna Nurmi, Katri-Maria Järvinen & Pia Vuolanto. 2024. Trust and the public vaccine debate in Finland before and during the COVID-19 pandemic. In Lars Borin, Mia-Marie Hammarlin, Dimitrios Kokkinakis & Fredrik Miegel (eds.), *Vaccine hesitancy in the Nordic countries: Trust and distrust during the COVID-19 pandemic*. London: Routledge.

Le Page, Robert B. & Andrée Tabouret-Keller. 1985. *Acts of identity: Creole-based approaches to language and ethnicity*. Cambridge: Cambridge University Press.

Miegel, Fredrik. 2024. Civic side effects. In Lars Borin, Mia-Marie Hammarlin, Dimitrios Kokkinakis & Fredrik Miegel (eds.), *Vaccine hesitancy in the Nordic countries: Trust and distrust during the COVID-19 pandemic*. London: Routledge.

Milroy, James & Lesley Milroy. 1985/2012. *Authority in language: Investigating standard English*. 4th edn. London: Routledge.

O'Hare, Ryan. 2020. Crunching the numbers for coronavirus. *Imperial College London News* (2020-03-13). https://www.imperial.ac.uk/news/196137/crunching-numbers-coronavirus/

Ødemark, John, Vetle Hove, Trine Krigsvoll Haagensen & Tony Sandset. 2024. "Infections without properties": Trust and cultural asymmetries in the Norwegian public debate about minorities and COVID-19. In Lars Borin, Mia-Marie Hammarlin, Dimitrios Kokkinakis & Fredrik Miegel (eds.), *Vaccine hesitancy in the Nordic countries: Trust and distrust during the COVID-19 pandemic*. London: Routledge.

Putnam, Robert D. 1993. *Making democracy work: Civic traditions in modern Italy*. Princeton: Princeton University Press.

Putnam, Robert D. 2000. *Bowling alone: The collapse and revival of American community*. New York: Simon & Schuster.

Ricknell, Emma. 2024. Where the fringe and mainstream meet: Discussions on vaccine hesitancy among public radio listeners on Facebook. In Lars Borin, Mia-Marie Hammarlin, Dimitrios Kokkinakis & Fredrik Miegel (eds.), *Vaccine hesitancy in the Nordic countries: Trust and distrust during the COVID-19 pandemic*. London: Routledge.

Rönnerstrand, Björn. 2024. Distrust and COVID-19 vaccine hesitancy in Sweden. In Lars Borin, Mia-Marie Hammarlin, Dimitrios Kokkinakis & Fredrik Miegel (eds.), *Vaccine hesitancy in the Nordic countries: Trust and distrust during the COVID-19 pandemic*. London: Routledge.

Rosanvallon, Pierre. 2008. *Counter-democracy: Politics in the age of distrust*. Cambridge: Cambridge University Press.

Rothstein, Bo. 2007. *Den sociala tilliten* [Social trust]. Det nya Sverige [SOM-rapport 41]. Göteborg: Göteborgs universitet, SOM-institutet.

Rothstein, Bo. 2013. Corruption and social trust: Why the fish rots from the head down. *Social research* 80(4): 1009–1032.

Rothstein, Bo & Dietlind Stolle. 2003. Introduction: Social capital in Scandinavia. *Scandinavian Political Studies* 26(1): 1–26.

Sandberg, Siv. 2023. The role of administrative tradition in government responses to crises: A comparative overview of five Nordic countries. In Bengt Johansson, Ihlen Øyvind, Jenny Lindholm & Mark Blach-Ørsten (eds.), *Communicating a pandemic: Crisis management and Covid-19 in the Nordic countries*, 31–50. Gothenburg: Nordicom, University of Gothenburg. DOI: 10.48335/9789188855688-2

Santos, Henri C., Michelle N. Meyer & Christopher F. Chabris. 2022. Reports of the death of expertise may be exaggerated: Limits on knowledge resistance in health and medicine. In Jesper Strömbäck, Åsa Wikforss, Kathrin Glüer, Torun Lindholm & Henrik Oscarsson (eds.), *Knowledge resistance in high-choice information environments*, 148–165. London: Routledge. DOI: 10.4324/9781003111474-8

Shifman, Limor. 2014. *Memes in digital culture*. Cambridge: MIT Press.

Statistics Sweden. 2023. *Olika mått på överdödlighet ger liknande resultat för Sverige* [Different excess mortality measures yield similar results for Sweden]. https://www.scb.se/hitta-statistik/artiklar/2023/olika-matt-pa-overdodlighet-ger-liknande-resultat-for-sverige/. (Accessed on 29 March 2023).

Svedin, Glenn. 2017. Den svenska tillitens historiska vagga [The historical cradle of trust in Sweden]. *Statsvetenskaplig tidskrift* 119(4): 781–801.

Sverdljuk, Jana & Bastiaan Bruinsma. 2024. COVID-19 vaccine discussion on Twitter: Topics of controversy and generalised trust. In Lars Borin, Mia-Marie Hammarlin, Dimitrios Kokkinakis & Fredrik Miegel (eds.), *Vaccine hesitancy in the Nordic countries: Trust and distrust during the COVID-19 pandemic*. London: Routledge.

Trägårdh, Lars. 2013. The historical incubators of trust in Sweden: From the rule of blood to the rule of law. In Marta Reuter, Filip Wijkström & Bengt Kristensson Uggla (eds.), *Trust and organizations: Confidence across borders*, 181–203. New York: Palgrave Macmillan. DOI: 10.1057/9781137368812

Part I

Nordic societal trust under stress

2 Apollonian and Dionysian trust in vaccination

Mikael Klintman

Introduction

Background

There is a widespread worry about vaccination hesitancy. The World Health Organization defines vaccination hesitancy as "delay in acceptance or refusal of vaccines despite availability of vaccination services" (World Health Organization 2015). Among those who worry about vaccination hesitancy, two different understandings of such hesitancy seem to be particularly common. The first is that vaccination hesitancy, especially the more stubborn kind, is irrational – a term sometimes used as a synonym for "emotional". For instance, the psychologists Zatti and Riva state that

> [i]t is … reasonable to think that the apparently irrational attitude of the so-called No Vax rests on a more archaic emotional rationality in which the bodily self opposes its defences to sub-microscopic attacks, entrenching itself on the principle of inviolability and integrity of one's body
>
> (Zatti & Riva 2022: 1)

However, if stubborn vaccination hesitancy were simply irrational, vaccination-hesitant people given additional scientific facts about the health benefits or risks of vaccination would change their beliefs about vaccinations only non-randomly, or not at all. On the contrary, experiments on vaccination hesitancy and other culturally or ideologically polarised issues, such as climate change or GMOs, indicate that polarised groups are not randomly influenced by additional scientific findings (Kahan et al. 2012). Between groups polarised on vaccination, more scientific facts contending that the benefits outweigh the risks of vaccination and that the risks are negligible for healthy people, either have a nonrandom effect of no change in the level of endorsement or hesitancy, or an increasingly polarising effect (Kupferschmidt 2017). Groups of people that are neutral or not highly hesitant to vaccination either stick to their position or become even more favourable to vaccination by such additional science-based information. However, groups of people who, on the other hand,

DOI: 10.4324/9781003305859-3

are initially very hesitant and whose social identity is connected to their view on vaccination also stick to their position or become even more hesitant with more scientific facts. Amit Aharon and colleagues, who from their research draw a similar conclusion of increased polarisation, state that

> the price of having a [highly] health-literate public is that some individuals, in this case, parents of infants, can show a high level of vaccine hesitancy and decide not to vaccinate their children based on their view that they are capable of making health decisions autonomously, albeit against the recommendations of the medical establishment.
>
> (Amit Aharon et al. 2017: 773)

The second understanding of vaccination hesitancy of the stubborn kind that leads people to avoid vaccination is that it can be best explained as a lack of relevant knowledge (cf. Motoki et al. 2021). However, this seems to be the case only among parts of the population, namely those initially neutral or somewhat negative to vaccination. On the other hand, people whose cultural, ideological, and group identity incorporates this hesitancy are likely to become even more hesitant once exposed to additional scientific findings indicating that vaccination is safe. Put differently, the "knowledge deficiency model" (criticised by, for instance, Rayner 2012) contending that more and better knowledge input makes all or most of the difference, is valid only among parts of the population whose hesitancy is moderate or low, and not deeply rooted in their identity.

How, then, can we better understand negative – and positive – vaccination sentiments and actions in a way that makes sense of the non-random but also non-linear influence that scientific findings have on people's vaccination sentiments and actions?

Aim and proposition

This chapter aims to develop such an understanding. It does this by integrating insights from sociology and evolutionary thought. By letting these insights provide us with a more nuanced conceptualisation of trust, some paradoxical findings about vaccination hesitancy can be turned into a deeper understanding. The proposition in this chapter is that vaccination-related distrust and trust are primarily adaptations to the social environments in which people find themselves rather than random irrationality or mere knowledge deficiency. To concretise this proposition, this chapter gives examples from the Nordic countries, mainly Denmark and Sweden. Whereas they are similar in terms of cultural and social structures, the Nordic countries have taken approaches that partly differ in what type of trust they have aimed at concerning trust in the management of the COVID-19 pandemic. It is beyond the scope of this chapter to make systematic comparisons between the countries' strategies, let alone make causal claims about their outcomes. The national examples mainly serve as illustrations. The rest of this chapter provides arguments and empirical evidence that help us assess this proposition's validity.

Structure of this chapter

The chapter continues by briefly exploring vaccination as a phenomenon. I highlight how vaccination goes against our human intuition in various ways. To understand and deal with these challenges to trust, we need to dig a bit deeper into the nuances of trust. This leads me to distinguish between – and explain – what I call Apollonian and Dionysian trust. Crucially, this is not a distinction between a "rational" and an "emotional" trust. Instead, it is a distinction between different kinds of rationality in which emotions must be intertwined. I hold that actors and organisations promoting vaccination programmes have so far focused primarily on enhancing only one of these two dimensions. This limitation has probably failed not just at reducing vaccination hesitancy among some groups; it may even have increased vaccination hesitancy among groups whose hesitancy is rooted in their cultural and ideological identity. To shed further light on how vaccination hesitancy (and its opposite) can be fruitfully understood as social adaptations, I then apply the principles of Apollonian and Dionysian trust to three vaccination concerns. These concerns, formulated as questions, highlight how crucial it is that vaccination programmes incorporate ways of stimulating convergence and integration of the two dimensions of trust among all socio-economic, ideological, and cultural groups when organising and communicating the programmes. The last section discusses ways for research, policymaking, and vaccination programmes to develop these insights further.

There's something odd about vaccination

When we try to understand why certain health and environmental topics seem more likely to be more controversial than others, it is sometimes worthwhile to reflect on how well the issues converge with our human intuition. This is particularly valuable concerning vaccination.

Consider the practice of sticking a needle into a perfectly healthy, innocent person – often a cute baby – and injecting a contaminated substance into her. Perhaps it's no coincidence that a vaccination injection is metaphorically called a "shot", and the injected substance is called an "enemy" substance. It's a bit like an armed invader infiltrating our camp (Klintman 2019: 114). Some argue that its counter-intuitive character is why misinformation about vaccination is easily spread and believed (Loomba et al. 2021). Intriguingly, the Danish Prime Minister, the Danish Medicines Agency, and the Danish Health Authority constructed an equally bellicose counter-frame of vaccines: people's weapon for defending themselves against the enemy, the disease. These politicians and authorities have called vaccines the "super weapon" and a "weapon arsenal, for instance" (á Rogvi & Hoeyer 2024, chapter 6, this volume). Elsewhere, counter-frames – albeit less aggressive – have been shown to influence some groups of vaccination-hesitant people significantly. There, the vaccination substance has been reframed to a benevolent agent strengthening the body's intelligence service (see Klintman 2019: 106).

Contamination and exposure to harmful substances is something humans are hardwired to learn quickly to avoid in the specific environment where we find ourselves. Even those who aren't hypochondriacs avoid the food they suspect is rotten, an avoidance that usually follows from a cringing face. This genetic hardwiring stems from million years ago – even before we became Homo sapiens. The brain systems that evolved to avoid contamination before becoming Homo sapiens evolved into preparedness to also distinguish between contaminated and uncontaminated people (cf. Douglas 1978). Moreover, evolution has also expanded this hardwired ability and inclination into a capacity to learn and act upon this distinction metaphorically. People, usually from an "out-group", a group other than our own, whom, in issues far beyond contamination, we sense don't deserve our trust, can give rise to a sense of aversion similar to spoiled food (Schnall et al. 2008; Skarlicki et al. 2013). This becomes highly relevant when discussing the significance of Apollonian and Dionysian trust for vaccination hesitancy and acceptance.

Consider, moreover, that this contaminated substance has been produced far away by complete strangers to us, strangers who operate in organisations whose main objective is to maximise the revenue for their shareholders spread around the globe. On top of this, the authorities who are responsible for controlling the safety of vaccines might – to be sure – be benevolent. But can't the multinationals pressure them to compromise with their scrutiny when they and the country they represent receive enormous financial carrots and sticks from the pharmaceuticals – threats of leaving the country?

Apollonian and Dionysian trust

The distinction between the gods Apollo and Dionysus is rooted in Greek mythology. It has several versions; the most well-known one was developed by Nietzsche (1872/2010).

Apollo's character is self-constraint, consciousness, long-term planning, and informed decision-making (Klintman 2012). In my interpretation, Apollo has an issue-rational drive. He wishes to assess knowledge claims systematically and without biases before deciding which option resolves the explicit issue at stake. It could, for instance, concern health, environment, personal comfort, private, financial gain, or peace on earth – anything where his goal is well defined and explicit. Importantly, Apollo is a visionary god with strong emotions and grand hopes for a better world. He pays his principal attention to the individual level – such as the individual's integrity to think independently – as well as the global, universal level of humankind, such as the need for worldwide morality, universal human rights, and so forth (Klintman 2018; cf. Kingsbury & Jones 2009). The middle level – consisting of the community, special groups, and sub-cultures people belong to and share their identities with, is largely irrelevant from an Apollonian outlook.

Apollonian trust, then, is the trust that we hold in the solid knowledge basis and issue-specific problem-solving potential of a specific arrangement, practice, recommendation, or obligation. In a world where single individuals cannot fully assess many short- and long-term risks they and others are exposed to, Apollonian trust is often directed towards people and organisations with particular expertise. Accordingly, they have access to the best available, science-based knowledge on preventing infections in a population.

But there is also the other trust dimension, the Dionysian, at least in pre-Nietzschean thought. It is a trust that subscribing to a specific belief, arrangement, practice, or recommendation and trusting those who represent this will benefit our inclusion and bonding with the groups we identify with (Kourvetaris 1997). At least as importantly, Dionysian trust is a trust that the beliefs, arrangements, practices, and recommendations we subscribe to benefit our distinction from groups we don't identify with.

The deeply social basis of Dionysian trust stems from the ancient Greek portrayal of Dionysus – the half-brother (or half-sister) of Apollo – as prioritising group identity over individual integrity and universal, grand ideals. It also means that Dionysus prioritises group identity and cohesion over Apollonian ideals of unbiased truth-seeking and systematically resolving explicit issues.

As some readers may note, the mental model of Apollo and Dionysus is partly similar to Daniel Kahneman's distinction between thinking slow (cf. Apollo) and thinking fast (cf. Dionysus) (Kahneman 2011). One similarity is the recognition that thinking fast and the Dionysian dimension are associated with increased activity in the older parts of our brains. The Apollonian side is instead associated with the more recently evolved parts of our brains, such as the prefrontal cortex (Reyna & Zayas 2014).

One difference between Kahneman's model and the Apollo-Dionysus model is that Kahneman, concerning the mode that he calls "thinking fast", largely overlooks the deeply social – indeed, "socially rational" – character of many impulses and intuitions (Klintman 2012). Since resolving explicit, substantive issues – such as preventing infections being what "ought to be" one of people's main concerns – he typically categorises "thinking fast" as simply irrational. In this chapter, however, I try to show how Dionysian trust can be better understood as a key part of what I call "social rationality" (see also Klintman 2018). Another difference is that Kahneman often portrays the role and function of "thinking slow" as correcting our irrational fast thinking so that we make more issue-rational decisions (Kahneman 2003). Such corrections occur now and then, to be sure, as when we go home and reconsider an overly spontaneous, expensive, and unnecessary item for our home. However, this Kahnemanesque process fails to explain how many people who identify as vaccination hesitant stick to their position or become even more hesitant after getting scientific information with overwhelming evidence of how the benefits far outweigh the risks of vaccination. Instead, what seems to take place is that we use our slow,

Apollonian thinking to find arguments and indications confirming that our Dionysian intuition was plausible and correct in the first place (cf. Mercier 2013). As I will explain, such confirmation, although not necessarily moving us closer to resolving the substantive issue at stake, has greatly benefited our social bonding with our groups, enabling cooperation and protection against enemy out-groups.

We have so far touched upon Dionysian trust's fundamental character and function. Still, it's fair to say that the standard strategy among governmental bodies to make us trust vaccination programmes is to appeal to and try to strengthen only our "Apollonian trust" in these arrangements, something that I will discuss later.

The following section will apply the principles of Apollonian and Dionysian trust to three common vaccination concerns. As the reader shall see, understanding and responding to them fully requires we use both Apollonian and Dionysian ways of thinking. These concerns highlight how crucial it is that vaccination programmes incorporate ways of stimulating convergence and integration of Apollonian and Dionysian dimensions of trust.

Three issues of vaccination concern

"What if the vaccine isn't completely safe?"

This question might run through the minds of most of us when we're faced with new recommendations – or even requirements – for getting vaccinated. After all, "if it ain't broken, don't fix it" is an age-old heuristic that has served people well in many areas of life. Furthermore, with the counter-intuitive character of vaccination, not least for our healthy and precious offspring, we may be forgiven for apprehending most practices that don't seem 100% risk-free.

Nor is it surprising that some people try to translate past, actual vaccination complications into significant risks with COVID-19 vaccines. An example of this is the swine flu vaccine. A decade before the COVID-19 pandemic, the swine flu vaccine Pandemrix was considered to have caused long-term side effects in the form of narcolepsy in rare cases. In their comparative media analysis of news media framing of the swine flu vaccine and COVID-19 vaccine in Sweden, Larsson and Kelly (2021) argue that a more significant proportion of news articles about COVID-19 vaccines mention the side effect issue. This is probably a response to the association people make between these very different types of vaccines.

What would Apollonian responses look like if their goal is to strengthen our trust in vaccination? A vulgar and dishonest answer is, "Vaccination is completely safe – don't worry!" A slightly more ambitious response is to provide people with a large, scale statistical picture contending that in the case of COVID-19, only, for instance, one in millions of people – and only people with previous risk factors – have gotten sick from the vaccine in question. However, as we know from the fear of flying, such statistics – if not increasing the fear – at least fail to reduce it (Clark & Rock 2016). After all, we can't escape the risk of being more significant than zero.

An Apollonian strategy that follows up on this recognition is to help us put vaccination risks in proportion. Proportionality is a crucial trait in the Apollonian dimension, as we can see in, for instance, classicist aesthetics. Applied to vaccination risks, the Apollonian strategy would be to make two kinds of comparisons. The first type is to compare the vaccination risks with the benefits to ourselves and others. The other type would be to compare vaccination risks with the risk levels of our other activities. It would soon become apparent that, for instance, moving around in urban traffic regardless of travelling mode is statistically more dangerous. The same is true with many other practices, from our eating and drinking habits to spending excessive time on social media, taking a short trip on a moped, or taking a horse ride (Epstein 2021). The idea is that providing people with such risk comparison will adjust their concern about vaccination so that it becomes proportionate to their concerns – or non-concerns – about the other habits. As a medical expert, the Finnish professor in medicine, Juhani Knuuti, claimed, for instance, that one is more likely to die from a lightning strike than to get a blood clot from a COVID-19 vaccine (Fagerström 2021).

Dionysian responses to reduce vaccination hesitancy would instead focus on our deeply rooted social concerns. Whereas the Apollonian strategy involves signalling what people ought to do, a Dionysian approach would focus more on "descriptive norms": what others like ourselves do (John et al. 2014). To some extent, the health authorities in the Nordic countries used descriptive norms to encourage people to do the right thing to prevent the spread of COVID-19. They used "social proofing" to promote the idea that most people were taking the necessary precautions and following the advice of health authorities. This included using pictures and video footage of people wearing masks, washing their hands, and getting vaccinated. However, the authorities used fewer directly group-specific, descriptive norms directed to particular age groups, ethnic groups, and so forth. Instead, descriptive norms of specific groups were more often implicitly communicated via, for instance, "ambassadors" in local areas, speaking the native language of the minorities in question. In Oslo, for example, such ambassadors not only translated factual information from healthcare professionals, but also collaborated with NGOs to build a sense of trust among the immigrant residents based on, among other things, a shared ethnic background (Brekke 2022).

Indirectly, group-specific, descriptive norms were signalled through specific practical arrangements. For instance, by placing vaccination buses in housing areas or next to large workplaces, vaccination becomes more convenient. It also makes it more visible that others like ourselves stand in line to get vaccinated. The COVID-19 vaccination buses and hubs visited residential areas in the northern and southern parts of the city of Malmö (Rämgård & Sjögren-Forss 2023). These areas are home to many minority groups and are close to public transportation hubs. This way could make people gain their Dionysian trust and a sense of belonging with those in line with whom we share many cultural and socio-economic characteristics. Another Dionysian strategy is to provide arguments that resonate with our particular loyalty to and priority of our family, friends, and small community: "You should think of your family and friends", said the Head of the Danish Health Authority, Søren Brostrøm, in his call for solidarity at all levels of society (Statsministeriet [The Danish Prime Minister's Office] 2021b). The concern for family and friends is typically mentioned with the addition that, unless we get vaccinated, we cannot visit the parts of our circle of friends that are older adults and ill (Abramson 2021).

"What if we act on current recommendations for vaccination that must be revised later?"

Whereas the previous question about absolute safety implies that the benefits and risks of vaccination can be correctly assessed by science, the second question refers to the fallibility of knowledge claims, including scientific ones. Most of us have probably experienced some science-based recommendations that have had to change, sometimes extensively. Areas of health and medicine are no exception (see also Klintman 2018).

Apollonian efforts in turning distrust into trust and endorsement of vaccination face an enormous change. In light of our deeply rooted binary sentiments mentioned earlier – of what or who puts us in danger or safety – the unique nature of science is complicated to get across to the part of the public that is initially very hesitant towards vaccination. Scientific claims about vaccination share a fundamental trait with all knowledge claims: They can, in principle, later turn out to be inaccurate. Therefore, a vulgar and dishonest response to this second concern would be similar to the first concern: "It's a fact that vaccination is safe, and far safer than not getting vaccinated – so don't worry!" More sophisticated, Apollonian efforts at turning distrust into trust must go much deeper than this. Here we need to explain that science, on which vaccination is based, is not about providing truth but about identifying probabilities while rejecting what is false. If scientific claims weren't, in principle, falsifiable, they couldn't be classified as scientific – only pseudoscientific (Popper 1959). The health authorities in the Nordic countries have been actively communicating to the public that science on COVID-19 is, and must be, probabilistic, and that decisions may need to be revised as new information becomes available. For example, in Sweden, the Public Health Agency has emphasised that their recommendations are based on *current* knowledge and the best *available* knowledge. This implies that science-based recommendations can change as new evidence emerges. In Finland, the national health agency has also highlighted the probabilistic nature of science and that decisions may be revised as further information becomes available. The Apollonian reason we should trust scientific claims, for instance, about vaccination is that it is our most trustworthy knowledge-generating *process*. Accordingly, science has the most knowledgeable people and organisations on medicine and health issues. When done correctly and without corruption, science is a continuously self-correcting process (Ophir & Jamieson 2021). The scientific community constantly scrutinises scientific claims, rejecting, modifying, or refining them through systematic processes according to universal scientific principles and norms. The appeal to Apollonian trust in science would hold that rival vaccination claims from religious or ideological groups, populist politicians, and so forth are instead based on opposite processes of confirmation bias, misleading claims, and so on.

The Dionysian response to the concern about scientific fallibility would, for instance, move beyond the abstract, systemic mode of statistics and scientific principles. Instead, the answer would occur in the so-called narrative mode (van Bavel & Gaskell 2004). Narratives, personal stories, and anecdotes align with our deeply rooted Dionysian dimension (Luna 2020). Throughout human evolution, we have survived by learning from stories, anecdotes, rumours, and gossip. Moreover, this has strengthened our group bond and helped us signal that we share norms and values with our groups and are trustworthy (Dunbar 2014).

"Why should we let others pressure us to be vaccinated?"

The third and final concern, contending that we don't wish that others put soft or hard pressure on us regarding vaccination, is even more multifaceted than the first two (Hausman 2019). How can it be answered from an Apollonian perspective? The standard Apollonian response would be that vaccination and vaccination programmes have been developed by knowledge-authoritative scientists and organisations that deserve our trust. An additional, Apollonian argument rests on universal morality and the democratic duty of the public. The former Swedish Prime Minister, Stefan Löfvén, said: "To all those who are now being offered time to get vaccinated, I really want to urge you: take your vaccine. Take your responsibility. The vaccine protects you, but it also protects your fellow human beings. Taking the vaccine is an act of solidarity" (Löfvén 2021).

The Danish Prime Minister's version had even more normative intensity: "[in] my eyes, there is no excuse – no moral excuse either – for not getting vaccinated … I can't highlight enough the unfairness in that a few [unvaccinated] potentially ruin it for most of us" Statsministeriet [The Danish Prime Minister's Office] 2021a; in á Rogvi & Hoeyer 2024, chapter 6, this volume).

The scientific expertise and the democratically elected political institutions and government organisations that take their advice from these experts must have the power to put at least soft pressure on us to prevent the spreading of infections. In such serious issues, the authorities need at least to ensure we don't cause unnecessary health risks to others. Intrinsic arguments against this kind of pressure are irrelevant from this Apollonian perspective. Such intrinsic value arguments would include attempts at adducing a natural right of complete individual independence (Koerth-Baker 2016) or rejection of vaccination based on its "unnaturalness".

The Dionysian response, instead, would focus on the word "others" in the stated concern. Accordingly, the basis for vaccination hesitancy tied to this concern is not a lack of knowledge and competence in the scientific community. Instead, it's the extensive distance people sense between themselves (in the groups they identify as their in-groups) and the institutions (out-groups) that research, develop, market, lobby for, regulate, and control vaccination and its various programmes. A significant part of this concern has to do with the institutions that are responsible for regulating and controlling the safety of vaccination. Some previous failings in fulfilling this responsibility – sometimes in other health issues, such as food safety – may also have created public distrust that spills over to vaccination (Falcone et al. 2022). The Dionysian response would be to turn the public sense of "others" closer to "us". One way is to use role models whom people feel are group members sharing their identity. Role models should be popular and well-respected among the vaccination-hesitant groups. Their message should be that they used to share the same concerns and hesitation as the people in this group, but they learned about some concrete cases of the devastating consequences of not getting vaccinated. These cases should be told as personal stories and narratives. Another Dionysian strategy is to develop programmes where citizens or organisations representing them – such as patient organisations – participate (cf. Klintman et al. 2022). There, non-scientific, ordinary people or their representatives could learn and participate in parts of the vaccination programmes, spreading their experiences to others in groups that share their socio-economic level and cultural identity. Something similar has occurred in southern Sweden, in residential areas, with many people born outside the Nordic countries. There, local governments have worked with non-medical community organisations and religious leaders to help spread accurate information about the vaccines and address any concerns or questions people may have. NGOs known and trusted by the local population from previous contacts on different issues have helped extend that trust to include vaccination (Rämgård & Avery 2022). A final Dionysian strategy would involve family doctors or clinics where patients go repeatedly and get to know the nurses and doctors. In the Nørrebro neighbourhood in Copenhagen, the government established vaccination clinics staffed by healthcare workers who speak the same languages as the local residents. Evidence indicates that people whose initial mistrust of vaccination can be turned to its opposite if nurses or doctors offer them vaccination they know from repeated previous visits (Greyson & Bettinger 2022).

Implications

Vaccination themes have traditionally been promoted with mainly or only Apollonian trust in mind. Apollonian strategies focus on the "substantively relevant" basis for trust in vaccination and the people and organisations involved. Examples include medical scientists in the Nordic countries comparing vaccination risks with other everyday ones, the latter of which is intended to be perceived as ridiculously negligible. A further example is campaigns that argue that we should vaccinate for the sake of *all* our fellow human beings, not just for the sake of people's community.

However, vaccination's counter-intuitive characteristics make it quickly become a polarised, controversial health issue. Such polarisation creates a need to share one's view on vaccination with one's identity group(s), a view distinct from those of one's out-groups. This makes it essential to follow the recommendations of Sturgis and colleagues, namely

> of looking beyond individual-level correlates of vaccine confidence to incorporate a consideration of how norms of trust and mistrust of science are produced and maintained in different social contexts.
>
> (Sturgis et al. 2021: 1533)

A simplistic conclusion would be rejecting Apollonian strategies and promoting only Dionysian ones. Dionysian strategies instead focus on "substantively irrelevant" factors. They include using personal anecdotes, bringing in non-expert role models, and reframing vaccination from a "shot" of an "enemy substance" into a "friendly intelligent service" placed in our bodies to protect us from new, enemy substances (as described by Klintman 2019). One problem with putting all efforts into Dionysian strategies is that this is already done by unscientific and populist attempts at increasing and spreading vaccination distrust (Pepping et al. 2021). Without working on earning Apollonian trust, through the health authorities' improved science communication and public scientific engagement, it would become impossible for the public to distinguish between unscientific and science-based signalling, and hence impossible to make the most well-informed decisions about vaccination.

Moreover, the Apollonian strategies have several features that help strengthen the Dionysian ones. These include the recognition that an isolated, scientific factual claim can always be false, whereas the process of science is self-correcting. Being a self-correcting process makes science superior to scattered and purely anecdotal claims about vaccination risks. The image of science as a self-correcting process is relatively easy for people to translate into sound, social interaction, an image that can become more widespread and transparent if we allow for greater public involvement in scientific processes in the health sector. The goal, then, ought to be a combined Apollonian and Dionysian trust that the processes of developing vaccination and vaccination programmes should not be blindly trusted. A better attitude to science would be a reflective trust in the process (cf. Boström & Klintman 2017): incessantly self-correcting, publicly engaging, transparent – imperfect, but the best knowledge process we have.

References

á Rogvi, Sofie & Klaus Hoeyer. 2024. Trust, mistrust, and data narratives about COVID-19 vaccines in Denmark: How people reflect on the past, present, and future when navigating the pandemic. In Lars Borin, Mia-Marie Hammarlin, Dimitrios Kokkinakis & Fredrik Miegel (eds.), *Vaccine hesitancy in the Nordic countries: Trust and distrust during the COVID-19 pandemic* (Chapter 6, this volume). London: Routledge.

Abramson, Ashley. 2021. Vaccine wars: How the decision not to get the shot is tearing loved ones apart. *The Guardian*, 28 August 2021. https://www.theguardian.com/us-news/2021/aug/28/vaccine-wars-decision-vaccine-tearing-loved-ones-apart

Amit Aharon, Anat, Haim Nehama, Shmuel Rishpon & Orna Baron-Epel. 2017. Parents with high levels of communicative and critical health literacy are less likely to vaccinate their children. *Patient Education and Counseling* 100(4): 768–775. https://doi.org/10.1016/j.pec.2016.11.016

Amin, Avnika B., Robert A. Bednarczyk, Cara E. Ray, Kala J. Melchiori, Jesse Graham, Jeffrey R. Huntsinger & Saad B. Omer. 2017. Association of moral values with vaccine hesitancy. *Nature Human Behaviour* 112: 873. https://doi.org/10.1038/s41562-017-0256-5

Boström, Magnus & Mikael Klintman. 2017. Can we rely on "climate-friendly" consumption? *Journal of Consumer Culture* 19(3): 359–378. https://doi.org/ 10.1177/1469540517717782

Brekke, Jan-Paul. 2022. Informing hard-to-reach immigrant groups about COVID-19: Reaching the Somali population in Oslo. *Journal of Refugee Studies* 35(1): 641–661. https://doi.org/10.1093/jrs/feab053

Clark, Gavin I. & Adam J. Rock. 2016. Processes contributing to the maintenance of flying phobia: A narrative review. *Frontiers in Psychology* 7. https://doi.org/10.3389/fpsyg.2016.00754

Douglas, Mary. 1978. *Purity and danger: An analysis of the concepts of pollution and taboo*. London: Routledge & Kegan Paul.

Dunbar, Robin. 2014. *Thinking big: How the evolution of social life shaped the human mind* (1st edn). London: Thames and Hudson Ltd.

Epstein, David. 2021. I'm vaccinated. I can't stop double-masking and wearing safety goggles. *Slate*, 15 June 2021. https://slate.com/podcasts/how-to/2021/06/how-to-cope-with-pandemic-trauma

Fagerström, Niklas. 2021. Rädslan för Astra Zenecas coronavaccin är kraftigt överdriven, påpekar expert – större risk att dö av ett blixtnedslag än att få blodpropp av vaccinet. *Svenska Yle*, 13 April 2021. https://svenska.yle.fi/a/7-1528045

Falcone, Rino, Alessandro Ansani, Elisa Colì, Marco Marini, Alessandro Sapienza, Cristiano Castelfranchi & Fabio Paglieri. 2022. Trusting COVID-19 vaccines as individual and social goal. *Scientific Reports* 12(1): 9470. https://doi.org/10.1038/s41598-022-13675-3

Greyson, Devon & Julie A. Bettinger. 2022. How do mothers' vaccine attitudes change over time? *SSM – Qualitative Research in Health* 2: 100060. https://doi.org/10.1016/j.ssmqr.2022.100060

Hausman, Bernice L. 2019. *Anti/Vax: Reframing the vaccination controversy*. Ithaca: ILR Press.

John, Peter, Michael Sanders & Jennifer Wang. 2014. The use of descriptive norms in public administration: A panacea for improving citizen behaviours? Available at SSRN 2514536. http://papers.ssrn.com/sol3/papers.cfm?abstract_id=2514536

Kahan, Dan M., Ellen Peters, Maggie Wittlin, Paul Slovic, Lisa Larrimore Ouellette, Donald Braman & Gregory Mandel. 2012. The polarizing impact of science literacy and numeracy on perceived climate change risks. *Nature Climate Change* 2(10): 732–735. https://doi.org/10.1038/nclimate1547

Kahneman, Daniel. 2003. A perspective on judgment and choice: Mapping bounded rationality. *American Psychologist* 58(9): 697–720. https://doi.org/10.1037/0003-066X.58.9.697

Kahneman, Daniel. 2011. *Thinking, fast and slow* (Reprint edition). New York: Farrar, Straus and Giroux.

Kingsbury, Paul & John Paul Jones III. 2009. Walter Benjamin's Dionysian adventures on Google Earth. *Geoforum* 40(4): 502–513. https://doi.org/10.1016/j.geoforum.2008.10.002

Klintman, Mikael. 2012. *Citizen-consumers and evolution: Reducing environmental harm through our social motivation*. London: Palgrave Pivot.

Klintman, Mikael. 2018. *Human sciences and human interests: Integrating the social, economic, and evolutionary sciences*. London: Routledge.

Klintman, Mikael. 2019. *Knowledge resistance: How we avoid insight from others*. Manchester: Manchester University Press. http://www.manchesteruniversitypress.co.uk/9781526135209

Klintman, Mikael, Anna Jonsson, Maria Grafström & Petra Torgilsson. 2022. Academia and society in collaborative knowledge production towards urban sustainability: Several schemes – Three common crossroads. *Environment, Development and Sustainability*. https://doi.org/10.1007/s10668-022-02564-4

Koerth-Baker, Maggie. 2016. Anti-vaccination might be rational, but is it reasonable? *Aeon Magazine*, 16 February 2016. https://aeon.co/essays/anti-vaccination-might-be-rational-but-is-it-reasonable

Kourvetaris, George A. 1997. The Dionysian and Apollonian dimensions of ethnicity: A convergence model. *International Review of Sociology* 7(2): 229–237.

Kupferschmidt, Kai. 2017. Can skeptical parents be persuaded to vaccinate? *Science | AAAS*. http://www.sciencemag.org/news/2017/04/can-skeptical-parents-be-persuaded-vaccinate

Larsson, Andreas & Joel Kelly. 2021. *Pandemrix – en brytpunkt? En komparativ studie om nyhetsmedias gestaltning av vaccin under två pandemier* [Bachelor's thesis]. Uppsala University.

Löfvén, Stefan. 2021. Facebook post, 14 May 2021. https://www.facebook.com/stefanlofven/photos/a.649223008451930/5882448555129323/?type=3

Loomba, Sahil, Alexandre de Figueiredo, Simon J. Piatek, Kristen de Graaf & Heidi J. Larson. 2021. Measuring the impact of COVID-19 vaccine misinformation on vaccination intent in the UK and USA. *Nature Human Behaviour* 5(3): Article 3. https://doi.org/10.1038/s41562-021-01056-1

Luna, Rafael E. 2020. The art of scientific storytelling: Framing stories to get where you want to go. *Nature Reviews Molecular Cell Biology* 21(11): 653–654. https://doi.org/10.1038/s41580-020-00293-y

Mercier, Hugo. 2013. Using evolutionary thinking to cut across disciplines. In Thomas R. Zentall & Philip H. Crowley (eds.), *Comparative decision making*, 279–304. Oxford: Oxford University Press. http://www.oxfordscholarship.com/view/10.1093/acprof:oso/9780199856800.001.0001/acprof-9780199856800-chapter-10

Motoki, Kosuke, Toshiki Saito & Yuji Takano. 2021. Scientific literacy linked to attitudes toward COVID-19 vaccinations: A pre-registered study. *Frontiers in Communication* 6. https://www.frontiersin.org/articles/10.3389/fcomm.2021.707391

Nietzsche, Friedrich. 1872. *The birth of tragedy*. Whitefish, MT: Kessinger Publishing, LLC.
Ophir, Yotam & Kathleen Hall Jamieson. 2021. The effects of media narratives about failures and discoveries in science on beliefs about and support for science. *Public Understanding of Science* 30(8): 1008–1023. https://doi.org/10.1177/09636625211012630
Pepping, Thijs, Menno Doorn & Sander Duivestein. 2021. *Real fake: Playing with reality in the age of AI, deepfakes and the metaverse*. Ludibrium Publishers.
Popper, Karl Raimund. 1959. *The logic of scientific discovery*. New York: Psychology Press.
Rämgård, Margareta & Helen Avery. 2022. Lay health promoters empower neighbourhoods: Results from a community-based research programme in southern Sweden. *Frontiers in Public Health* 10: 703423. https://doi.org/10.3389/fpubh.2022.703423
Rämgård, Margareta & Katarina Sjögren-Forss. 2023. *Erfarenheter av en lokalt förankrad vaccinationsstrategi i Skåne under Covid19-pandemin: Befolkningsgrupper som är svåra att nå*. Länsstyrelsen i Skåne. https://www.lansstyrelsen.se/publikation?entry=1397&context=18
Rayner, Steve. 2012. Uncomfortable knowledge: The social construction of ignorance in science and environmental policy discourses. *Economy and Society* 41(1): 107–125. https://doi.org/10.1080/03085147.2011.637335
Reyna, Valerie F. & Vivian Zayas. 2014. Introduction to The neuroscience of risky decision making. In Valerie F. Reyna & Vivian Zayas (eds.), *The neuroscience of risky decision making*, 3–8. Washington, DC: American Psychological Association. http://ludwig.lub.lu.se/login?url=http://search.ebscohost.com/login.aspx?direct=true&db=pzh&AN=2013-29104-001&site=eds-live&scope=site
Schnall, Simone, Jonathan Haidt, Gerald L. Clore & Alexander H. Jordan. 2008. Disgust as embodied moral judgment. *Personality and Social Psychology Bulletin* 34(8): 1096–1109. https://doi.org/10.1177/0146167208317771
Skarlicki, Daniel P., Joandrea Hoegg, Karl Aquino & Thierry Nadisic. 2013. Does injustice affect your sense of taste and smell? The mediating role of moral disgust. *Journal of Experimental Social Psychology* 49(5): 852–859.
Statsministeriet [The Danish Prime Minister's Office] 2021a. Pressemøde den 8. november 2021 [Press Conference, 8 November 2021]. https://www.stm.dk/presse/pressemoedearkiv/pressemoede-den-8-november-2021/
Statsministeriet [The Danish Prime Minister's Office] 2021b. Pressemøde mandag den 23. august [Press conference Monday, 23 August]. https://www.stm.dk/presse/pressemoedearkiv/pressemoede-mandag-den-23-august/
Sturgis, Patrick, Ian Brunton-Smith & Jonathan Jackson. 2021. Trust in science, social consensus and vaccine confidence. *Nature Human Behaviour* 5(11): Article 11. https://doi.org/10.1038/s41562-021-01115-7
van Bavel, René & George Gaskell. 2004. Narrative and systemic modes of economic thinking. *Culture & Psychology* 10(4): 417–439. https://doi.org/10.1177/1354067X04042892
World Health Organization. 2015. *Vaccine hesitancy A growing challenge for immunization programmes*. 18 August 2015. https://www.who.int/news/item/18-08-2015-vaccine-hesitancy-a-growing-challenge-for-immunization-programmes
Zatti, Alberto & Nicoletta Riva. 2022. Anguish and fears about attitude towards Covid-19 vaccines: Contrasts between yes and no vax. *Discover Psychology* 2(1): 26. https://doi.org/10.1007/s44202-022-00038-2

3 Civic side effects

Fredrik Miegel

Introduction

One of the most common fears and uncertainties regarding vaccines is the risk of side effects. These are usually taken to be the unforeseen medical consequences besides the ones intended with the vaccine. Even though they can be beneficial, the term usually refers to unwanted outcomes of a more or less harmful nature. Alongside such medicinal side effects, mass vaccination campaigns like the one carried out during the COVID-19 pandemic also affect society and culture in different ways. My aim in this chapter is to broaden the notion of side effects so that it captures also unintended social epistemic and civic processes resulting from the public's management of a major societal issue such as the pandemic and the mass vaccination strategy used to fight it. Just like the medical ones, the civic side effects can be advantageous as well as undesirable, but analogous to the predominant negative connotations regarding the former, it is the potentially problematic outcomes of the latter that I use the term to refer to in this chapter. This conceptual expansion has become increasingly important in today's media-saturated society, in which information of all degrees of truth and falsity is spread among people in and between the various social networks and communities they are part of. Metaphorically, the public engagement in debates regarding vaccination and vaccination policies can be seen as a civic side effect with consequences for the public deliberations citizens engage in, and hence for the status of democracy. The main purpose of this chapter is, thus, to suggest an extended framework for understanding the consequences of the sentiments expressed in civic debates on the internet regarding matters experienced as contentious by the public.

I start with a brief discussion about trust in certain knowledge pretensions as a key property of the engagement in communities on the internet dedicated to the vaccine and vaccination question. The epistemic aspect of vaccine-hesitant engagement is then elaborated in a section inspired by a pragmatist view that the ambition to eliminate doubt and uncertainty constitutes a crucial motive for participating in communities and forums trying to bring order in ambiguous matters. Thereafter, I proceed to two Swedish examples of organised civic engagement regarding the COVID-19 vaccines

DOI: 10.4324/9781003305859-4

and vaccination policies and discuss the social epistemological and civic implications they may have. The analysis of the two cases is followed by a reflection based on the academic discussion about the effects of an increasingly unstable concept of knowledge for democracy and its future. I conclude by identifying three crucial civic side effects spawned by public engagement in complex social matters.

Civic culture, knowledge, and trust

The nature and content of popular engagement in public matters constitute what Dahlgren (2003, 2009) calls the civic culture of society. According to him, it is a multidimensional concept of knowledge and skills, values, trust, practices, and identities (see Dahlgren 2003). Although to some extent I will touch upon all five dimensions as they are interrelated, my prime focus is on the epistemological aspect of them in relation to trust.

Taking this path means entering the realm of social epistemology, that is broadly speaking, the idea that there is an essential community aspect of knowledge (e.g., Goldman 1999; Fuller 2002; Brady & Fricker 2016; Fricker et al. 2020). Since people base their convictions and opinions on what they perceive as knowledge, the social epistemological dimension of civic culture is crucial for fully understanding the public debates and disputes regarding COVID-19 vaccination. As Hausman (2019) points out, vaccine hesitancy is not primarily a medical controversy in the public sphere. It cannot, therefore, simply be informed away with scientific knowledge by medical or other experts. Problematising the ways in which the COVID-19 pandemic was framed as, and reduced to, a primarily medical issue in most countries, Mormina (2022) argues that an epistemic injustice (Fricker 2007) is done to the complexity of an issue that involves equally important social, cultural, political, and economic factors. Neglecting the importance of these factors when trying to make sense of vaccination-sceptical sentiments expressed in the public debates is, as Hausman (2019: 2) perspicaciously points out, to misunderstand a social controversy as a medical one, with consequences for how the scepticism towards vaccines and vaccination is addressed.

> [A] social controversy is something that must be addressed by social means – by social interaction, by community decision-making, by democratic deliberation and lawmaking, for example. It cannot be addressed by scientific or biomedical data dumped into the public sphere – it represents a problem in society that requires a social solution.
>
> (Hausman 2019: 2)

Similarly, the vaccination-critical attitudes voiced in the public discussions cannot be explained away as resulting from missing or flawed medical or scientific knowledge. As a social phenomenon, knowledge depends heavily on trust among the members of a community. To persist, such trust must be rooted in communal knowledge (Milner 2002: 39). Therefore, these two dimensions of civic culture are virtually inseparable, as Hardwig (1991) points out:

> [T]hose who do not trust cannot know; those who do not trust cannot have the best evidence for their beliefs. In an important sense, then, trust is often epistemologically even more basic than empirical data or logical arguments: the data and the arguments are available only through trust. If the metaphor of foundation is still useful, the trustworthiness of members of epistemic communities is the ultimate foundation for much of our knowledge.
>
> (Hardwig 1991: 693–694)

The communities in which knowledge is generated, sustained, and disseminated can, as Goldman (1999: 4) argues, be everything from small groups of friends or colleagues to an entire society. What is important is the dimension of sociality of the collaborative social paths that lead to what we take as knowledge, how information and/or misinformation are distributed among the members of a community Goldman (1999: 4).

In today's media saturated society, the possibilities to establish epistemic communities of various types are virtually unlimited. Since in principle all humankind was affected by the pandemic and the various measures taken by governments and other authorities to reduce the harm it caused individuals as well as society, it was a source of immediate concern for most people's daily lives. Unsurprisingly, it soon incited heated debates and discussions on social media platforms like Twitter and Facebook and on forums such as Reddit and the Swedish equivalent Flashback. Whereas the content in many of the forum threads dedicated to vaccine and vaccination matters is momentary, disorganised, unstructured, and disjointed, more enduring, organised, and cohesive endeavours to both promote and oppose the vaccine as such, as well as the applied vaccination policies, have also emerged. Although both types of engagement are civically valuable, the impact of the latter on the public debate and thus on the civic culture is deliberate and more profound. Such engagement constitutes forms of networked social movements (cf. Castells 2012) with explicit agendas and knowledge claims. It involves recruiting members and supporters, opposing the current state of affairs, participating in public debates and discussions, and so on. Thereby it contributes to shape and define the content, form, and direction of the public discourse regarding the issue and, in the long run, civic talk in general. It is in this capacity that civic engagement in social matters such as vaccines and vaccination policies can be understood as civic side effects. Needless to say, the willingness of the public to critically engage in public debates on political, social, and cultural matters is a characteristic of a vital and well-functioning democracy, and engagement in the vaccination debate is no exception in that respect.

Theoretical points of departure

The debates between adherents and opponents to vaccination is about trust or lack thereof in the dominant scientific as well as public opinion regarding the matter. That shared views on a substantial set of "truths" is a prerequisite for the social cohesion of a society or community is a sociological commonplace. The trust in such factual truths, as they are commonly called, is, according to several contemporary social scientists, exposed to increasing threats owing to the abilities of the internet to momentarily reach multitudes of people with true as well as false assertions. As a result, society moves in a more sceptical direction, Sunstein claims (2014b); becoming increasingly a society of mistrust with populism as the most rapidly growing ideology, Rosanvallon argues (2008, 2021); and where adherents of alternative facts challenge for political dominance, McIntyre fears (2018). Instead of taking mistrust and belief in false assertions or alternative facts as the opposite of trust in the prevailing knowledge, the concept of doubt is arguably better suited to capture the many facets of vaccination-sceptical sentiments.

The concept of doubt is epistemologically important precisely because it is a fundamental aspect of how we conceive of reality. The core of this idea was formulated by Charles Sanders Peirce (1877/1992), who suggested that our conceptions, or knowledge, of reality principally consist of beliefs that have become fixed within a community as a result of systematic inquiry and communication of ideas perceived as facts. In brief, he argued that doubt constitutes unpleasant and annoying states of mind, which urge people to try to get rid of it and substitute it with a state of belief. The annoyance caused by doubt thus sparks the kind of inquiry he saw as the sole function of our thinking. Human beings pursue this kind of inquiry until a new belief becomes fixed and settles the irritation caused by doubt. Since thinking, according to Peirce, is always done within a community presupposing continuous communication between the single thinkers, the beliefs we settle on are always the product of a collective effort aiming to solve and help us cope with the actual problems we encounter in our lives. Herein lies implicitly also the idea that doubt management is a profoundly communicative process. Peirce insisted that doubt management is not about the hypothetical questioning of everything à la Descartes, but concern actual doubts (1877/1992).

This emphasis on the communicative endeavours of eliminating actual doubts remains a cornerstone in pragmatist epistemology. The societal implications of the pragmatist idea of communicative doubt management are apparent in, for instance, Habermas's (1985) *Theory of Communicative Action*, when he argues that social order results and depend on the ability of the citizens to acknowledge and consider each other's viewpoints (see also Selk and Jörke 2020). Most prominently, however, the civic importance of communicative doubt management and its relation to knowledge formation is expressed by John Dewey (1916/1966: 5) when he argues that "[n]ot only is social life identical with communication, but all communication (and hence all genuine social life) is educative".

Since our actions are motivated by knowledge, or the lack thereof, the relation between doubt and knowledge is, thus, essential to study if we want to understand what is going on in the vaccine debates on the internet. Following Dewey (1910/1991: 39), we can see the ongoing vaccine debate as an intellectual discussion with the function and "power to start and direct significant inquiry and reflection". To use a concept that he favoured in his moral theory, intelligence in inquiry is a question of "conscientiousness", that is the proficiency in judging the significance of what we are doing and to use that judgement to direct what we do (Goldman 2012: 20).

When using a combination of Peirce's and Dewey's pragmatist perspective on the vaccination debates, we can understand them as strategies for managing the irritating doubt surrounding a real and living matter for people. The discussions taking place on various internet forums are from this perspective communicative inquiries aimed at resolving the irritation which the doubts about the vaccine question cause in people. The view of knowledge as "a function of association and communication" among both experts and the public, as Dewey (1927/1991: 158) puts it, is the epistemological starting point of this article.

Pointing out, like Dewey, the democratic aspect of a modern concept of knowledge, also the knowledge sociology of Mannheim (1956: 182) emphasises its insistence that "everything could be different", and its inclination to "explain phenomena in terms of contingency rather than essence". This view is also embraced by contemporary pragmatists like Rorty (1989), for whom contingency is an essential aspect of all knowledge.

The point of invoking Mannheim's perspective on the sociology of knowledge is that he already in the 1930s pointed out and warned about the democratic consequences of an increasingly unstable concept of knowledge, in terms similar to the comparable discussions of today: that is, the rise of populist movements, the impugning of established knowledge authorities, contempt for intellectuals, and "its demand for unrestricted publicity" (Mannheim 1956: 185). In a similar vein as the pragmatists, he also argued that all knowledge production takes place within communicative communities, i.e., milieus in which thinking and knowledge formation take place (Mannheim 1936a: 234). The internet today obviously constitutes a crucial such communicative milieu where ideas held as knowledge are being produced and propagated, and where established beliefs are being questioned and doubted, as expressed by Rosanvallon in relation to our time:

> The Web is not only a true political form but also a social form in the fullest sense of the word. What is more, it is a social form of a new type, in that it plays a part in efforts to build unprecedented kinds of communities.
>
> (Rosanvallon 2008: 67)

Two Swedish cases

Perhaps the most informative Swedish case of civic engagement regarding vaccines and vaccinations is the internet magazine Vaccin.me. It has at the time of writing been around for more than a decade and has collected a large amount of material supporting the editors' aversions against vaccination. The nature of the material linked and referred to varies from personal narratives from readers of the journal to actual research on the matter. The common denominator of the material is that it either supports or is interpreted in a way that endorses the view that vaccines are generally harmful and unnecessary. Established science and research are systematically questioned and criticised with back up from alternative experts and sources. Authorities like the Swedish Medical Products Agency (Läkemedelsverket), the Public Health Agency of Sweden (Folkhälsomyndigheten), and the pharmaceutical industry are depicted as untrustworthy and dishonest. The site contains a clearly social epistemic element in addition to its explicit educational ambition to inform and enlighten the public about the real truths about vaccines. They describe their editorial policy and objective as follows:

- We want to work for a medical democracy and for people to see more sides of a question.
- We welcome comments but the comment field is primarily for those who really want to know more about the topic, share/and or conduct a dialogue. Our time is limited.
- We think it is important to take peoples' experiences seriously.
- We allow advertising since we work voluntarily. The advertisements do not necessarily coincide with the personal views of the editors.
- We want to bring forth the backside with vaccination since we do not get comprehensive information from official sources.
- Vaccin.me is a non-profit internet magazine.

https://vaccin.me/redaktion (2023-02-07, my translation)

Vaccin.me gives the impression of being a serious resource about vaccines and vaccinations, providing, as they state, articles, analyses, and reportage about vaccine risks. The people behind Vaccin.me appear strongly committed to their mission. The site is professionally designed and has an editor in chief as well as a responsible editor. They are active also on Facebook and Twitter.

Vaccin.me, thus, exhibits many of the characteristics of the networked social movements pointed out by an increasing number of social scientists researching contemporary civic engagement. In its persistent and systematic critical scrutiny of political and other authorities and its questioning of established knowledge, the website displays several of the counter-democratic features Rosanvallon (2008, 2011) identifies as characteristic of present-day civic engagement. It expresses a growing gap between the public and the authorities in power, marking a transition from ideologically based politics towards a society and politics of distrust (Rosanvallon 2008: 181). It is also a manifestation of how politics is increasingly defined by the citizens' surveillance of society and its institutions. By publishing stories of human suffering caused by the side effects of vaccines experienced by the member of the site as well as articles about both past vaccine tragedies, like the narcolepsy cases caused by the swine flu vaccine, the site appeals to people's emotions, which further contributes to sowing seeds of doubt about the effectiveness and safety of the vaccines and the trustworthiness and intentions of experts, authorities, and politicians. Vaccin.me in this practice also illustrates how distrust and doubt are constitutive features of democratic life and the dissolution of legitimacy and trust its main challenge, as Rosanvallon (2006: 237–238) contends.

Yet another way to nourish the doubt in well-established scientific knowledge is to capitalise on the innate cautiousness of science when interpreting its results. Oreskes and Conway (2012: 75) show how this tactic, to emphasise the unfinishedness of all science as an argument that more research is needed, has been successfully employed by economic interests such as the tobacco and oil industries to fight threats of restrictions and regulations. In a similar way, the uncertainties inherent in the ongoing scientific studies on COVID-19, its mutations, and the vaccines developed to fight the disease are interpreted as a general lack of scientific support for the vaccines and as a cause for doubting them. Paired with the often-invoked so-called fairness doctrine – that is, the view that we must pay equal attention to all sides in a controversy – it is easy to see how civic engagement of the kind represented by Vaccin.me and its adherents under the right circumstances can have significant social epistemological consequences.

> History shows us clearly that science does not provide certainty. It does not provide proof. It only provides the consensus of experts, based on the organized accumulation and scrutiny of evidence. Hearing "both sides" of an issue makes sense when debating politics in a two-party system, but there's a problem when that framework is applied to science.
>
> (Oreskes & Conway 2012: 268)

Rosanvallon and Oreskes and Conway are both examples of influential contemporary theoreticians occupied with analyses of the consequences of public civic engagement in major social issues. Both are concerned about the outcome of such engagement. Rosanvallon's focus is on social explanations of the engagement, and from his perspective Vaccin.me can be understood as one of many expressions of a general development of contemporary civic participation, increasingly characterised by scepticism towards authorities, politicians, and officials. Oreskes and Conway instead emphasise the problems resulting from inadequate or insufficient knowledge among the civically engaged, thus running the risk of reducing a social problem to a primarily epistemological one.

Returning to Mannheim's theories of knowledge and democratisation, we can there find a clue as to why the kind of engagement epitomised by Vaccin.me thrives today and why so many social scientists worry about it (an issue I will return to in the concluding part of the chapter). He noted that more people tend to become actively engaged in public discussions in times when society undergoes major changes, motivated by a need to express their personal interpretations of reality (Mannheim 1956: 189). A global pandemic is certainly among the kind of dramatic social and cultural occurrences Mannheim had in mind, and the digital shift is the sort of comprehensive societal change that he discussed. Acknowledging the democratically desirable in an increased inclination among the public to engage in civic deliberation, he at the same time warned that these processes could provide fertile soil for doubt and mistrust to grow, and for new alternative "truths" to establish and win supporters. Also, more contemporary thinkers have arrived at similar double-edged conclusions as Mannheim, noting how citizens are increasingly driven by passion and attracted to alternative forms of democracy, and thus changing how political participation is exercised, not least on the internet (e.g., Dahlgren 2013; Rosanvallon 2008, 2011; Sunstein 2014b).

Since they rest on different assumptions and trust different sources, there are good reasons to believe that the belief systems created on communities on the internet also will come into conflict with one another. An illuminating example of such a clash is the fundamental disagreement regarding the Swedish vaccination strategy between two campaigns arranged by members of the public. The first one was initiated by the association for communications agencies, *Komm!*, a trade association organising about 240 bureaus working within communications, advertising, public relations, and the like (https://komm.se/om-oss20220302). In 2021, the association initiated the campaign #KavlaUpp (#roll up the sleeve) to appeal to the Swedish population to get vaccinated in order to reach as high a vaccination coverage as possible (https://kavlaupp.se/kampanj). They did it by engaging about a hundred Swedish celebrities from different areas and letting them pose on images and in videos with their sleeves rolled up and ready to take the shot. The message was:

> The Corona virus is probably the first time in world history when all people around the world are affected by the same thing, at the same time.
>
> Now we at last face the opportunity to leave the worst behind us. Together we can regain a world where we can move freely. And even touch each other again. To reach there, we all need to roll up a sleeve.
>
> We roll up the sleeve not just to keep ourselves healthy. We do it for each other.
>
> Get vaccinated when it is your turn.
>
> (https://kavlaupp.se 20230302, my translation)

This campaign supported the official Swedish vaccination strategy, and thus clearly relied basically on the same belief system that was communicated by the Public Health Agency of Sweden, the Swedish Medical Products Agency, the Swedish Contingencies Agency, and other authorities and experts.

As a direct answer to the #KavlaUpp initiative, a countercampaign was instigated by a group of initially anonymous citizens. This campaign was called #KavlaNer (# roll down the sleeve) and appealed to people not to get vaccinated against COVID-19. Just as the former, the latter campaign is present also on social media like Facebook and Instagram but was banned from Twitter soon after the campaign started. The initiators argue for their cause based on the view that mass vaccination, in combination with the restrictions implemented to constrain disease transmission, in practice made it resemble involuntary medical experiments, and in effect violated human rights. On their website they describe themselves and their cause as follows:

> *Why roll down*
>
> We cherish our human right to ourselves decide in which medical experiments to participate. For this there is support in the Nuremberg Convention and in Article 7 of the UN Universal Declaration of Human Rights.
>
> *About us*
>
> This campaign is economically, religiously and politically independent and is managed by engaged citizens who worry about the authoritarian development we see with the more or less imperative mass vaccination as an alarming aspect.
>
> (https://kavlaner.se 20230302, my translation)

When reading the texts on their platforms, it soon becomes clear that the two campaigns rest on profoundly different social epistemologies. As previously mentioned, the beliefs of #KavlaUpp harmonises with the view of the authorities and the majority of the medical and epidemiological expertise, whereas #KavlaNer turns to both other sources and alternative interpretations of the same sources that their counterparts rely on.

Just as for Vaccin.me, the occurrence of side effects constitutes an essential part of the argumentation, and among the material on the website, there are counters keeping track of the official number of all side effects, the number of serious side effects, the number of deaths caused by the COVID-19 vaccines reported to the Medical Products Agency, and the number of cases which are examined/handled, and the number waiting to be dealt with by the same agency. The site also provides links to other material from a variety of sources on side effects present on the internet. A substantial part of this material refers to official sources like the Public Health Agency of Sweden, the Swedish Medical Products Agency, the Swedish Contingencies Agency, newspapers, medical journals, and the like, but also to social media accounts dedicated to personal stories by people experiencing side effects from the COVID-19 vaccines. Irrespective of the sources, the material is carefully chosen and presented so that it fits the agenda of the site, which is to instil doubt and mistrust in the vaccine and the mass vaccination strategy as well as in the authorities and experts involved.

There are, of course, many more examples than the ones I have discussed here, but these suffice to show how there is an imperative social epistemic aspect involved in civic engagement. The internet forums, social media threads, blogs, websites, and all other places where the engagement takes place unavoidably produce and strengthen the beliefs necessary for people to join forces with them. They become communities of knowers, so to speak, for those who believe in the "correct" truths. On the website of #KavlaNer there is even a facetious test one can do to find out whether one is informed and smart for real or stupid and dangerous for real. Unsurprisingly, for one to fall into the former category one has to share the social epistemics of those who roll down the sleeve.

The point is that the internet provides virtually unrestricted opportunities to diffuse apparently plausible disinformation and misinformation, which according to a growing number of researchers can have seriously detrimental effects on civic literacy, on civic culture, and in the end on democracy (cf. Brennan 2017; Galeotti & Meini 2022; Giusti & Piras 2021; Loveless 2021; Milner 2002; Piras 2021; Rosanvallon 2021).

The civic side effects

The concern among researchers regarding the consequences of the spread of falsehoods, untruths, disinformation, and lies on the internet is easily observable by the increasing number of books and academic journal articles on the topic. Knowledge resistance, fake news, science denial, post truths, populism, pseudoscience, echo chambers, information cocoons, and conspiracies are but a few terms and concepts used to capture the matter (cf. Farkas & Schou 2020; Klintman 2019; McIntyre 2018, 2020, 2021; Mohammed 2012; Oreskes 2021; Oreskes & Conway 2012; Sunstein 2007, 2014a, 2014b, 2017). In research about vaccination hesitancy, the interpretations and analyses of it are often made in terms of these and related concepts. My point in this chapter is that the phenomena which these concepts aim to capture in themselves can be understood as symptoms of what I call civic and epistemic side effects of how major social occurrences are managed by powerholders and experts. In the end the discourses created around the COVID-19 pandemic, the measures taken to fight it, the mass vaccination strategy, and the vaccines themselves are a democratic matter.

The relation between the knowledgeability of the citizenry and the quality of the civic and democratic culture of a society has since long been a central theme in political and social theory, not least within the pragmatist perspective used in this chapter. Especially John Dewey (1916/1966) identified democracy with the constantly growing knowledge among all members of society, because knowledge enables people to critically reflect and make well-grounded autonomous choices on social and political matters. His democratic ideal was a community of well-informed citizens taking part in free and equal communication (cf. Habermas 1985). He therefore emphasised the importance of mass education for furthering and improving democracy, and as one of the essential aims of science to facilitate a more democratic, just, and equal society. The democratic role that Dewey ascribes to science makes the public debates on the COVID-19 vaccines and vaccination policies highlight the social epistemic aspect of the civic engagement regarding the matter. It furthermore makes an increasing number of social scientists and political philosophers concerned about the development:

> If political fake news represents a serious concern for democratic politics, no less worrisome is scientific news with patently distorted content, for it affects individual and social behavior with serious consequences for human health and the environment, as the recent pandemic crisis has well brought to light. Besides, the spread of scientific misinformation also affects public policies thus impacting the political sphere as well.
>
> (Galeotti & Meini 2022: 703)

The kind of knowledge alluded to in this quote is a crucial part of what is sometimes called civic literacy, that is, the knowledge and competences needed for adequate civic engagement and participation. In a comparative study of several western democracies, Milner (2002) shows how the more knowledgeable the citizens, the better democracy works. At the same time, he notices signs of a decline in civic literacy in several of the countries included in the study and warns that only societies with a high degree of civic literacy among its citizens will be able to handle the future challenges of society effectively and justly.

Rosanvallon (2021: 5) argues that populism is the rising ideology of the 21st century, based partly on a cognitive distance between the worldview maintained by the authorities and the actual experiences of people. Acknowledging this epistemic gap is a key to understanding the growing distrust in the authorities resulting in the kind of negative civic engagement, which he sees as characteristic of populist expressions of disagreement. The availability on the internet of a constant flow of information has facilitated not only the diffusion of disinformation and falsehoods, but also of growing possibilities of producing apparently credible alternative interpretations of correct and proven knowledge, as in the two Swedish cases referred to in the previous section. The network character of the internet constitutes an ideal milieu for attracting followers of populist alternative knowledge and expressions of discontent based on emotions of resentment and fear. The growth of communities of followers who share these beliefs and sentiments is a sign of the vulnerability of democracy in our time, Rosanvallon argues (2021: 46f).

For Milner and Rosanvallon, as for Dewey before them, the way ahead is to strengthen democracy by improving the level of civic literacy and closing the epistemic gap between the authorities and the citizens. Not everybody draws the same conclusion, but some scholars instead express a fundamental distrust in the ability and eligibility of the citizens to participate in democratic practices, and therefore question democracy as the best form of governance in contemporary society. Arguably the most influential among these thinkers is the American political philosopher Jason Brennan, who in his book with the provocative title *Against Democracy* (2017) argues in favour of substituting democracy with what he terms an epistocratic form of government. The point Brennan makes is that most citizens are too uninformed or uninterested in politics, and that therefore they often vote against not only their own interest, but more importantly, against the best interest of other citizens and society at large, with potentially harmful consequences:

> In civil society, most of my fellow citizens are my civic friends, part of a great cooperative scheme. One of the repugnant features of democracy is that it transforms these people into threats to my well-being. My fellow citizens exercise power over me in risky and incompetent ways. This makes them my civic enemies.
>
> (Brennan 2017: 245)

Therefore, Brennan wants to disqualify the most uninformed and unknowledgeable citizens from voting in political elections. Brennan's radical ideas are of course contested by many (e.g., Van Bouwel 2023), but the point is that they are showing up alongside other analyses of what is going on with democracy at a time when major social events like the COVID-19 pandemic and the strategies to fight it spur increased civic engagement among citizens. That is also what I have intended with the concept of civic side effects: to highlight the social epistemic and civic processes resulting from people's engagement in issues that concern them, and the wider social and political consequences of these processes.

Conclusion

I have in this chapter argued that the mass vaccination strategy to fight the COVID-19 pandemic has spawned an intense civic engagement on the internet, with potential consequences for civic culture and democracy. These consequences I have called civic side effects, since they can be seen as unintended outcomes of people's engagement in matters related to the vaccines and mass vaccination campaigns employed to fight it. These consequences are of different kinds. Firstly, there are the actual civic engagement and formation of communities of adherents to different beliefs regarding the vaccine and vaccination campaigns, as illustrated by the cases of Vaccin.me and #KavlaUpp and #KavlaNer. Secondly, there are the academic reactions to this engagement in the form of the discussion among researchers about what such engagement means for civic culture and democracy, as illustrated by the arguments of contemporary as well as previous theoreticians and researchers. Thirdly, there is the dawning questioning of democracy as an adequate political system in our time, as illustrated by Brennan's arguments against democracy in favour of epistocracy. Finally, there is the social epistemic question underlying all of the other civic side effects, illuminated by the theories about the relation between knowledge and democracy. The side effects are mutually related and have in the end to do with the democratic consequences of the kind of civic engagement and communities of alternative beliefs about vaccine and vaccination created on the internet.

Therefore, it might be worthwhile to return yet again to Mannheim's (1956) insights from the interwar period about how people in times of major social transformations tend to become more actively engaged in public discussions, motivated by an urge to express their personal interpretations of reality. The democratic consequences of the increasingly varied concept of knowledge and the questioning of intellectuals and traditional knowledge authorities promoted the emergence of populist movements in the form of Nazism and fascism with disastrous consequences for democracy. Even if the situation today in many ways differs from that of the time Mannheim (1936a, 1936b, 1956) wrote about, there are enough similarities that his knowledge-sociological analyses provide a still-valid argument for paying close attention to the social epistemological aspect of civic engagement for also diagnosing our own time.

References

Brady, Michael S. & Miranda Fricker (eds.). 2016. *The epistemic life of groups: Essays in the epistemology of collectives*. Oxford: Oxford University Press.

Brennan, Jason. 2017. *Against democracy*. Princeton and Oxford: Princeton University Press.

Castells, Manuel. 2012. *Networks of outrage and hope: Social movements in the internet age*. Cambridge: Polity Press.

Dahlgren, Peter. 2003. Reconfiguring civic culture in the new media milieu. In J. Curran & D. Pels (eds.), *Media and the restyling of politics: Consumerism, celebrity and cynicism*, 151–170. London: Sage.

Dahlgren, Peter. 2009. *Media and political engagement: Citizens, communication, and democracy*. Cambridge: Cambridge University Press.

Dahlgren, Peter. 2013. *The political web: Media, participation and alternative democracy*. Cambridge: Cambridge University Press.

Dewey, John. 1910/1991. *How we think*. Amherst, NY: Prometheus Books.

Dewey, John. 1916/1966. *Democracy and education*. New York: The Free Press.

Dewey, John. 1927/1991. *The public and its problems*. Athens: Ohio University Press.

Farkas, Johan & Jannick Schou. 2020. *Post-truth, fake news and democracy*: London: Routledge.

Fricker, Miranda. 2007. *Epistemic injustice: Power and the ethics of knowing*. Oxford: Oxford University Press

Fricker, Miranda, Peter J. Graham, David Henderson & Nikolaj J. L. L. Pedersen (eds.). 2020. *The Routledge handbook of social epistemology*. London: Routledge.

Fuller, Steve. 2002. *Social epistemology*. Bloomington and Indianapolis: Indiana University Press.

Galeotti, Anna Elisabetta & Cristina Meini. 2022. Scientific misinformation and fake news: A blurred boundary. *Social Epistemology* 36(6): 703–718.

Giusti, Serena & Elisa Piras (eds.). 2021. *Democracy and fake news: Information manipulation and post-truth politics*. London and New York: Routledge.

Goldman, Alvin I. 1999. *Knowledge in a social world*. Oxford: Oxford University Press.
Goldman, Loren. 2012. Dewey's pragmatism from an anthropological point of view. *Transactions of the Charles S. Peirce Society* 48(1): 1–30.
Habermas, Jürgen. 1985. *The theory of communicative action. Volume two. Lifeworld and system: A critique of functionalist reason*. Boston: Beacon Press.
Hardwig, John. 1991. The role of trust in knowledge. *Journal of Philosophy* 88(12): 693–708.
Hausman, Bernice L. 2019. *Anti/Vax: Reframing the vaccination controversy*. Ithaca and London: Cornell University Press.
Klintman, Mikael. 2019. *Knowledge resistance: How we avoid insight from others*. Manchester: Manchester University Press.
Loveless, Matthew. 2021. Information and democracy: Fake news as an emotional weapon. In Serena Giusti & Elisa Piras (eds.), *Democracy and fake news: Information manipulation and post-truth politics*. London and New York: Routledge.
Mannheim, Karl. 1936a. *Essays on the sociology of knowledge*. London: Routledge.
Mannheim, Karl. 1936b. *Ideology & utopia: An introduction to the sociology of knowledge*. New York: Harvest/HBJ.
Mannheim, Karl. 1956. *Essays on the sociology of culture*. London: Routledge & Kegan Paul.
McIntyre, Lee. 2018. *Post truth*. Cambridge: MIT Press.
McIntyre, Lee. 2020. *The scientific attitude: Defending science from denial, fraud, and pseudoscience*. Cambridge: MIT Press.
McIntyre, Lee. 2021. *How to talk to a science denier: Conversations with flat earthers, climate deniers, and others who defy reason*. Cambridge: MIT Press.
Milner, Henry. 2002. *Civic literacy: How informed citizens make democracy work*. Hanover: University Press of New England.
Mohammed, Shaheed Nick. 2012. *The (dis)information age: The persistence of ignorance*. New York: Peter Lang.
Mormina, Maru. 2022. Knowledge, expertise and science advice during COVID-19: In search of epistemic justice for the "wicked" problems of post-normal times, *Social Epistemology* 36(6): 671–685.
Oreskes, Naomi. 2021. *Why trust science?* Princeton: Princeton University Press.
Oreskes, Naomi & Eric M. Conway. 2012. *Merchants of doubt: How a handful of scientists obscured the truth on issues from tobacco smoke to global warming*. London: Bloomsbury.
Peirce, Charles Sanders. 1877/1992. The fixation of belief. In Nathan Houser & Christian Kloesel (eds.), *The essential Peirce. Selected philosophical writings. Volume 1 (1867–1893)*. Bloomington and Indianapolis: Indiana University Press.
Piras, Elisa. 2021. Inequality in the public sphere: Epistemic injustice, discrimination, and violence. In Serena Giusti & Elisa Piras (eds.), *Democracy and fake news: Information manipulation and post-truth politics*. London and New York: Routledge.
Rorty, Richard. 1989. *Contingency, irony, and solidarity*. Cambridge: Cambridge University Press.
Rosanvallon, Pierre. 2006. *Democracy past and future*. New York: Columbia University Press.
Rosanvallon, Pierre. 2008. *Counter democracy: Politics in an age of distrust*. Cambridge: Cambridge University Press.
Rosanvallon, Pierre. 2011. *Democratic legitimacy: Impartiality, reflexivity, proximity*. Oxford: Princeton University Press.

Rosanvallon, Pierre. 2021. *The populist century*. Cambridge: Polity.
Selk, Veith & Dirk Jörke. 2020. Back to the future! Habermas and Dewey on democracy in capitalist times. *Constellations* 27: 36–49.
Sunstein, Cass. 2007. *Republic.com 2.0*. Princeton: Princeton University Press.
Sunstein, Cass. 2014a. *Conspiracy theories and other dangerous ideas*. New York: Simon & Schuster.
Sunstein, Cass. 2014b. *On rumors: How falsehoods spread, why we believe them, and what can be done*. Princeton and Oxford: Princeton University Press.
Sunstein, Cass. 2017. *#Republic: Divided democracy in the age of social media*. Princeton: Princeton University Press.
Van Bouwel, Jeroen. 2023. Strengthening the epistemic case against epistocracy and for democracy. *Social Epistemology* 37(1): 110–126.

4 Distrust and COVID-19 vaccine hesitancy in Sweden

Björn Rönnerstrand

The rapid development of vaccines against COVID-19 was a great accomplishment for the biomedical sciences (Fauci 2021). In Sweden, vaccinations began in late December 2020 and were rolled out to the entire population during the spring of 2021. First out were the older people and people with different medical risk factors. Thereafter, the vaccine was gradually offered to the entire adult population and, during the autumn of 2021, also to children over 12 years.[1]

The benefits of COVID-19 vaccines are scientifically undisputed. High uptake protects risk groups, limits health care costs, and reduces overall morbidity and mortality. However, the ability of societies to secure these important ends require that people take the vaccine. A paramount question for the social and behavioural sciences is therefore what can motivate people to vaccinate.

The focus of this chapter is the link between distrust and vaccine hesitancy. Vaccine hesitancy is "delay in acceptance or refusal of vaccination despite availability of vaccination services" (MacDonald 2015). Social trust can be defined as a stereotypic perception that other people can be trusted (Sønderskov 2011). This chapter defines distrust as the opposite – the perception that other people cannot be trusted. Distrust comes with many problems. This negative outlook on other people makes cooperation difficult. In fact, trust among people is argued to be key for the solution of many collective action problems, i.e., situations that require many people to cooperate to solve a common problem (Boix & Posner 1998; Ostrom 1998).

The containment of communicable disease is a quintessential collective action problem. It requires that many people implement potentially costly efforts to control disease transmission, which is a collective goal that everyone benefits from. Theory would thus predict that social trust promotes vaccine acceptance, because high-trusting individuals want to contribute to the solution of the collective dilemma posed by disease transmission. Correspondingly, theory predicts distrust to spur vaccine hesitancy, one reason being that "low-trusting" individuals distrust that other people will do their fair share in the collective struggle to halt disease transmission and will therefore not cooperate themselves (Rönnerstrand 2015).

In the scholarship on vaccine acceptance, a few studies focus on trust in the vaccine, or the producer and supplier. Some prior studies have also investigated

DOI: 10.4324/9781003305859-5

the role of social trust (Larson et al. 2018). For example, social trust was found to be linked to the 2009 A(H1N1) pandemic vaccine uptake in Sweden. In a study of intention to receive the pandemic vaccine, a higher likelihood of vaccine was found among people with high social trust, also when controlling for demographics, risk factors, and trust in health care (Rönnerstrand 2013). These individual-level findings were supported by studies indicating a positive association between contextual levels of social trust in U.S. states and A(H1N1) vaccine uptake. The higher vaccine uptake was found in states where the level of social trust was higher (Rönnerstrand 2014, 2016).

In line with findings from the 2009 A(H1N1) pandemic, studies have also found individual COVID-19 vaccine acceptance to be linked to higher levels of social trust (Ahorsu et al. 2022; Eisnecker et al. 2022; Sekizawa et al. 2022). Furthermore, a large-scale study of country-level uptake of the vaccine against COVID-19 found both institutional and social trust (called interpersonal trust in the study) to be significant predictors of vaccine coverage in middle- and high-income countries, with higher vaccine uptake in countries with higher levels of trust (Bollyky et al. 2022).

However, it is fair to say that when it comes to the link between social trust and vaccine acceptance, the result in prior research is rather mixed. Some studies have found only weak associations between social trust and vaccine acceptance (Gerretsen et al. 2021), or the absence of associations (Edwards et al. 2021; Jennings et al. 2021; Kerr et al. 2021). Furthermore, a study of vaccine-hesitant groups in Sweden found that distrust was a defining characteristic of hesitant groups, but also that some groups combine low social trust with moderate or low levels of hesitancy (Lindvall & Rönnerstrand 2022).

The mixed results motivate and inspire to further theoretical and empirical scrutiny of the link between social trust and vaccine uptake, which is the ambition of this chapter. The argument developed is that while there are theoretical reasons to expect a positive link between distrust and vaccine hesitancy, this link may be subject to moderation by risk-related predictors (Eisnecker et al. 2022; Lindvall & Rönnerstrand 2022). As will be developed in this chapter, one core mechanism linking social trust and vaccine acceptance is altruistic considerations in the vaccine decision (Rönnerstrand 2015). Since altruistic considerations are likely to be a relatively more important driver of vaccine uptake among people outside risk groups, this chapter hypothesises a stronger link between distrust and vaccine hesitancy among people who are of lower risk of contracting a severe COVID-19 infection.

To empirically test these theoretical predictions, Swedish cross-section data from two nationally representative surveys from 2021 are being used, which include both questions about vaccine intention/acceptance as well as questions to measure respondents' level of social trust (n = 6,303).

As the Results section will demonstrate, a significant link between social trust and vaccine acceptance is identified. Controlling for potential confounders, the predicted level of hesitancy is around 8% in the group with the lowest level of trust and only around 1% in the group with the highest level of trust. However, the moderating effect of personal risk on the link between social trust and vaccine hesitancy is only partly supported. Social trust is found to be more strongly linked to vaccine hesitancy among people who consider themselves to be of low risk of being affected severely by the coronavirus, as compared to those who believe themselves to be at risk. But the objective indicator of risk – age – is not a significant moderator of the social trust and vaccine acceptance link.

The following section will elaborate on the theoretical claim that social trust spurs collective action, discuss the implications for the relationship between distrust and vaccine hesitancy, and formulate hypotheses derived from theory. After that, the data and method will be presented, followed by the results. The chapter ends with a discussion of the empirical findings and what they mean for the vaccine hesitancy literature and theories about the behavioural consequences of social trust.

Social trust, collective action, and immunisation against transferable disease

Building on the early work of Alexis de Tocqueville (1805–1859), pathbreaking publications by scientist Robert D. Putnam paved the way for a renewed interest in research about social capital and how it can improve democratic governance. Putnam defines social capital as features of social organisation such as trust, norms, and networks that promote collective action for the common good (Putnam et al. 1994). In *Making Democracy Work* (1994), he traced the deep historical roots of the north-south divide in social capital in Italy and demonstrated how social capital shapes the workings of modern-day democracy.

Despite the influence of Putnam's theory of social capital, a recurring point of critique concerns the definition of the concept. Firstly, what is often argued to be the outcome of social capital – collective action – is included as a function in Putnam's definition (Portes 1998). Secondly, what is claimed by Putnam to be an important feature of social capital – trust – should be treated as a separate concept (Bjørnskov & Sønderskov 2013). Thus, while social capital provides the overarching theoretical foundation for this chapter, it will focus on the narrower concept of social trust, and how it is linked to collective action.

Social trust is known to correlate with many highly valued outcomes, including prosocial behaviours (Bjørnskov 2021; Uslaner 2002), economic activity and development (Bjørnskov 2022; Knack & Keefer 1997), and population health (Kawachi 2018). The great value of trust has also been pointed out in relation to the management of the COVID-19 pandemic. Estimations say the global COVID-19 infection rate could have been reduced by 40% if all countries had the same level of trust as Denmark (Bollyky et al. 2022).

One core question in the literature is why trust produces all these normatively highly valued outcomes, and correspondingly, why distrust results in the opposite (Nannestad 2008). Many scholars maintain that trust is important for the success of societies because it promotes cooperation in collective action dilemmas, which are situations in which there is a conflict between individual and collective benefit (Boix & Posner 1998; Ostrom 1998; Uslaner 2002).

Collective action dilemmas permeate human social interaction. One prominent example is the management of natural resources. In Garrett Hardin's famous article "The Tragedy of the Commons", the conflict between individual and collective rationality is illustrated by herdsmen's overuse of a piece of grassland. The dilemma is that for the individual herdsman, it is rational to use the grasslands as much as possible, but this may lead to the collapse of this common resource (Hardin 1968). Elinor Ostrom and her co-workers make a case for trust as solution to the commons' dilemma. If the users of the resource trust each other, groups of people can overcome the free-rider problem and sustain common resources, even in the absence of formal authority (Ostrom 1990). One reason is that trust makes an investment in collective objectives less of a risk, which lay the foundation for reciprocity strategies, and rational cooperation for mutual benefit (Ostrom 1998).

While sharing the same underlying conflict between individual and collective utility, the small-scale local collective action dilemma described by Hardin and studied by Elinor Ostrom differ greatly from many of the most pressing global challenges of today (Dietz et al. 2003). However, the value of trust is not confined to small-scale interaction, rather also relevant for collective action characterised by a large number of actors, anonymity, and complexity (Jagers et al. 2020). Findings also suggest social trust to be linked to individual-level cooperation in collective action in relation to a diverse set of behaviours, such as recycling behaviour (Sønderskov 2011), tax-paying (Scholz & Lubell 1998), charity (Uslaner 2002), or collective action in relation to health behaviours (Rönnerstrand & Andersson Sundell, 2015). The underpinning trust mechanism is based on the normative logic of "conditional cooperation". People generally accept contributing to the solution of collective problems if they trust that most other people will do the same (Kollock 1998; Levi 1997; Rothstein 2000).

The theorised and empirically verified effect of trust on cooperation in larger-scale collective action has implications for what this chapter denotes as *the collective action dilemma of immunisation*. The question is, how can people outside risk groups be convinced to vaccinate if they do not perceive themselves subject to risk of a severe infection?

What makes this question relevant is the collective aspect of vaccines against transferable disease. One reason why vaccines against transferable disease are among the most effective medical treatments available is that they provide a dual protection. They convey protection to the person taking the vaccine, and they also contribute to the provision of the public good of community protection, or herd immunity. If enough people vaccinate against a disease, it will no longer be able to circulate in society, and in some cases, the disease can be completely eradicated. One prominent example is the eradication of smallpox, which has been called the most important public good ever produced (Barrett 2007).

The collective aspects of vaccines have consequences. Research shows that altruistic consideration in vaccination decisions is an important driver of vaccine acceptance for some people, as they are motivated by the other-regarding consequence of vaccinations (Loomba et al. 2021; Pfattheicher et al. 2021; Vietri et al. 2012). Getting vaccinated against infectious diseases is thus not just a way to protect yourself. It is also an opportunity to contribute to a reduction in disease transmission, for the benefit of the community.

The collective aspect of vaccines is both a blessing and a potential curse. If many people vaccinate, this opens the door for free-riding strategies among people who would like to avoid the potential side-effects or the practical "costs" of the vaccine. The extent to which people use free-riding strategies is disputed in the literature, but some studies actually indicate that this may play a role in the vaccination decision for some people (Agranov et al. 2021; Betsch et al. 2013; Caserotti et al. 2022).

The essence of the collective action dilemma of immunisation is those factors that can move peoples' motives away from free-riding strategies to altruism in the vaccination decision.[2] This question connects the vaccine dilemma to the broader literature about social trust and collective action. In theory, trust may stimulate vaccine acceptance because high-trusting individuals are more willing to contribute to the solution of the collective action dilemma posed by disease transmission. Correspondingly, distrusting people are less likely to be willing to contribute in collective action to fight disease transmission. This is the rationale for the first hypothesis tested in the empirical investigation:

> **H1:** *Distrust in other people is linked to COVID-19 vaccine hesitancy.*

For many diseases, the stakes are different in different groups. For example, younger people are at lower risk of a severe COVID-19 infection. This has implication for collective action in relation to the vaccine dilemma. The collective aspect of the vaccination decision is more relevant for people who do not fear the disease themselves. Those who do not see themselves as being vulnerable to a COVID-19 infection are likely to perceive the individual benefit from the vaccine as lower, which leaves room for altruistic considerations in the vaccination decision. Hence, there are theoretical reasons to expect that the effect of distrust on vaccine hesitancy is moderated by risk-related factors.

> **H2:** *The link between distrust and COVID-19 vaccine hesitancy is stronger among people with perceived low risk of a severe infection.*

Data and methods

This chapter makes use of data from two nationally representative surveys conducted by the Society, Opinion and Media (SOM) Institute at the University of Gothenburg. The first was the *Corona SOM survey*, distributed to a random sample of the Swedish population between 22 March and 31 May 2021. The second, also distributed to a random sample of the Swedish population, was in field between 20 September and 30 December the same year (the *National SOM survey*).

The net response rate was 48% in the Corona SOM survey and 47% in the National SOM survey. These rates are quite respectable, not least in the light of the overall trend towards declining mail survey response rates noticed (Groves 2006). It is nevertheless important to consider the risk of nonresponse bias in survey estimates. One problem is that the main independent variable in the study – social trust – is likely to be linked to a higher probability of responding to the survey. This means that the point-estimate of the level of social trust might be overestimated, as compared to the "true" level of social trust in Sweden. However, it is not very likely that nonresponse bias influences the association between social trust and vaccine willingness in a considerable way.

Dependent variable

In the analysis of data, we make use of a dichotomised indicator of vaccine hesitancy, combining data from the two surveys into one variable. The response alternatives included in the hesitancy group are marked by (H).

The Corona SOM asked: "Will you get vaccinated against the Corona virus". Six response alternatives were used: "Yes, absolutely", "Yes, probably", "No, probably not" (H), "No, absolutely not" (H), "Do not know", and "Have already been vaccinated".

The 2021 National SOM asked the same vaccine question as the Corona SOM survey, but with different response alternatives. They were "Yes, I have had two doses", "Yes, I have had one dose", "No, but I will get vaccinated", "No, I do not want to get vaccinated" (H), and "No, for some other reason".

Focal independent variable

The question wording to measure social trust was: "According to your view, to what extent is it possible to trust people in general?" Respondents were asked to answer on a 0–10 scale, where the 0 means that "it is not possible to trust people in general", and 10 that "it is possible to trust people in general". The 11-point scale has important advantages as compared to binary indicators of social trust (Lundmark et al. 2016).

Moderation variables

To be able to test the hypothesis that risk-factors moderate the association between distrust and vaccine hesitancy, this empirical analysis makes use of two variables measuring subjective and objective risk. The subjective measure is based on a question asking respondents about the extent to which they are concerned about the consequences of the coronavirus for themselves. The question wording was: "How worried are you about the coronavirus and its consequences for yourself?" The response alternatives were "Very worried", "Rather worried",

"Not particularly worried", and "Not worried at all". In the analysis of data, the variable was dichotomised into "Worried" and "Not worried".

The objective risk indicator is age, with three different age groups distinguished: lower, medium, and higher age.

Control variables

To minimise the risk of confounding, the models included several control variables. Firstly, apart from age and personal worry, two additional risk-related variables used were self-rated health and place of residence (city/outside city). Socioeconomic control variables included gender, education, and born in the Nordics/outside the Nordics. One news media variable was used. This variable is an index from 0 to 3 measuring the extent to which people regularly consume (1) public television news, (2) radio news, and (3) local television news.

Statistics

To test the hypotheses presented in this chapter, logistic regression models were used. To estimate the predicated probability of vaccine hesitancy in different subgroups and the interaction between trust and the risk-related predictors, the margins command was used. The analyses of data were implemented using the STATA 17 statistical software.

Results

Let us first consider vaccine hesitancy in the sample. The approach described in the previous section leaves us with 96.7% in the vaccine acceptance group and 3.3% in the vaccine hesitancy group. The mean level of social trust is 6.5 on the scale from 0 to 10. This value can be compared to results from a 2013 country-comparative study by Eurostat using a similar question wording and response scale, where the Swedish score was 6.8. The Swedish social trust score was higher than the EU average (5.8) but lower as compared to Denmark (8.3), Finland (7.4), Norway (7.3), and Iceland (7.0).[3]

The mean age in the sample is 53 years, and the share of respondents who are worried/not worried about the coronavirus for themselves are 39% and 61%, respectively.

Now, returning to the first hypothesis, it says that distrust should be linked to vaccine hesitancy. Figure 4.1 shows the predicted vaccine hesitancy as a function of social trust, when the confounders age, place of residence, self-rated health, sex, education, born outside the Nordics and media use are controlled for.[4] It shows that the predicted likelihood of hesitancy is related to social trust. The predicted share of hesitancy is 8.3% in the group with the lowest level of trust, and less than 1% in the group with the highest level of trust. Thus, while the level of hesitancy is also rather low among low-trusting people, there is a

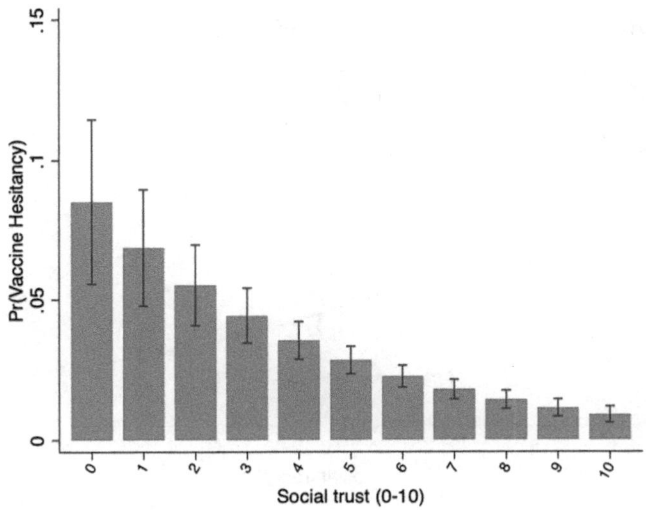

Figure 4.1 Predicted probabilities of vaccine hesitancy as a function of social trust, percentage (2021).

very large difference in hesitancy compared to "high-trusters". The results from the logistic regression model thus provide support for the first hypothesis (see Table 4.1 in Appendix A for the full model).

But let us now consider the second hypothesis. It says that the effect of distrust on vaccine hesitancy should be stronger among people who do not fear the disease personally. The first indicator of risk is subjective worry about being affected by the Corona pandemic. As illustrated by Figure 4.2, the link between distrust and vaccine hesitancy depends upon the personal worry about the virus.[5] Among people who are worried about the virus personally, level of vaccine hesitancy is predicted to be equal (and low) across the 11-point trust scale. In this group, hesitancy levels are in the interval from 1% to 2.5% across the board. This means that distrust does not seem to go hand in hand with hesitancy if the personal risk of the coronavirus is perceived to be high.

In contrast to this, the level of hesitancy among people who do not worry about the coronavirus varies markedly depending upon levels of social trust. Among people who do not worry about the virus but have the highest level of social trust (10 on the 11-point scale), the level of hesitancy is predicted to be around 1.3%. This can be compared to the level of hesitancy among low-trust individuals without personal worry. The share being hesitant is around 15% among people who combine the lowest level of trust (0 on the 11-point scale) with the absence of worry about the coronavirus. The moderation effect is illustrated in Figure 4.2 and confirmed formally by the significant interaction

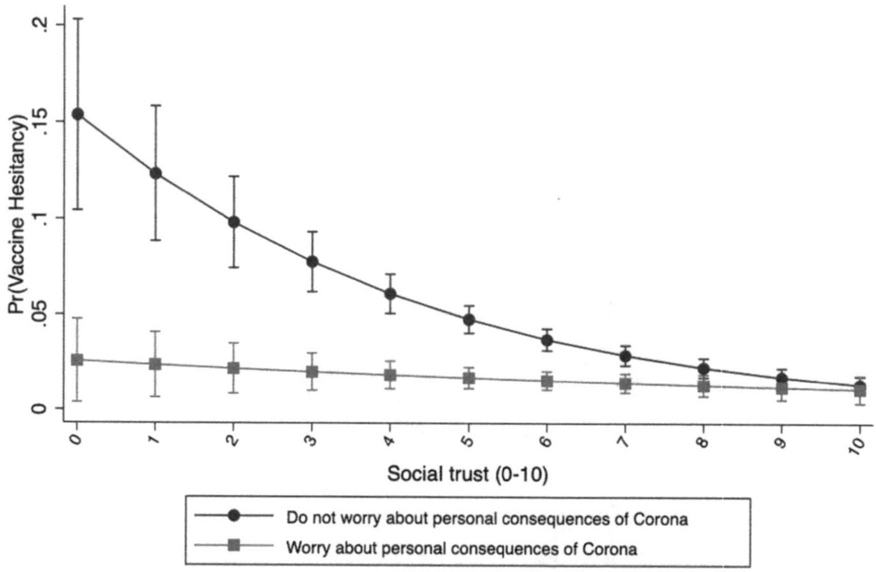

Figure 4.2 Predicted probabilities of vaccine hesitancy over social trust divided by personal worry about the coronavirus, percentage (2021).

effect between social trust and personal worry (see the regression model in Table 4.2 in Appendix A).

Now let us turn to the objective indicator of risk, age, and investigate if the same interaction can be observed as we saw when we used the subjective risk indicator. Figure 4.3 plots the predicted likelihood of vaccine uptake across three different age groups: (1) lower age = one standard deviation below the sample mean age (about 35 years), (2) medium age = the sample mean age (about 53 years), and (3) higher age = one standard deviation above the sample mean age (about 71 years).[6] The same tendency as we saw in Figure 4.2 can be observed, with the difference that the confidence interval around the predicted probabilities of vaccine hesitancy overlap. As indicated by Figure 4.3 and confirmed by the logit model (see Table 4.3 in Appendix A), we cannot say that the association between distrust and vaccine is significantly stronger in any of the three different age groups.

The results leave us with mixed support for the second hypothesis. The link between distrust and vaccine hesitancy is significantly stronger among people who do not fear the coronavirus personally, as compared to those who themselves are concerned about the virus. But a similar moderation effect could not be verified for the objective indicator of risk. The association between distrust and hesitancy was not significantly different among people in low, medium, or high age.

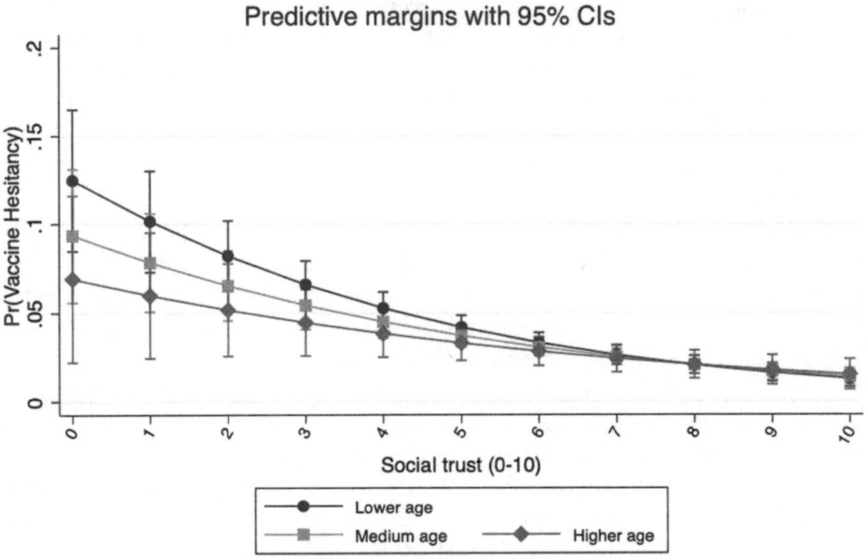

Figure 4.3 Predicted probabilities of vaccine hesitancy over social trust divided by age, percentage (2021).

Discussion

This chapter concerns the link between distrust and COVID-19 vaccine hesitancy in Sweden. The theoretical argument presented was that transferable disease poses a collective challenge that requires large-scale cooperation to be resolved effectively. Based on theories about the role of social trust in collective action, distrust was hypothesised to spur vaccine hesitancy, and that this link should be more pronounced among people who perceive themselves to have little to gain from accepting the vaccine personally.

The analysis of data from two cross-section surveys in Sweden shows that distrust is linked to vaccine hesitancy. People who distrust other people are more likely to be hesitant against the COVID-19 vaccine, also when controlling for potential confounding from risk factors, socio-economic variables, and media use. This is in line with previous research, both as regarding the COVID-19 pandemic and the 2009 A(H1N1) pandemic.

The current study was not designed to explore the mechanisms linking social trust and vaccine attitudes. However, the previous literature provides room for several different interpretations. One reason could be that social trust generally goes hand in hand with a positive outlook on life (Uslaner 2002), which makes high-trusting people less likely to think that the vaccine will bring about side effects. But if the trust effect on vaccine attitudes is only about positivity, this could equally well result in vaccine reluctance, because of low perceived risk of contracting a serious infection.

One other mechanism that may account for some of the association between social trust and vaccine uptake may be that social trust is linked to institutional trust, which is a factor strongly linked to vaccine uptake. But since previous research found social trust to be linked to pandemic vaccine uptake, also under control for trust in health care (Rönnerstrand 2013), the potential confounding effect of institutional trust is unlikely to account for all the association.

The focus of this chapter has been on altruism as potential mechanism linking social trust to vaccine willingness. The logic behind this argument is that social trust brings about a willingness to contribute to the solution of collective problems, and that this manifests itself in altruistic considerations in the vaccination decision. Thus, one reason while high trust individuals vaccinate is that they want to avoid transmitting the disease to other people and contribute to a reduction in disease transmission in society. Correspondingly, distrustful people do not feel obliged to contribute to this common objective.

The chapter also theorised that the effect of distrust on vaccine hesitancy would be stronger among people who do not perceive themselves to be at risk, since the relative value of altruistic considerations are stronger when the personal health is not at stake. In line with results from a similar study with survey data from Germany (Eisnecker et al. 2022), the empirical investigation provided only partial support for this hypothesis. The link between distrust and vaccine hesitancy was found to be significantly stronger among people who do not believe themselves to be subject to risk of being affected severely by the coronavirus. One way of interpreting this finding is that distrustful people who do not think they are subject to risk of a serious COVID-19 infection lack both personal and other-regarding motivations to vaccinate. They do not fear the disease, and they do not feel obliged to contribute to the collective goal of herd immunity. However, there were no significant interaction effects when it comes to the objective indicator of risk. The association between distrust and vaccine hesitancy was not significantly stronger among younger people, as compared to people of average age in the sample, or older people.

Despite the mixed results, it is interesting to discuss the interaction between subjective risk, social trust, and vaccine hesitancy in greater detail. The finding that distrust seems to evoke the strongest effect on vaccine hesitancy among people who are not personally worried about the coronavirus pandemic puts the previous literature in new light. It may explain the mixed results found in previous studies. For example, if the level of concern is very high in the population, most people will accept the vaccine based on pure self-interest. This may require a different kind of trust – trust in the vaccine, the producer, and decision-making bodies (Larson et al. 2018) – but may not involve altruistic considerations, and hence not social trust. Many previous studies have found this kind of "vertical trust" to be strongly linked to vaccine acceptance (Lazarus et al. 2021; Prati 2020).

If social trust is more important when risks are perceived to be low, one may draw the (premature) conclusion that social trust matters most when it is needed the least. However, central to handling of the vaccine dilemma is to reach immunisation coverage rates closer to the social optimum. This requires that people outside risk groups can be motivated to take the vaccine, not least since non-risk groups, such as young people, are responsible for a large part of disease transmission in society. If social trust can motivate people to take collective action to limit disease transmission, such as accepting vaccines, this may explain the remarkable negative country-level association between trust and COVID-19 infections found in earlier research (Bollyky et al. 2022).

Vaccination against transferable disease is an example of a broader category of problems related to the provision of public goods (Rönnerstrand 2015). Many previous studies have found trust to be important in relation to, for example, environmental collective action (Jagers et al. 2020). The benefit of investigating the role of trust in relation to the collective action problem of vaccination is that it is possible to compare groups with different personal stakes involved. Along with the theoretical predictions, this study provided partial support for the view that trust matters most for collective action when the individual benefit from the behaviour is low. This also demonstrates that this kind of research can further the theoretical understanding of trust and its link to behaviour, with important applications far beyond the public health sphere.

Appendix A

Table 4.1 Logistic regression of vaccine hesitancy over personal worry about coronavirus, age, place of residence, self-rated health, sex, education, born outside the Nordics, media use, and social trust (2021)

Variables	*Regression coefficients and t statistics*	
Personal worry about Corona	−0.972***	(−5.08)
Age	−0.00625	(−1.30)
Live in city	−0.394*	(−2.26)
Self-rated health	0.0583	(1.54)
Sex	−0.393**	(−2.65)
Low education	0.228	(1.52)
Born outside the Nordics	0.641*	(2.42)
News media consumption	−0.549***	(−5.56)
Social trust	−0.229***	(−7.08)
Constant	−1.672***	(−4.75)
N	6303	

t statistics in parentheses
* $p < 0.05$
** $p < 0.01$
*** $p < 0.001$

Table 4.2 Logistic regression of vaccine hesitancy over personal worry about Corona, age, place of residence, self-rated health, sex, education, born outside the Nordics, media use, social trust and interaction between social trust and worry about Corona (2021)

Variables	*Regression coefficients and t statistics*	
Personal worry about Corona	−1.890***	(−3.64)
Age	−0.00617	(−1.28)
Live in city	−0.392*	(−2.24)
Self-rated health	0.0592	(1.56)
Sex	−0.396**	(−2.66)
Low education	0.226	(1.51)
Born outside the Nordics	0.641*	(2.41)
News media consumption	−0.548***	(−5.55)
Social trust	−0.258***	(−7.31)
Social trust × Personal worry about Corona	0.167*	(1.99)
Constant	−1.520***	(−4.25)
N	6303	

t statistics in parentheses
* $p < 0.05$
** $p < 0.01$
*** $p < 0.001$

Table 4.3 Logistic regression of vaccine hesitancy over personal worry about Corona, age, place of residence, self-rated health, sex, education, born outside the Nordics, media use, social trust and interaction between social trust and age (2021)

Variables	*Regression coefficients and t statistics*	
Personal worry about Corona	−0.965**	(−5.04)
Age	−0.0188	(−1.78)
Live in city	−0.393*	(−2.25)
Self-rated health	0.0589	(1.55)
Sex	−0.382*	(−2.56)
Low education	0.226	(1.50)
Born outside the Nordics	0.643*	(2.42)
News media consumption	−0.558**	(−5.64)
Social trust	−0.203**	(−5.37)
Social trust × age	0.00238	(1.35)
Constant	−1.830**	(−4.87)
N	6303	

t statistics in parentheses
* $p < 0.05$
** $p < 0.001$

Appendix B Survey questions and response alternatives in Swedish

Corona SOM survey 2021

Kommer du att vaccinera dig mot coronaviruset?

Ja, absolut
Ja, förmodligen
Nej, troligen inte
Nej, absolut inte
Vet ej
Har redan vaccinerat mig

National SOM survey 2021

Är du vaccinerad mot coronaviruset?

Ja, har fått två doser
Ja, har fått en dos
Nej, men jag ska ta vaccinet
Nej, vill inte ta vaccinet
Nej, av annan anledning

Corona SOM survey National SOM survey 2021

Enligt din mening, i vilken utsträckning går det att lita på människor i allmänhet?

0. Det går inte att lita på människor i allmänhet
1.
2.
3.
4.
5.
6.
7.
8.
9.
10. Det går att lita på människor i allmänhet.

Corona SOM survey National SOM survey 2021

Hur oroad är du för coronaviruset och dess konsekvenser för: Dig själv.

Mycket oroad
Ganska oroad
Inte särskilt oroad
Inte alls oroad

Notes

1 https://www.folkhalsomyndigheten.se/smittskydd-beredskap/utbrott/aktuella-utbrott/covid-19/vaccination-mot-covid-19/ (Accessed 19 September 2022)
2 I define altruism as accepting a net cost to oneself in order to benefit others (Fehr & Schmidt 2006). The literature on vaccine acceptance sometimes makes use of the notion of vaccine solidarity, referring to vaccination "as an act of civic responsibility" (Kapadia 2022). I use the notion of altruism because the focus of the chapter is on behaviour rather than on motivations for or the moral underpinnings of behaviour.
3 https://ec.europa.eu/eurostat/databrowser/view/ilc_pw03$DV_310/default/table?lang=en (Accessed 3 January 2023)
4 The figure describes the estimated likelihood of vaccine hesitancy over social trust. It is based on a logit model with vaccine hesitancy as dependent variable. The independent variables in the model are personal worry about Corona, age, place of residence, self-rated health, sex, education, born outside the Nordics, media use and social trust. The bars are predicted probabilities of vaccine uptake; the lines are 95% confidence intervals around the estimated likelihoods. Data: The *Corona SOM survey 2021* and the *National SOM survey 2021*.
5 The figure describes the estimated likelihood of vaccine hesitancy over social trust, divided by personal worry about the coronavirus. It is based on a logit model with vaccine hesitancy as dependent variable. The independent variables in the model are personal worry about Corona, age, place of residence, self-rated health, sex, education, born outside the Nordics, media use, and social trust. The bars in the graph are predicted probabilities of vaccine uptake; the lines are 95% confidence intervals around the estimated likelihoods. For the full model, see Appendix. Data: The *Corona SOM survey 2021* and the *National SOM survey 2021*.
6 The figure describes the estimated likelihood of vaccine hesitancy over social trust, divided by age group. It is based on a logit model with vaccine hesitancy as dependent variable. The independent variables in the model are personal worry about Corona, age, place of residence, self-rated health, sex, education, born outside the Nordics, media use, and social trust. The bars in the graph are predicted probabilities of vaccine uptake; the lines are 95% confidence intervals around the estimated likelihoods. For the full model, see Appendix A. Data: The *Corona SOM survey 2021* and the *National SOM survey 2021*.

References

Agranov, Marina, Matt Elliott & Pietro Ortoleva. 2021. The importance of social norms against strategic effects: The case of COVID-19 vaccine uptake. *Economics Letters* 206: 109979.

Ahorsu, Daniel Kwasi, Chung-Ying Lin, Rafat Yahaghai, Zainab Alimoradi, Anders Broström, Mark D. Griffiths & Amir H. Pakpour. 2022. The mediational role of trust in the healthcare system in the association between generalized trust and willingness to get COVID-19 vaccination in Iran. *Human Vaccines & Immunotherapeutics* 18(1): 1–8.

Barrett, Scott. 2007. The smallpox eradication game. *Public Choice* 130(1): 179–207.

Betsch, Cornelia, Robert Böhm & Lars Korn. 2013. Inviting free-riders or appealing to prosocial behavior? Game-theoretical reflections on communicating herd immunity in vaccine advocacy. *Health Psychology* 32(9): 978–985.

Bjørnskov, Christian. 2021. Civic honesty and cultures of trust. *Journal of Behavioral and Experimental Economics* 92: 101693.

Bjørnskov, Christian. 2022. Social trust and patterns of growth. *Southern Economic Journal* 89(1): 216–237.

Bjørnskov, Christian & Kim Mannemar Sønderskov. 2013. Is social capital a good concept? *Social Indicators Research* 114(3): 1225–1242.

Boix, Carles & Daniel N. Posner. 1998. Social capital: Explaining its origins and effects on government performance. *British Journal of Political Science* 28(4): 686–693.

Bollyky, Thomas J., Erin N. Hulland, Ryan M. Barber, James K. Collins, Samantha Kiernan, Mark Moses, David M. Pigott, Robert C. Reiner Jr, Reed J. D. Sorensen & Cristiana Abbafati. 2022. Pandemic preparedness and COVID-19: An exploratory analysis of infection and fatality rates, and contextual factors associated with preparedness in 177 countries, from Jan 1, 2020, to Sept 30, 2021. *The Lancet* 399(10334): 1489–1512.

Caserotti, Marta, Teresa Gavaruzzi, Paolo Girardi, Alessandra Tasso, Chiara Buizza, Valentina Candini, Cristina Zarbo, Flavia Chiarotti, Sonia Brescianini & Gemma Calamandrei. 2022. Who is likely to vacillate in their COVID-19 vaccination decision? Free-riding intention and post-positive reluctance. *Preventive Medicine* 154: 106885.

Dietz, Thomas, Elinor Ostrom & Paul C. Stern. 2003. The struggle to govern the commons. *Science* 302(5652): 1907–1912.

Edwards, Ben, Nicholas Biddle, Matthew Gray & Kate Sollis. 2021. COVID-19 vaccine hesitancy and resistance: Correlates in a nationally representative longitudinal survey of the Australian population. *PLoS ONE* 16(3): e0248892.

Eisnecker, Philipp Simon, Martin Kroh & Simon Kühne. 2022. The role of generalized trust in COVID-19 vaccine acceptance. *PLoS ONE* 17(12): e0278854.

Fauci, Anthony S. 2021. The story behind COVID-19 vaccines. *Science* 372: 109–109.

Fehr, Ernst & Klaus M. Schmidt. 2006. The economics of fairness, reciprocity and altruism–experimental evidence and new theories. In Kolm, Serge-Christophe & Jean Mercier Ythier (eds.), *Handbook of the economics of giving, altruism and reciprocity*, 615–691. Amsterdam: Elsevier.

Gerretsen, Philip, Julia Kim, Fernando Caravaggio, Lena Quilty, Marcos Sanches, Samantha Wells, Eric E. Brown, Branka Agic, Bruce G. Pollock & Ariel Graff-Guerrero. 2021. Individual determinants of COVID-19 vaccine hesitancy. *PLoS ONE* 16(11): e0258462.

Groves, Robert M. 2006. Nonresponse rates and nonresponse bias in household surveys. *Public Opinion Quarterly* 70(5): 646–675.

Hardin, Garrett. 1968. The tragedy of the commons. *Science* 162(3859): 1243–1248.

Jagers, Sverker C., Niklas Harring, Åsa Löfgren, Martin Sjöstedt, Francisco Alpizar, Bengt Brülde, David Langlet, Andreas Nilsson, Bethanie Carney Almroth, Sam Dupont & Will Steffen. 2020. On the preconditions for large-scale collective action. *Ambio* 49(7): 1282–1296.

Jennings, Will, Gerry Stoker, Hannah Bunting, Viktor O. Valgarðsson, Jennifer Gaskell, Daniel Devine, Lawrence McKay & Melinda C. Mills. 2021. Lack of trust, conspiracy beliefs, and social media use predict COVID-19 vaccine hesitancy. *Vaccine* 9(6): 593.

Kapadia, Farzana. 2022. Vaccine solidarity requires social justice: A public health of consequence, February 2022. *American Journal of Public Health* 112(2): 202–203.

Kawachi, Ichiro. 2018. Trust and population health. In Uslaner, Eric (ed.), *The Oxford handbook of social and political trust*, 447–470. New York: Oxford University Press.

Kerr, John R., Claudia R. Schneider, Gabriel Recchia, Sarah Dryhurst, Ullrika Sahlin, Carole Dufouil, Pierre Arwidson, Alexandra L. J. Freeman & Sander van der Linden. 2021. Correlates of intended COVID-19 vaccine acceptance across time and countries: results from a series of cross-sectional surveys. *BMJ Open*: 11(8): e048025.

Knack, Stephen & Philip Keefer. 1997. Does social capital have an economic payoff? A cross-country investigation. *The Quarterly Journal of Economics* 112: 1251–1288.

Kollock, Peter. 1998. Social dilemmas: The anatomy of cooperation. *Annual Review of Sociology* 24: 183–214.

Larson, Heidi J., Caitlin Jarrett, Elisabeth Eckersberger, David M. D. Smith & Pauline Paterson. 2018. Measuring trust in vaccination: A systematic review. *Human Vaccines & Immunotherapeutics* 14(7): 1599–1609.

Lazarus, Jeffrey V., Scott C. Ratzan, Adam Palayew, Lawrence O. Gostin, Heidi J. Larson, Kenneth Rabin, Spencer Kimball & Ayman El-Mohandes. 2021. A global survey of potential acceptance of a COVID-19 vaccine. *Nature Medicine* 27(2): 225–228.

Levi, Margaret. 1997. *Consent, dissent, and patriotism*. Cambridge: Cambridge University Press.

Lindvall, Johannes & Björn Rönnerstrand. 2022. Challenges for public-service delivery: The case of Covid-19 vaccine hesitancy. *Journal of Euvropean Public Policy* 30: 1–22.

Loomba, Sahil, Alexandre de Figueiredo, Simon J. Piatek, Kristen de Graaf & Heidi J. Larson. 2021. Measuring the impact of COVID-19 vaccine misinformation on vaccination intent in the UK and USA. *Nature Human Behaviour* 5(3): 337–348.

Lundmark, Sebastian, Mikael Gilljam & Stefan Dahlberg. 2016. Measuring generalized trust: An examination of question wording and the number of scale points. *Public Opinion Quarterly* 80(1): 26–43.

MacDonald, Noni E. 2015. Vaccine hesitancy: Definition, scope and determinants. *Vaccine* 33(34): 4161–4164.

Nannestad, Peter. 2008. What have we learned about generalized trust, if anything? *Annual Review of Political Science* 11(1): 413–436.

Ostrom, Elinor. 1990. *Governing the commons: The evolution of institutions for collective action*. Cambridge: Cambridge University Press.

Ostrom, Elinor. 1998. A behavioral approach to the rational choice theory of collective action: Presidential address, American Political Science Association, 1997. *The American Political Science Review* 92(1): 1–22.

Pfattheicher, Stefan, Michael Bang Petersen & Robert Böhm. 2021. Information about herd immunity through vaccination and empathy promote COVID-19 vaccination intentions. *Health Psychology* 41(2): 85.

Portes, Alejandro. 1998. Social capital: Its origins and applications in modern sociology. *Annual Review of Sociology* 24(1): 1–24.

Prati, Gabriele. 2020. Intention to receive a vaccine against SARS-CoV-2 in Italy and its association with trust, worry and beliefs about the origin of the virus. *Health Education Research* 35(6): 505–511.

Putnam, Robert D., Robert Leonardi & Raffaella Y. Nanetti. 1994. *Making democracy work: Civic traditions in modern Italy*. Princeton: Princeton University Press.

Rönnerstrand, Björn. 2013. Social capital and immunisation against the 2009 A(H1N1) pandemic in Sweden. *Scandinavian Journal of Public Health* 41(8): 853–859.

Rönnerstrand, Björn. 2014. Social capital and immunization against the 2009 A(H1N1) pandemic in the American States. *Public Health* 128(8): 709–715.

Rönnerstrand, Björn. 2015. *Generalized trust and the collective action dilemma of immunization*. Göteborg: Göteborg Studies in Politics, 139.

Rönnerstrand, Björn. 2016. Contextual generalized trust and immunization against the 2009 A(H1N1) pandemic in the American states: A multilevel approach. *SSM - Population Health* 2: 632–639.

Rönnerstrand, Björn & Karolina Andersson Sundell. 2015. Trust, reciprocity and collective action to fight antibiotic resistance: An experimental approach. *Social Science & Medicine* 142: 249–255.

Rothstein, Bo. 2000. Trust, social dilemmas and collective memories. *Journal of Theoretical Politics* 12(4): 477–501.

Scholz, John T. & Mark Lubell. 1998. Trust and taxpaying: Testing the heuristic approach to collective action. *American Journal of Political Science* 42(2): 398–417.

Sekizawa, Yoichi, Sora Hashimoto, Kenzo Denda, Sae Ochi & Mirai So. 2022. Association between COVID-19 vaccine hesitancy and generalized trust, depression, generalized anxiety, and fear of COVID-19. *BMC Public Health* 22(1): 126.

Sønderskov, Kim Mannemar. 2011. Explaining large-N cooperation: Generalized social trust and the social exchange heuristic. *Rationality and Society* 23(1): 51–74.

Uslaner, Eric M. 2002. *The moral foundations of trust*. Cambridge: Cambridge University Press.

Vietri, Jeffrey T., Meng Li, Alison P. Galvani & Gretchen B. Chapman. 2012. Vaccinating to help ourselves and others. *Medical Decision Making* 32(3): 447–458.

5 "Read the room Sweden"

Memes, trust, and vulnerability in pandemic engagement

Joanna Doona

Memes and public health

In March 2021, a Stockholm regional-government agency website on COVID-19 vaccination made international headlines after unwittingly using a stock-photo-turned-meme, often referred to as "Hide the pain Harold".[1] Harold's popularity seems rooted in his facial expression: a smile combined with "sad, pained eyes" (Fulton 2021). Upon realising Harold's celebrity, officials removed the image and stated this had not hurt public trust in COVID-19 vaccines (Fulton 2021). Despite extensive vaccine promotion, there was real albeit short-lived worry that it could impact vaccination rates.

Humorous internet memes are ubiquitous in digital culture. As influential meme researcher Limor Shifman points out, "meme" as a term originates from biologist Richard Dawkins "to describe small units of culture that spread from person to person by copying or imitation" (Shifman 2014: 2). Dawkins included cultural artefacts like melodies, catchphrases, and fashion, and "abstract beliefs (for instance, the concept of God)" (Shifman 2014: 9). His ideas are relevant to the contemporary understanding of memes: insofar as they compete for hosts' attention; their survival and spread hinge on suiting a given "sociocultural environment"; and that groups of so-called "coadaptive memes tend to be replicated together – strengthening each other in the process" (Shifman 2014: 9). A key difference, however, is the use of biology metaphors. Memes as "virus" implies that internet user "hosts" are passive and helpless to their spread. As media and cultural scholars have long argued (and proved), comparing sociocultural and natural phenomena underestimates and undermines individual critical abilities (Shifman 2014); "reducing culture to biology narrows and simplifies complex human behaviors" (2014: 11f). In this chapter, humorous internet memes (hereafter memes) are understood in relation to users' active engagement: as potential emerging spaces of political communication (Coleman 2013b) characterised by "polyvocal expression" (Shifman 2014: 123). Specifically, memes are defined as:

DOI: 10.4324/9781003305859-6

> (a) a group of digital items sharing common characteristics of content, form, and/or stance, which (b) were created with awareness of each other, and (c) were circulated, imitated, and/or transformed via the Internet by many users.
>
> (Shifman 2014: 41)

The COVID-19 pandemic boosted memes' prevalence (Murro & Vicari 2021) as pandemic life increased digital media use; making citizens aware of political issues related to pandemic strategy and vaccination. Based on processes of civic bonding (Newton et al. 2022), I argue that memes can be understood as an unruly, unorganised civic resistance to elite pandemic discourse; and related issues of trust that citizens place in each other and governing institutions. Often repeated in relation to public health, generalised trust is key to vaccination and pandemic policies. Here conceptualised as dependent on processes of social and cultural bonding (Klintman 2019; Klintman 2024, chapter 2, this volume), trust relates to the "implicit imbalance of power" associated with information asymmetry, "where trusting individuals accept a vulnerable position in relation to a trusted party" (Larson et al. 2018: 1599).

While intrinsic to representative democracy (Coleman 2013a; Dahlgren 2009) such asymmetry is associated with discursive and emotional issues related to "experiences of being represented, misrepresented, acknowledged, ignored, spoken for and spoken to" by elites (Coleman 2013a: 233). As theorised by Hariman (2008), political humour and parody counters such asymmetry, aiding processes of evening out imbalance in the context of public debate. Motivated by a theoretical interest in memes' civic potential in the pandemic context, the present chapter uses memes found in meme-sharing communities on the platform Reddit[2] that comment on or refer to Sweden's pandemic and vaccination strategies – Sweden is used as an example and focal point for transnational pandemic engagement, allowing for a deeper theoretical inquiry and contextualisation. By emphasising social bonds, elite knowledge, and emotional expressions of vulnerability, the chapter's aim is to contribute to the theoretical understanding of how memes and associated processes of symbolic levelling construct institutional and interpersonal trust or distrust.

Several studies describe the proliferation of vaccine-hesitant content before and during the pandemic across Reddit (Brady et al. 2021; Kwon & Park 2023). However, the differences between communities (so-called subreddits) are vast (Wu et al. 2021). The initial phase of this study uncovered that the large meme-sharing communities on the platform included few vaccination-themed memes – seemingly depending on community-specific rules, moderation, and culture. This is discussed further in the coming sections, as it prompted a broader focus on pandemic strategy.

Humorous pandemic memes' relation to trust

Memes as expressions of civic institutional and interpersonal trust have not been explored much, especially not in the Swedish or Nordic "high trust" context. Interest lies in what memes on Swedish vaccination and pandemic strategy reflect, not as sources of information but as expressions of symbolic levelling. During the pandemic, memes became "resource[s] for solace, social ritual and ontological security" (O'Boyle 2022: 458), constituting participatory media that aid oblique political communication (O'Boyle 2022). A growing field of study, meme research explores technical, communicative, educational, aesthetic, and social dimensions. By drawing on such research alongside theoretical approaches to humorous, ironic, and satirical media, memes are explored as expressions of civic trust and distrust.

The "alien perspective" established through humour is equally valued and feared (Critchley 2002: 62). For some, such distanced perspectives risks creating distrustful, disingenuous and/or cynical political subjects. However, this again implies passive and easily manipulated users, and conflates irony and poking fun with "smirking cynicism" and political disengagement (Day 2011: 28). For sure, memes can be used to market, relativise, hide political intentions, or otherwise manipulate (Askanius & Keller 2021). Yet research must be context-aware and avoid oversimplification regarding civic expression: allowing for the potential of humorous and ironic expression reflecting critically inclined active civic subjects. Context is imperative: humorous and ironic intent and interpretation might vary greatly (Hutcheon 1994). Irony, as "the superimposition or rubbing together of … meanings (the said and the plural unsaid) with a critical edge created by a difference in context" (1994: 19) allows it to be "transideological" (1994: 10) – a possible tool for any kind of ideology or position of power.

As humour is communicatively complex, humorous expressions of civic criticism continues to be overlooked (Rossing 2016). These humorous expressions' relation to trust needs further attention: in this chapter, understood as closely associated with civic vulnerability (Larson et al. 2018). During the pandemic such vulnerability was intensified: the dynamic of information asymmetry between citizens and elites impacted trust and ontological security, as experts expressed unusual levels of uncertainty (Giddens 1991; Holmberg & Rothstein 2020). Characterising much of civic discourse, issues of pandemic strategy and vaccination were associated with scientific knowledge and knowledge loyalty – the "defence of … knowledge claims that dominate in a given community" (Klintman 2019: 44).

Meme's context is not easily pinned down: they move across digital space and are "powerful – yet often invisible – agents of globalization" (Shifman 2014: 153), representing diverging communities' sentiment and taken-for-granted truths (Milner 2012). And while national borders closed, global media scrutinised strategies, reported on vaccine development, and tallied different countries' death tolls, hospitalisations, and vaccination rates.

Civic engagement in the Swedish COVID-19 response is particularly interesting with regard to trust: no strict lockdown or comparatively forceful measures rewarding vaccination[3] were imposed. Schools mostly stayed open, and social distancing was recommended over stay-at-home-mandates. The strategy rested heavily on individual responsibility: to limit social contacts and travel, work from home if possible, and get vaccinated. When debated domestically and internationally, Trägårdh and Özkırımlı made the often-repeated point that these measures depended on comparatively high levels of trust: "respect[ing] citizens as responsible, ethical beings, equal in their contributions" (2020). While there is undisputed societal value in high trust (Holmberg & Rothstein 2020), excessive trust can be problematic democratically speaking (Dahlgren 2009). The coming section explains the study's methodological perspective and approach, followed by the main section, where examples are used to support the theoretical argumentation.

Memes on Reddit: methodological approach and ethical considerations

The chapter argues for a theoretical and methodological framework that emphasises exploration and contextualisation. The selection and analysis method used for the chapter's empirical examples are described in this section.

Purposeful selection and thematic analysis

Based on a theoretically informed purposive criterion-based sample of memes about the Swedish strategy and vaccination, the approach is inspired by Nørgaard Kristensen and Mortensen (2021). It covers March 2020–June 2022 and aims for a quantity appropriate to thematic analysis. Importantly, the sampling of memes cannot reach saturation, since "ephemerality is a key genre trait" (Nørgaard Kristensen & Mortensen 2021: 2450). This argues for a case-based approach that allows for analytical generalisation. After initial exploration, sampling was limited to Reddit as one of the most popular spaces for memes globally. Reddit's anonymity norm (enforced through rules of conduct, moderation, and infrastructure) obscures sourcing, which has ethical value as it protects single users' privacy. This anonymity and platform infrastructure, where users subscribe to specific interest-focused communities, potentially attracts forms of symbolic levelling not represented elsewhere.

Searches of memes were carried out in two ways: first, using specific terms in various combinations (*Sweden, meme, vaccine, vaxx, COVID, corona*); second, studying specific meme-sharing communities (including but not limited to r/meme, r/coronamemes, r/unket).[4] Then, further selection was based on aim-related criteria, referring to Sweden's vaccination and/or pandemic policies. This resulted in 43 memes, some of which share images but include different texts.[5] Such images are often referred to as image macros, which are recurring images that most internet users recognise, that express a certain attitude or emotion, such as the aforementioned "Hide the pain Harold". After thematic coding, representative examples from each were analysed more closely.

The thematic method allows for synthesising analytical observations of memes (Nørgaard Kristensen & Mortensen 2021). Concretely, this meant mapping and coding for discursive and visual similarities and differences, identifying distinguishable types. This balances diversity and generalises interpretations, prioritising retention over reduction (Bazeley 2013).

First, an inductive familiarisation noting observations and analytical reflections was carried out; second, topical labels (like *Sweden atypical*, *lockdown/freedom*) alongside emotional labels (like *denial* or *sadness*) were created. These were clustered, sometimes reflecting oppositions (such as *denial/arrogance/cockiness*, *silliness/sarcasm*, *death/darkness/gallows*). From here, analytical themes were created through a back-and-forth process "between initial observations and defining/naming/renaming themes" (Nørgaard Kristensen & Mortensen 2021: 2450); using key concepts like vulnerability, knowledge loyalty, and humorous directionality/targeting (Kuipers 2011). Focusing on clusters was motivated by memes' polysemy; this final phase was loosely inspired by Stuart Hall's encoding/decoding model, wherein dominant, negotiated, and oppositional readings were adapted. While Hall's reading positions relate to hegemony (1996), the highly contested nature of transnational pandemic discourse meant that different readings related to the competing paradigms of vaccination mandates and lockdowns. In the coming section, the chapter's theoretical themes and contribution are presented using the representative examples.

Memetic ambiguous bonding and trust

Memes lack narrative clarity, inviting potentially opposing interpretations. Adding complexity is their obscured authorship and audience alongside their intertextual elements (Shifman 2014). This, however, allows for broad appeal, as memes reflect shared feelings and encourage "alignment around a collective identity" (Newton et al. 2022: 1). Hence, the present approach reveals clustered interpretations which pinpoint memes as social forms: shared references imply (but cannot guarantee) common understanding and bonding.

While professionally produced satire attracts mostly middle-class audiences (Friedman 2014), memes are widely accessible and easy to recognise, create, and circulate (O'Boyle 2022). In digital spaces like Reddit, differences in humour culture, knowledge loyalties, and civic inclinations deserve scholarly recognition and consideration (Dahlgren 2009). When facing vulnerability, memes create communicative protection, as they can "always be subsequently disavowed as humor" (Soh 2020: 1119). Their non-committal feature is especially interesting in spaces like Reddit, where anonymity is the norm.

Community moderation and culture

To complicate matters further, platforms' infrastructures and cultures differ, as well as how users "experience and respond [to them]" (Dyer & Abidin 2023: 170). Reddit has a content policy that pertains to issues like respecting user privacy and safety; spamming; and non-consensual and/or child-related explicit sexual content (Reddit 2022a). Beyond that:

> every community … is defined by its users. Some of these users help manage the community as moderators … [t]he culture of each community is shaped explicitly, by the community rules enforced by moderators, and implicitly, by the upvotes, downvotes, and discussions of its community members.
>
> (Reddit 2022a)

Explicit rules – clearly visible in each community – regulate moderation. The studied communities' rules include no explicit banning of vaccine-related content, yet ban "misinformation that [is not] clearly satirical" (Reddit 2022b); "political squabble or agenda-pushing" (Reddit 2022c; author's translation); "pushing politics/propaganda" (Reddit 2022d); and "medical advice without expertise" (Reddit 2022e). Here, vaccination seems to be considered "more" political than pandemic strategy, requiring tougher moderation of vaccine-related memes. Over time, scarcity of such memes drives vaccine-interested users to other communities and platforms. While there is no definitive way of knowing if this is what causes the absence of vaccine-related memes here, such implicit community-specific culture might play a greater role than moderation does; and the two are not entirely possible to separate.

In memes problematising Swedish pandemic strategy or vaccination, an initial reading of humorous directionality seems to target the country and its inhabitants – elites and regular citizens – often in terms of permissiveness. Strategy-defenders are portrayed as duped or manipulated by narrow-minded scientific perspectives; societal institutions are made to be arrogant, obstinate, or even cruel.

A common image macro named "Some of you may die" (Know your meme 2022) comes from the 2001 animated film *Shrek* and a scene with antagonist character Lord Farquaad speaking to his knights. (The original quote is "Some of you may die, but it's a sacrifice I am willing to make".) In two different memes from Swedish-speaking meme-sharing community r/unket, Farquaad's face has been replaced with that of then Prime Minister Stefan Löfvén. They reflect a common theme of insensitivity and even callousness ascribed to Swedish authorities at the time. Yet other readings are likely to occur. In *Shrek*, Farquaad is evil, and as this is an image macro, many users are familiar with this. However, if looking only at the image, Farquaad might be interpreted as more heroic. To some, the Swedish strategy could be understood as brave, not budging despite massive criticism. Stating that some may die could be understood as realistic in relation to a pandemic, making the object of ridicule overly naïve strategy critics.

Here, context provides clues. While many questioned the Swedish strategy as risky, Swedes' opinions varied, ranging from very positive to less so between 2020 and 2021. High institutional trust correlated with positive opinions, while interpersonal trust mattered less (Jönsson & Oscarsson 2021). The Public Health Agency enjoyed high trust, dropping from 81% in 2020 to 65% a year later (Andersson 2021). Of course, Reddit users' relationship to this is unknown – it might be fair to assume that Swedish-speaking communities include mostly Swedish users – yet their trust and politics are unknown.

Another recurring image macro called "Roll Safe" depicts a smiling actor, Kayode Ewumi. He is pointing to his temple and looking straight into the camera (Know your meme 2022). In one iteration, the text reads, "Confirmed infections won't increase if we stop testing people". Here, the obvious reading places callous elite as the object of ridicule. Another reading would be that limited testing is a clever response to continued criticism. A third ridicules sincerity in any form, meaning it does not matter much, that this is "only" a funny idea.

The use of irony as it relates to memetic polysemy must be considered too – not only on the level of individual memes, but as part of platform culture. As memes can be understood as simultaneously mocking elite authority and strategy critics, the third apolitical position must be considered, related to the aforementioned moderation rules banning explicitly political and/or argumentative memes. These memes could then be understood as mocking worry, earnestness, or conflict. In this third position, there is no serious argument. Instead, the darkness associated with sacrifice or callous calculations create distance and comedic offence. In line with certain types of digital culture, "

> the more myopic one's gaze, the easier it is to laugh at whatever might be in one's direct line of sight. Just a clever punchline. Just a funny still image" (Phillips & Milner 2017: 120); creating a "fetishized distancing between *text* ... and *context*.
>
> (2017: 120, emphasis in original)

Memes as ironic space

As several readings are valid simultaneously, memes are here conceptualised as ironic space. A core civic value of satire is the allowance of a politically, morally, socially, and affectively charged uncertainty and distance (Combe 2015). Irony is "a form of not being perfectly sure" (Lear 2011: 6) – a "peculiar form of committed reflection" (2011: 21). Here, myopia is part of a process rather than a static state. Hence, ironic space concerning pandemic strategy and vaccination allows for multifaceted forms of engagement rather than disengagement. From this perspective, the Reddit community moderators' banning of misinformation, agenda-pushing, propaganda, and activism becomes a commitment to protect ironic space.

Ironic space allows for double-speak, where two or more things are true and false at once (Bakhtin 1987). For instance, reduced testing *did* mean less reliable data on infection rates; however, that was most probably not the actual motivation. In a situation where the strategy was questioned repeatedly by plenty of actors, we might assume a certain level of civic fatigue or annoyance related to it – be it questioning, criticism, or praise. Media's persistent comparing of strategies, death tolls, and vaccination rates became commonplace and were rarely problematised.[6] In the "Roll Safe" meme, Ewumi is not just smiling. His temple-pointing and his looking straight into the camera creates the effect of looking straight onto the viewer. The combination of gaze and gesture indicates mutual understanding; communicating "I see what you did there", or "we both know what this means" – signalling users being "in" on the joke, argument, or the revealing of someone else's crime. Being "in" becomes more important than agreeing about the meaning of the joke. Memes as ironic space is hence more about a loosely formed sense of community based on humorous ambiguity, than about the political opinions communicated.

Humorous ambiguity can be understood as therapeutic. Satirical irony attracts those who enjoy sharing uncertainty with others: a form of solidarity built on the uncomfortable unstableness of ontological insecurity. Here, irony is a form of detachment, not from commitment, but from social pretence (Lear 2011: 19). Detaching from social pretence with other users has a paradoxical social orientation: commitment becomes directed slightly differently than in non-ironic space. People who regularly enjoy memes to the extent that they subscribe to meme-communities on Reddit belong to this group, wherein sincerity and stable meaning are rejected, yet at the same time, always present too. Issues of pandemic strategy and vaccination instructions were so highly contested they permeated news and interpersonal agendas. Opposition on vaccination and strategies became impossible to bridge, fraught with conflict based on knowledge beliefs and "fundamentalist certainty" (Coleman 2013b: 383), impacting social bonds across all levels: from family and friend groups to global relations. This kind of situation creates a need for ironic space: Klintman (2019: 54) argues that "unquestionable beliefs might feel like a straitjacket for some individuals"; for others, they provide an equally important "comfort zone" in such uncertain times.

This does not mean that ironic space automatically translates into earnest engagement in politics or civic life, but rather, that it cannot be disregarded as obviously overly distanced. There are plenty of spaces dedicated to memes that do not address pandemic strategy or vaccination, or that address them in non-ironic, more earnest ways.

Connecting memefied Sweden to pandemic Sweden

As evident, popular culture references are common in memes (Shifman 2014), appearing often in the gathered material. Two similar memes from the English-language community r/CoronavirusMemes use images from the popular American horror film *Midsommar* (2019). It follows a young American woman travelling with her anthropology-student boyfriend and his friends to a fictitious Swedish village, to celebrate the summer tradition of Midsummer.[7] At first, the village seems friendly and beautiful, decorated with colourful summer flowers; but slowly, the villagers turn out to be cult members engaged in blood sacrifice – including the sacrifice of older villagers.

To many, the most evident reading would be that the film's scenes (depicting elders being forced to jump off a high cliff) are metaphoric of the Swedish strategy's officially admitted neglect of seniors (Öhman & Ridderstedt 2021). Another, darker oppositional reading could be that these memes side with the fictitious cult: that old people are vulnerable and might have to be sacrificed (like in the *Shrek* meme referred to earlier). The more myopic reading – shying away from seriousness and context – considers the thematic similarities between real-world events and the film's focus on sacrifices of older people serendipitously amusing. Here, enjoyment is found in the comparison: between a famous popular film and pandemic discourse.

The first meme example shows three images. On the top left-hand side is the high cliff, with older villagers, reading "elderly Swedes", and the rest of the villagers standing below reading "Other Swedes"; on the top right-hand side are the cult leaders holding an oversized club and the text "Anders Tegnell");[8] on the bottom right-hand-side are the American characters looking shocked, with the text "Expats in Sweden" and "Every other country". In the film, this is the moment the American characters understand they are witnessing a sacrifice. The second meme example includes the image on the top-right-hand side, of village leaders holding the large club. Here they are surrounded by other determined-looking young and middle-aged villagers, with the text "Sweden's covid strategy".

In the first example, specific groups critical of the strategy (expats, other countries) are mentioned explicitly. Even when applying the perspective of rational pragmatism impervious to emotional peer pressure from other countries or expats, the film's horror is used to create humour. A form of gallows humour, often found in the horror film genre, seems fitting to the horrors of the pandemic. Considering such dark humour, as characteristic of ironic space, makes it clear that the meme community's group orientation is constructed through detachment and uncertainty as well as committed reflection. As humour scholars theorise, dark humour implores us to engage momentarily "with the experience of loss" (Murray 2016: 55). As such, gallows humour is not superficial, but an ongoing "attempt to articulate the impact of grief and ascribe meaning to loss" (Murray 2016: 55). The fact that a popular yet somewhat niche American film pinpointed the dynamic of Swedish young and middle-aged impatience with elders only a year before a pandemic that harmed elderly, seems serendipitous. In the ironic space of memes, the intertextual connection is too tempting to ignore: the mere connection between plot and perceived reality is simultaneously funny and scary. Hence, even a myopic reading focusing on intertextuality can be understood contextually: as connected to the pandemic, where cruel humour involves "a widely shared desire or need" of coping with death (Lewis 1997: 253).

Ironic space in the context of the pandemic further illustrates how digital storytelling – like all storytelling, really – is collective. Memes have a ritualistic quality, as O'Boyle (2022) uses Carey (1989) to argue. Digital culture's ambivalent kind of collectivism (Phillips & Milner 2017) means stories are formed by individuals alongside a "chorus", in a manner both "self-contained and densely referential" (Phillips & Milner 2017: 127). Memes as ironic space give room for ambivalence, where the ritual element can be understood as oscillating between different issues of belonging and values. This creates a form of openness, united through opposition to certainty and ideas of a unified subject (Hutcheon 1994). Hutcheon uses Burke's (1973) concept of symbolic acts to describe irony as the "*dancing of an attitude* ... set[ting] up a differential relationship between the said and the unsaid" which invites inference of meaning, attitude, and judgment (Hutcheon 1994: 39, emphasis in original). Groups formed through shared ironic space are connected not through one unified message or identity, but through the ritual practices of such inference and interpretation. Like irony in general, this is intellectually satisfying (Hutcheon 1994), free from Klintman's "straitjacket", and allowing for a collective yet implicit feeling of coping with the pandemic as an existential issue. The attraction of ironic space is subjective and superior in the sense that it involves finding pleasure in "one's own interpretative virtuosity" (Hutcheon 1994: 43) which might or might not be associated with a sense of superior detachment; but it is collective too, involving enjoyment of the participatory creativity and meaning making, "sharing in a collaborative process of evaluation" (Hutcheon 1994: 43).

A patchwork carnival

Beyond the rules, moderation, and associated culture set in each community, ironic space has no clear central organising principle. This chapter's final meme example is vaccination-themed, demonstrating digital collective storytelling as a patchwork of different media forms, by different actors. Here, the meme-posters' headline "Scientists in Sweden: how do we make this problem much worse?" is combined with a headline screenshot from a KATV website news article,[9] reading "Implanted microchip could be used to verify COVID-19 vax status" (Rogers 2021). Below the headline, a by-line identifying the image as a screenshot, and an X-ray image of a human hand with an implanted rice-sized microchip. The subject line of the post reads "Learn how to read the room Sweden".

Here, there is no recurring image macro; instead, focus is on tracking the meme's various elements. The textual cues allude to a recurring theme of Swedish scientists (and Sweden as a whole) as disaffected by the pandemic, unable to "read the room". This can be read ironically, or more seriously – in any case, context is key. This was a time when most governments attempted to get entire populations vaccinated, but in the meme, Swedish scientists were ignoring this context: including vaccination mandates, conspiracy theories about the COVID-19 vaccine containing microchips, and mainstream criticism of segregation based on vaccine status. The original news story focused on a tweet with a video from the *South China Morning Post*, about a Swedish start-up company explaining how their microchip could work as a "COVID-19 vaccine passport under a person's skin" (Rogers 2021). The video explains the potential repurposing of the chip – originally meant to replace keys, ID cards, business cards, and function as data storage (including passports and medical records; Rogers 2021).

In this digital patchwork storytelling, media reports, and media logics, parody and conspiracy culture all play a role. Understanding the meme is based on understanding its references, perhaps even the news story itself, as well as knowledge of certain conspiracy theory tropes and microchip tech. Several forces and layers make up "patches" of this storytelling: the startup's PR-strategy of opportunistically connecting product-marketing to current news; the spread and amplification associated with news media logics; the context of criticism and debate of the Swedish strategy as well as of vaccine passports; and conspiracy theories about vaccine contents and policies. In the context of this meme-sharing community on Reddit, the enjoyment seems to be related first and foremost to the timing-related incongruity between text and context, where amusement is derived from incongruity. The target of the joke is Sweden and its pandemic strategy; yet from a pro-vaccine perspective, it might as well be vaccine sceptics who believe in conspiracy. A third reading in this ironic space could be more conspiratorial readings.

Discussion: ironic pandemic trust

Hall's (1996) encoding/decoding model was originally conceptualised in relation to non-humorous forms of media; here, the "motivational complexity of humor" (Rossing 2016) is important too. The playfulness of memes and humour does carry an element of conflict and combativeness, as it cannot be isolated from other parts of (pandemic) life – especially not when they are created through a patchwork of different media, actors, and ideas. As such, the vaccination-themed meme represents what Rossing (2016) describes as a value of humour in civic life, as a method of deriving pleasure from struggle. To acknowledge such "inescapably mixed motives is to embrace serious purposes of knowledge creation and cultural formation that cannot be extricated from play and contest" (Rossing 2016: 12). From this perspective, such playfulness cannot and should not be seen as separable from action (Rossing 2016). Further, Rossing argues, this invites "oscillation among multiple perceptions of reality" which "amplif[ies] its constructive functions" (Rossing 2016: 13). Importantly, it is the tension between these actors, voices, and affective charges, rather than each one of them isolated, that characterises ironic digital space. For instance, opposition, distancing, and self-protection align with a "refusal to be pinned down" (Chambers 1991: 55), creating space wherein no one is responsible for understanding. Based on Goffman (1974), Hutcheon (1994) argues that irony is beyond dichotomies of ironic/literal, or ironic/earnest. Instead, it is "relational, inclusive, and differential" (Hutcheon 1994: 66).

Humorous expression is often analysed as carnivalesque (Bakhtin 1968). The constant production, distribution, and consumption of memes can be understood as part of a global chaotic online carnival (Sienkiewicz 2012); yet the temporal and spatial aspects of digital media makes it increasingly difficult to apply Bakhtin's original conceptualisation. The carnivalesque comic inversion inspiring Hariman's idea of symbolic levelling, where common people are united and allowed to laugh at the elite, was isolated in time and space, "to reinforce the notion that, when it ends, things must return to normal" (Sienkiewicz 2012: 115). In digital space such as meme-sharing communities on Reddit, the carnival is always ongoing. In other words, the elite has lost control of the carnival.

Ironic space as a digital carnival is still temporary for individual users, as most people use several platforms and do other things too. But in terms of space, the carnival has become permanent: Reddit is always open and has been since 2005. In Reddit communities, users are constantly made aware of each other, through clearly visible community user information (including number of subscribing members and number of members currently online). This alongside community rules and moderation counters the ambivalence of ironic space, creating some sense of order; at the same time, memes travel across communities and platforms, making individual memes into travelling carnivals. When users engage with them, it might still seem fleeting to them, yet memes' intertextual nature and patchwork storytelling constitute parts of social and cultural memory (Swiatek 2016). Hence, memes fixate collective civic sentiment over time, allowing users to keep and/or switch out elements that reflect current events, feelings, culture, and politics, which then shape and reshape them continually, connecting different moments of time and groups of people.

This longer-lasting aspect of meme culture represents a slightly more fixed set of civic sentiment, often directed at the elite. Reddit communities' rules and cultures similarly serve as limits for how such sentiment can be expressed in ironic space. The analysed memes expose a spectrum of sentiment: from accusations of cold and callous authorities to a sense of trust, insight, and bold pragmatism – with grinning myopia on its own axis. The potential message of pandemic and vaccination memes related to Sweden – non-dependent of reading – is that Sweden chose its own path.

A fundamental process of democratic societies is the interactive foundation, where networks of trust are integrated into politics (Tilly 2007). Excessive trust might stifle conflict and uphold oppressive relationships (Dahlgren 2009), which means a continuous balancing of trust and distrust best serves civic agency. Memes can be understood as community-specific negotiations of trust and distrust, illuminating some of the specifics of vaccination and pandemic strategy engagement.

The identified space between contradictory humorous directionality and knowledge loyalties is here understood as ironic space; begging the question of how ambiguity relates to trust in times of ontological insecurity. Here, community rules and moderation create some stability; users are (mostly) in charge of moderation and rules, wielding a type of editorial power. This kind of peer-power adds a layer of safety not always present in digital spaces, which strengthens a sense of social presence and protection in the face of vulnerability. These strictures combined with the range of possible readings arguably strengthen interpersonal trust: prioritising community over perspective, potentially allowing for a wider variety of users to feel a sense of belonging.

Protection here pertains to social, civic, and emotional integrity in a vulnerable context. User-generated satire "work[ed] against the backdrop of a range of feelings (anger, bitterness, disappointment, frustration, despair etc.)" formed in response to the pandemic and its political consequences (Ponton 2021: 767). It potentially serves to reduce uncertainty and tension and build trust (O'Boyle 2022). Social distancing meant being alone; beyond ontological insecurity, the new constraints to daily life as well as democratic process meant citizens experienced misrecognition, exclusion, inequality, or disrespect. While trusting others makes us vulnerable, ironic space reflects such vulnerability through ambivalence, representing affinity without demanding conformity.

In relation to institutional trust, the transnational aspect of memes and digital communities creates challenges for civically focused research. Does it matter if an American Reddit user distrusts the Swedish COVID-19 response? While these issues cannot be solved in the present chapter, similarly themed humour about the Swedish strategy and vaccination exists in Swedish- as well as English-speaking communities. Sweden became a symbol for a more liberal policy; further, not all Swedes trusted the Swedish strategy, and correspondingly, not all non-Swedes objected to it. In ironic space, two seemingly different things can be true at once, emphasising how "the *us* and *them* established by constitutive humor isn't much of a binary" (Phillips & Milner 2017: 126; emphasis in original). While the construction of *us* necessitates a corresponding construction of *them* (Hutcheon 1994); in digital spaces, "either *us* or *them* can facilitate constructive, prosocial engagement, just as either *us* or *them* can facilitate destructive, anti-social engagement" (Phillips & Milner 2017: 126).

Digital humour's inherent ambivalence can provide keys to understanding constructions of *normal* and *aberrant* (Phillips & Milner 2017). What unites the studied memes despite this ambiguity is their fixation on Sweden as outlier. This recurring theme of Swedish deviation becomes a meta-level focal point. On this level, users agree. The incongruity between Sweden's and other countries' approaches creates a foundation for humour: independent of perspective, the agreement on Sweden's deviance creates room for fun. Hence, humorous constructions of an *us* and *them* do not necessarily promote specific perspectives and interpretations of specific memes. The emotional range allowed through ambivalence – here found between opposing interpretations – keeps reiterating Sweden's deviation. Beyond that, individual users' inclination towards different interpretations relates to group-orientation, knowledge loyalties, and associated judgement of humorous directionality.

Consequentially, institutional trust is continually re-negotiated. Just as opinions about vaccination and pandemic strategies vary within ironic space, distance and proximity do too: ranging from the myopic, contextless reading done "just" for fun, to the analytically distanced, where "things can be shown and thus seen differently" (Hutcheon 1994: 49). Hutcheon refers to Chevalier, who argues that "the habit of making or perceiving incongruities has an impressive tendency to broaden the view, leading to the perception of incongruities on a wider and wider scale" (Chevalier 1932: 44). So as the myopic reading fetishises distancing between text and context, analytical distance afforded through irony does the opposite; the two can be understood as opposing forces countering each other. Considering gallows humour as existentially important in times of crisis, aiding our coming to terms with anguish and loss (Murray 2016), its representation in ironic space allows not only for diverging opinions, but also for diverging forms of distance.

One important aspect of humorous forms is their lack of goal orientation. While the collective efforts of these users can be understood as using ironic spaces to negotiate and level vulnerability, feelings, perspectives, knowledge, and, thereby, institutional and interpersonal trust, part of the attraction of such spaces is that "[w]hen we are being funny, the usual intentions, presuppositions and consequences of what we say are not in force" (Morreall 2005: 68). That does not mean ironic space does not house serious or instrumental reasoning too; but it does impact how users interact, and what expectations they have when they enter ironic spaces. Here, a key aspect is inclusivity: different kinds of users, including the apolitical or disillusioned, the worried or the confident, can feel invited (Hutcheon 1994; Phillips & Milner 2017).

Symbolic levelling is based on power asymmetry, most often understood as the discursive and material power imbalance inherent in all representative democratic societies, where elite actors make decisions for and on behalf of the population. The symbolic levelling of meme culture balances such power and influence, and in the pandemic context, public life was constricted in various new ways, for instance through temporary laws banning demonstrations and street protests. Humorous forms based on replication, like memes and parodies, are "profoundly social" (Hariman 2008: 262), making political discourse accessible for a wider audience. Replication, Hariman argues, includes inflection – here, based in "deep playfulness" which aids development and negotiation of individual subjectivity's relation to publics (Hariman 2008: 263). For Hariman, levelling through parody is hence associated with civic education, making citizens aware of the constructed nature of the contemporary mediated public sphere. Arguably, social distancing pushed this to its extreme, as an increasing proportion of public life went digital. "Hide the pain Harold" might not be fitting for public health information, but his and others' familiar memefied faces do represent, among other things, civic negotiations of trust. The recurring gallows humour touched upon our collective and relative powerlessness in facing COVID-19. Civic satirical memes posted in these moderated meme communities create ironic space that levels trust and distrust in a constantly ongoing, ritual negotiation and performance; a collective act that affirms social bonds around vulnerability, uncertainty, insecurity, and even existential dread.

Rituals remind us of our collectivities and their potential agency. The agency embedded in ironic spaces encompasses oppositional elements and readings, including broad ranges of emotions, perspectives, and knowledge beliefs, alongside differing levels of vulnerability. Through playful interaction, memes allow civic tackling of issues actualised by the pandemic as a new political situation, like vaccination – processing themes that connect the political with the personal as well as collective existential issues actualised: deviation, sacrifice, and death.

Conclusion

This chapter used humorous pandemic and vaccination memes in different meme-sharing communities on Reddit to understand how memes and their associated processes of civic symbolic levelling construct institutional and interpersonal trust or distrust. Due to memes' polysemy, several readings of each meme are possible; which means that memes establish ambiguity as a core value – here described as ironic space.

The chapter contributes an understanding of ironic space wherein uncertainty, in an existentially and socially pressing pandemic context, is what unites users. Beyond negotiating different opinions, identities, perspectives, emotions, and knowledge beliefs, ironic space opens up space to negotiate proximity – from myopia to analytical distance. This can be understood as shielding users' sense of vulnerability in a time of restricted social and democratic interaction. Users are united through memes in an ephemeral sense: the gallows humour's identification of Sweden as aberrant is something that users agree on, despite other potential differences. Civic pandemic vulnerability is conveyed, balancing trust and distrust – ready to shift if need be – thereby constituting parts of the complex web of civic networks that make up the interactive foundation of democratic trust. Importantly, the chapter argues that the study of memes necessitates the study of platform infrastructure, logic, politics, and culture. Further studies are needed in this direction, as memes are created and circulated within and across platforms.

As argued by scholars interested in irony, its transideological and ambiguous properties work invitingly, and conversely also exclusionary: all are welcome in ironic space, with a few caveats related to moderation and, implicitly, offense. To further the understanding of the exclusionary and inclusionary mechanics of ironic space, including their associated relations to civic levelling of trust and distrust, users and their practices deserve further attention.

Notes

1 Most of the meme images mentioned can be found through online search using the titles referred to.
2 One of the largest meme-sharing platforms (Statista 2022; Semruch 2022), Reddit houses 100,000 communities of different sizes, including a broad range of users, topics, languages, and discursive forms.

3 Vaccine passes indirectly rewarded vaccination; however, they were used only at events gathering large crowds for a limited amount of time. Beyond that, their main relevance was for foreign travel.
4 *Unket* is Swedish for 'dank'; a common label for memes that have lost or, ironically meant, gained comedic value due to repetition (Wells 2018; also see Klee 2017).
5 There were 10 memes in Swedish, and 1 mixing Swedish and English; the rest were in English.
6 The studied Reddit community r/Coronamemes rules included "No Wishing Death Upon Others" and "No Blaming any Particular Race for COVID", indicating problems with such content.
7 Midsummer (*midsommar* in Swedish) is a Swedish pagan-rooted holiday celebration around the time of summer solstice.
8 Anders Tegnell was state epidemiologist during the pandemic. He was often used as a symbol or metonymy of the Swedish strategy.
9 KATV is a local affiliate of ABC Television based in Little Rock, Arkansas, United States.

References

Andersson, Ulrika. 2021. *Myndighetsförtroende under coronapandemin. SOM-undersökningen om coronaviruset 2021* [Government agency trust during the corona pandemic. The SOM survey about corona virus 2021]. Gothenburg: The SOM-institute.

Askanius, Tina & Nadine Keller. 2021. Murder fantasies in memes: Fascist aesthetics of death threats and the banalization of white supremacist violence. *Information, Communication and Society* 24(16): 2522–2539.

Bakhtin, Mikhail. 1968. *Rabelais and his world*. Bloomington: Indiana University Press.

Bakhtin, Mikhail. 1987. Discourse in the novel. In Holquist, M. (ed.), *The dialogic imagination: Four essays*. Austin: University of Texas Press.

Bazeley, Patricia. 2013. *Qualitative data analysis*. London: Sage.

Brady, Miranda J., Erika Christiansen & Emily Hiltz. 2021. Good Karen, bad Karen: Visual culture and the anti-vaxx mom on Reddit. *Journal of Gender Studies*. https://doi.org/10.1080/09589236.2022.2069088

Burke, Kenneth. 1973. *The philosophy of literary form: Studies in symbolic action*. Berkeley: University of California Press.

Carey, James. 1989. *Communication as culture: Essays on media and society*. Winchester: Unwin Hyman.

Chambers, Ross. 1991. *Room for manoeuvre: Reading (the) oppositional (in) narrative*. Chicago: University of Chicago Press.

Chevalier, Haakon. 1932. *The ironic temper: Anatole France and his time*. New York: Oxford University Press.

Coleman, Stephen. 2013a. *How voters feel*. New York: Cambridge University Press.

Coleman, Stephen. 2013b. The internet and the opening up of political space. In John Hartley, Jean Burgess & Axel Bruns (eds.), *A companion to new media dynamics*, 377-384. Blackwell Publishing Ltd.

Combe, Kumar. 2015. Stephen Colbert: Great satirist, or greatest satirist ever? *The International Communication Gazette* 77(3): 297–311.

Critchley, Simon. 2002. *On humour*. Oxon: Routledge.

Dahlgren, Peter. 2009. *Media and political engagement*. New York: Cambridge University Press.

Day, Amber. 2011. *Satire and dissent*. Bloomington: Indiana University Press.

Dyer, Harry T. & Crystal Abidin. 2023. Understanding identity and platform cultures. In William Housley, Adam Edwards, Roser Benito-Montagut & Richard Fitzgerald (eds.), *The SAGE handbook of digital society*. London: SAGE Publications.
Friedman, Simon. 2014. *Comedy and distinction.*. Oxfordshire: Routledge.
Fulton, Colm. 2021. Internet's "Hide the Pain Harold" accidentally used by Swedish COVID-19 vaccine website. Reuters, 31 March. https://www.reuters.com/article/us-health-coronavirus-sweden-meme-idUSKBN2BN1RM (Accessed 15 September 2022).
Giddens, Anthony. 1991. *Modernity and self-identity: Self and society in the late modern age*. Cambridge: Polity Press.
Goffman, Erving. 1974. *Frame analysis: An essay on the organization of experience*. Cambridge: Harvard University Press.
Hall, Stuart. 1996. Encoding/decoding. In Paul Marris & Sue Thornham (eds.), *Media studies: A reader*. Edinburgh: Edinburgh University Press.
Hariman, Robert. 2008. Political parody and public culture. *Quarterly Journal of Speech* 94(3): 247–272.
Holmberg, Sören & Bo Rothstein. 2020. *Social trust – the Nordic gold? The Quality of Government Institute working paper series 2020:1*. Gothenburg: University of Gothenburg.
Hutcheon, Linda. 1994. *Irony's edge: The theory and politics of irony*. London: Routledge.
Jönsson, Erik & Henrik Oscarsson. 2021. *Den svenska coronastrategin: SOM-undersökningen om coronaviruset 2021* [The Swedish corona strategy: the SOM survey on the corona virus]. Gothenburg: The SOM institute and University of Gothenburg.
Klintman, Mikael. 2019. *Knowledge resistance: How we avoid insight from others*. Manchester: Manchester University Press.
Klintman, Mikael. 2024. Apollonian and Dionysian trust in vaccination. In Lars Borin, Mia-Marie Hammarlin, Dimitrios Kokkinakis & Fredrik Miegel (eds.), *Vaccine hesitancy in the Nordic countries: Trust and distrust during the COVID-19 pandemic*. London: Routledge.
Know Your Meme. 2022. https://knowyourmeme.com (Accessed 20 August 2022).
Kuipers, Giselinde. 2011. The politics of humour in the public sphere: cartoons, power and modernity in the first transnational humour scandal. *European Journal of Cultural Studies* 14(1): 63–80.
Kwon, Soyeon & Albert Park. 2023. Examining thematic and emotional differences across Twitter, Reddit, and YouTube: The case of COVID-19 vaccine side effects. *Computers in Human Behavior* 144. https://doi.org/10.1016/j.chb.2023.107734
Larson, Heidi J., Richard M. Clarke, Caitlin Jarrett, Elisabeth Eckersberger, Zachary Levine, Will S. Schultz & Pauline Paterson. 2018. Measuring trust in vaccination: A systematic review. *Human Vaccines & Immunotherapeutics* 14(7): 1599–1609.
Lear, Jonathan. 2011. *A case for irony*. Cambridge: Harvard University Press.
Lewis, Paul. 1997. The killing jokes of the American eighties. *Humor* 103: 251–283.
Milner, Ryan M. 2012. *The world made meme*. PhD thesis, University of Kansas.
Morreall, John. 2005. Humour and the conduct of politics. In S. Lockyer & M. Pickering (eds.), *Beyond a joke: The limits of humour*. Basingstoke: Palgrave Macmillan.
Murray, Kristen A. 2016. The last laugh: Dark comedy on US television. In Chiara Bucaria & Luca Barra (eds.), *Taboo comedy: Television and controversial humour*. London: Palgrave Macmillan.
Murro, Maria Francesca & Stefania Vicari. 2021. Memetising the pandemic: memes, covid-19 mundanity and political cultures. *Information, Communication & Society* 24(16): 2422–2441.

Newton, Giselle, Michele Zappavigna, Kerryn Drysdale & Christy E. Newman,. 2022. More than humor: Memes as bonding icons for belonging in donor-conceived people. *Social Media + Society* 8(1): 1–13. https://doi.org/10.1177/20563051211069

Nørgaard Kristensen, Nette & Mette Mortensen. 2021. "Don't panic people! Trump will tweet the virus away": Memes contesting and confirming populist political leaders during the COVID-19 crisis. *Information, Communication & Society*, 24(16): 2442–2458.

O'Boyle, Neil. 2022. WhatsAppening Donald: The social uses of Trump memes. *European Journal of Cultural Studies*, 25(2): 458–462.

Öhman, Daniel & Maira Ridderstedt. 2021. Tegnell: "Åtgärderna hade inte lika stor effekt som vi hoppats". Sveriges Radio. https://sverigesradio.se/artikel/tegnell-medger-overtro-pa-atgarder-i-aldreomsorg;https://sverigesradio.se/artikel/tegnell-medger-overtro-pa-atgarder-i-aldreomsorg (Accessed 25 February 2023).

Phillips, Whitney & Ryan M. Milner. 2017. *The ambivalent internet*. Cambridge and Malden: Polity.

Ponton, Douglas M. 2021. "Never in my life have I heard such a load of absolute nonsense. Wtf": Political satire on the handling of the COVID-19 crisis. *Russian Journal of Linguistics* 25(3): 767–788.

Reddit. 2022a. Reddit content policy. https://www.redditinc.com/policies/content-policy (Accessed 20 August 2022).

Reddit. 2022b. r/Coronamemes. https://www.reddit.com/r/Coronamemes/ (Accessed 20 August 2022).

Reddit. 2022c. r/Unket. https://www.reddit.com/r/unket/ (Accessed 20 August 2022).

Reddit. 2022d. r/CoronavirusMemes. https://www.reddit.com/r/CoronavirusMemes/ (Accessed 20 August 2022).

Reddit. 2022e. r/CovIdiots. https://www.reddit.com/r/CovIdiots/ (Accessed 20 August 2022).

Rogers, Zachary. 2021. Implanted microchip could be used to verify COVID-19 vax status. KATV, December 20. https://katv.com/news/coronavirus/implanted-microchip-could-be-used-to-verify-covid-19-vax-status (Accessed 25 March 2023).

Rossing, Jonathan P. 2016. A sense of humor for civic life. *Studies in American Humor* 2(1): 1–22.

Semruch. 2022. Top Websites. https://www.semrush.com/website/top/ (Accessed 23 March 2023).

Shifman, Limor. 2014. *Memes in digital culture*. Cambridge and London: MIT Press.

Sienkiewicz, Matt. 2012. Out of control: Palestinian news satire and government power in the age of social media. *Popular Communication* 10(1–2): 106–118.

Soh, Wee Yang. 2020. Digital protest in Singapore: The pragmatics of political internet memes. *Media, Culture & Society*, 42(7–8): 1115–1132.

Statista. 2022. Most popular websites worldwide as of November 2022, by total visits. https://www.statista.com/statistics/1201880/most-visited-websites-worldwide/ (Accessed 23 March 2023).

Swiatek, Lukasz. 2016. Constructing cultural memory: A memetic approach. *International Journal of Media & Cultural Politics* 12(1): 129–142.

Tilly, Charles. 2007. *Democracy*. New York: Cambridge University Press.

Trägårdh, Lars & Özkırımlı, Umut. 2020. Why might Sweden's COVID-19 policy work? Trust between citizens and state. *The Guardian*, 21 April 2020. https://www.theguardian.com/world/commentisfree/2020/apr/21/sweden-COVID-19-policy-trust-citizens-state (Accessed 2 October 2022).

Wu, Wei, Hanjia Lyu & Jiebo Luo. 2021. Characterizing discourse about COVID-19 vaccines: A Reddit version of the pandemic story. *Health Data Science*, https://doi.org/10.34133/2021/9837856

Part II

COVID-19 in Nordic public discourses

6 Trust, mistrust, and data narratives about COVID-19 vaccines in Denmark

How people reflect on the past, present, and future when navigating the pandemic

Sofie á Rogvi and Klaus Hoeyer

Introduction

Though vaccine hesitancy has long been associated with some form of knowledge deficit, not least in policy circles, recent research has suggested focusing instead on trust and trustworthiness in order to understand the choices people make (Goldenberg 2021; Warren et al. 2020). Inspired by this focus on trust, we explore processes through which trust and mistrust in COVID-19 vaccines have emerged in Denmark. We explore the narratives people make about vaccines, and we situate these narratives in a temporal arch of past, present, and future. Based on our analysis, we suggest that trust and mistrust interact with embodied and biographical ways of making sense of the world.

The COVID-19 pandemic, especially during its first months, was characterised by a high level of uncertainty. SARS-CoV-2, the virus causing COVID-19, was new and many aspects and characteristics about it were unknown (Hu et al. 2021; Kreps & Kriner 2020). Besides the uncertainty about what we may call the biology of the virus, people all over the world became affected by the uncertainties caused by interventions implemented to mitigate the spread of the disease. In some places, such as New York City in the United States, the pandemic acquired a visible presence in the form of ambulances and emergency graveyards (Martin 2021: xiii). In places like Denmark, however, people would for many months be more likely to experience the mitigation measures, such as lockdowns, than the disease itself. People needed to make sense of the pandemic threat in ways other than simple observation. They mostly depended on data.

The COVID-19 pandemic was inundated with data. Historically, epidemics have been known through data (Vandendriessche 2020), but this pandemic has been unprecedentedly data intense. Everything, from daily news and conversations over dinner to government press conferences and medical experts' communication, was flooded with numbers of infections, admissions to hospitals, and rates of death. Data were central to the sense-making strategies employed in most official communications about the disease, and data suffused everyday

DOI: 10.4324/9781003305859-8

living and debates about the new situation. However, data do not close conversations and debates. There can be multiple sources of data, and, in turn, manifold ways of reading them. Individuals need to decide which data and whose interpretations to trust before they can decide which path of action to take. When understanding how embodied and biographical ways of engaging the challenge of the pandemic interact with vaccine perception and behaviour, we see how even similar data can feature in very different narratives and lead to very different conclusions.

This chapter presents a case study about Denmark – a Scandinavian country which has managed the pandemic with relatively low death tolls, high vaccination rates, and a high level of satisfaction with the government's pandemic response (Devlin & Connaughton 2020; Mordecai 2020; Nielsen & Lindvall 2021; Petersen & Roepstorff 2021). While the Danish pandemic response was relatively swift, the lockdown measures were relatively soft. Denmark never, for example, implemented a curfew or limits to the right to take part in political street demonstrations. Denmark is known for high levels of generalised trust (Bjørnskov 2007; Petersen 2021; Petersen & Roepstorff 2021; Sønderskov & Dinesen 2014; Svendsen 2020), and references to trust were celebrated in the official political rhetoric during the pandemic (Statsministeriet [The Prime Minister's Office] 2020b, 2020c, 2021c, 2021d). However, some people, even in Denmark, did not trust the safety of the COVID-19 vaccines. Research even found a correlation between lack of trust in authorities and vaccine hesitancy (Lindholt et al. 2021; Petersen 2021). How did some people come to trust – and others mistrust – the health advice of the authorities? This question carries importance beyond understanding the COVID-19 pandemic, as it speaks to major challenges facing health services as people orient themselves towards new sources of authority in a digitally mediated world (Egher 2020; Petersen et al. 2022). We need to understand processes of trust to establish health services that work for all in a digital information age where expert authority cannot be taken for granted.

Making sense of – and with – trust

Trust can be understood as a hypothesis enabling "practical conduct" (Möllering 2001). Trust is necessary when information is incomplete, the future is uncertain, and the actions of others are uncontrollable. These elements arguably characterise most aspects of life, but rapid disruption of the type seen during the pandemic naturally augments them. Nooteboom (2002) has argued from an economic and organisational viewpoint that "the importance and nature of trust arise from the unpredictability, or radical uncertainty of human behaviour" (Nooteboom 2002: 5). For Nooteboom, uncertainty constitutes a lack of knowledge about the alternatives of choice. Still, trust cannot be replaced by knowledge. Trust has to do with relationships (Nooteboom 2002; see also Lewis & Weigart 1985): a subject trusting something or somebody. While this something or somebody may be considered the object of trust, this object acts as a subject as well. How this "other" reacts cannot be known with certainty. On a reading of Simmel's writings on trust, Möllering (2001) suggests that trust always involves a leap of faith – and form of "suspension" (*Aufheben*), which enables trust. Suspension is "the mechanism of bracketing the unknowable, thus making interpretative knowledge momentarily certain" (Möllering 2001: 403).

The sociologist Niklas Luhmann (1979) has conceptualised trust in functional terms. He has argued that trust is a way to reduce complexity. Trust works as a shortcut enabling action. Distrust is a functionally equivalent way of enabling action in a complex world. On distrust, he writes: "A person who distrusts both needs more information and at the same time narrows down the information which he feels confident he can rely on. He becomes *more* dependent on *less* information" (Luhmann 1979: 72, emphasis in original). Inspired by this functional equivalence and a long tradition of symmetry in social studies of science and technology (Lynch 2017), this chapter looks at trust and mistrust symmetrically.[1] Luhmann argues that trust involves some degree of order(ing) of the world (1979: 39). To act in the world, the world needs to be made meaningful, one way or the other.

If we accept that vaccine hesitancy is fundamentally a matter of (lack of) trust and cannot be explained as a knowledge deficit (Goldenberg 2021; Hausman 2019; Quinn et al. 2017), we can begin to explore how trust – in governance, institutions, and medical industry – builds up or is eroded. It is important, however, not to reproduce a deficit model of vaccine hesitancy now formulated as "lack of trust" instead of "lack of knowledge" (Leach & Fairhead 2007: 4). People do not "lack" the trust that others have, and there is no way to donate or transfer trust to those perceived as needing it. Hausman (2019) argues that we need to explore people's reasons in positive terms, rather than thinking that vaccine-hesitant people simply lack something other people possess. Vaccination choices are historically and socially situated acts (Goldenberg 2021). These choices become identity markers – and sometimes sources of political mobilisation (Hausman 2019; Leach & Fairhead 2007). Rather than focusing on knowledge deficits to understand vaccine hesitancy, we therefore need to understand how people make sense of the world around themselves during a period of heightened uncertainty.

To do so, we focus on embodied and biographical experiences. "Experience" has been criticised for being too loosely defined, not least when anthropologists write about their own experience in the field (Asad 1994). Still, experience remains an important category in phenomenological anthropology, where it serves as a way to avoid objectifying representations of people (e.g. Jackson 1996). Experience does not occur in a social, material, or political vacuum; it is socially constituted. While relational in nature (as is trust), experience is embodied and framed within biographies. These biographies become socially productive through narration. In our empirical material, narration takes the shape of interviews, speeches at street demonstrations, or posts and comments on social media. They always imply an audience. Narratives do not simply describe things as they are; rather, they structure experience. They are performative (Bruner 1986; Frank 2010) and affect "what people are able to see as real, as possible, and as worth doing or best avoided" (Frank 2010: 3). Through narratives, one person's experience becomes available to others (Bruner 1986). Narratives are generative of sociality; they can even mobilise social movements (Frank 2010: 3). Narratives are also a way to "alter the balance between actor and acted upon, thus allowing us to feel that we actively participate in a world that for a moment seemed to discount, demean, and disempower us" (Jackson 2002: 16). Stories help build communities of vaccine (mis)trust and (non) uptake, and they make some people distance themselves from others subscribing to different narratives. Stories "bring people together and they keep them apart" (Frank 2010: 2).

In the course of a data-intensive pandemic, data and discourses of science have become particular resources for narrative construction. Trust in data can reflect the degree to which one feels represented by the narratives the data are used to convey (Vandendriessche 2020). Still, trust is not just an analytical concept serving as a name of a particular mechanism or relational aspect. It is also a word featuring *in* these narratives, when individuals are positioning themselves in relation to others (Sheikh & Hoeyer 2018). Politicians, health authorities, and our interviewees all speak extensively about trust and mistrust. They reflect on the causes and consequences of trust and mistrust. As they speak about trust and mistrust, these actors build relationships and seek to affect their audiences in particular ways. They construct the relationships in which it is decided what counts as valid sources of knowledge. Therefore, reflections on what people are trying to *do* when talking about trust must form part of the methodology.

Methods – establishing three subsamples

The empirical material for this chapter builds on ethnographic fieldwork among, and interviews with, Danes on the subject of the COVID-19 pandemic. We collected material between March 2020 and July 2022. While there is no perfect method for any study, there are ways of reacting to the challenges encountered along the way. Indeed, this is what we had to do. We began with a qualitative interview study nested within a quantitative survey aimed at capturing views and experiences among a representative sample of the Danish population. The survey was distributed in the general population through a market research agency and carried out from the beginning of the pandemic (Clotworthy et al. 2021). We obtained a demographically balanced and thus ostensibly representative sample (based on the demographic traits geography, education, age, and gender). When answering the survey, respondents were invited to volunteer for an interview, and the agency selected representative candidates. Some were interviewed just once, others twice. We recruited 37 individuals through the survey, and we therefore call these the "survey-recruited subsample".

Gradually, however, we realised that this sample, while highly varied in a number of ways, did not count any voices strongly opposing the restrictions and the vaccines. Though demographically "representative", the sample seemed to represent mainly those with trust in the authorities. Yet we could see that opposition existed. We therefore had to rethink our sampling. We identified demonstrations and social media debates where views were articulated that clearly diverged from those in our previous interviews, and so we decided to recruit such opponents for interviews through street demonstrations and snowballing. We interviewed 11 individuals who identified themselves as critical towards the pandemic response in general. We call these interviewees the "restrictions resistance subsample". For this "resistance public", vaccines were not their main concern: they focused on restrictions. However, as vaccines became more widely rolled out, we gradually saw more and more people expressing vaccine hesitancy. Through Facebook's search function, observation of individual online posts which were critical of COVID-19 measures and street demonstrations, and based on recommendations from interviewees in the restrictions resistance subsample, we decided to follow three Danish Facebook forums debating the Danish COVID-19 response (restrictions and vaccines) and a former physician critical of the pandemic response (both vaccines and restrictions). One of these Facebook groups was established with the expressed purpose of critically debating vaccines. According to the group description, it is not "a radical anti-vaccine group" (our translation), but a place for discussing the risks involved in vaccines and the infections they are meant to prevent. People "totally pro-vaccines" (our translation) who only aim at counter-arguing are asked to go elsewhere by administrators. To understand the emerging mistrust of COVID-19 vaccines in depth, we recruited eight unvaccinated individuals from this vaccine-critical Facebook group for interviews. We call them the "unvaccinated subsample". In this way, we gained a strong basis for understanding both processes of trust and of mistrust. It made us able to compare very different positions: those who declare their trust, those who express mistrust towards the authorities and the pandemic response in general, and those who clearly have taken a stance against COVID-19 vaccines. Concomitantly, we followed the official political communication of the pandemic, including press conferences and press releases.

Figure 6.1 gives an overview of both the development of the Danish pandemic response from March 2020 to June 2022 and our fieldwork phases with the three subsamples (survey recruited, restrictions resistance, and unvaccinated).

All interviewees were informed about their right to withdraw participation at any time, and all gave informed consent before interviews. All names of interviewees are pseudonyms. Translations from Danish into English of both interviews and press conferences are by the authors. According to Danish law, this type of research is not subject to ethics approval, but ethics remains important and also intersects with analytical considerations. Since people enact relationships when discussing trust, we have had to be reflexive about our role as their audience. Many vaccine-hesitant people feel silenced. Our interviews

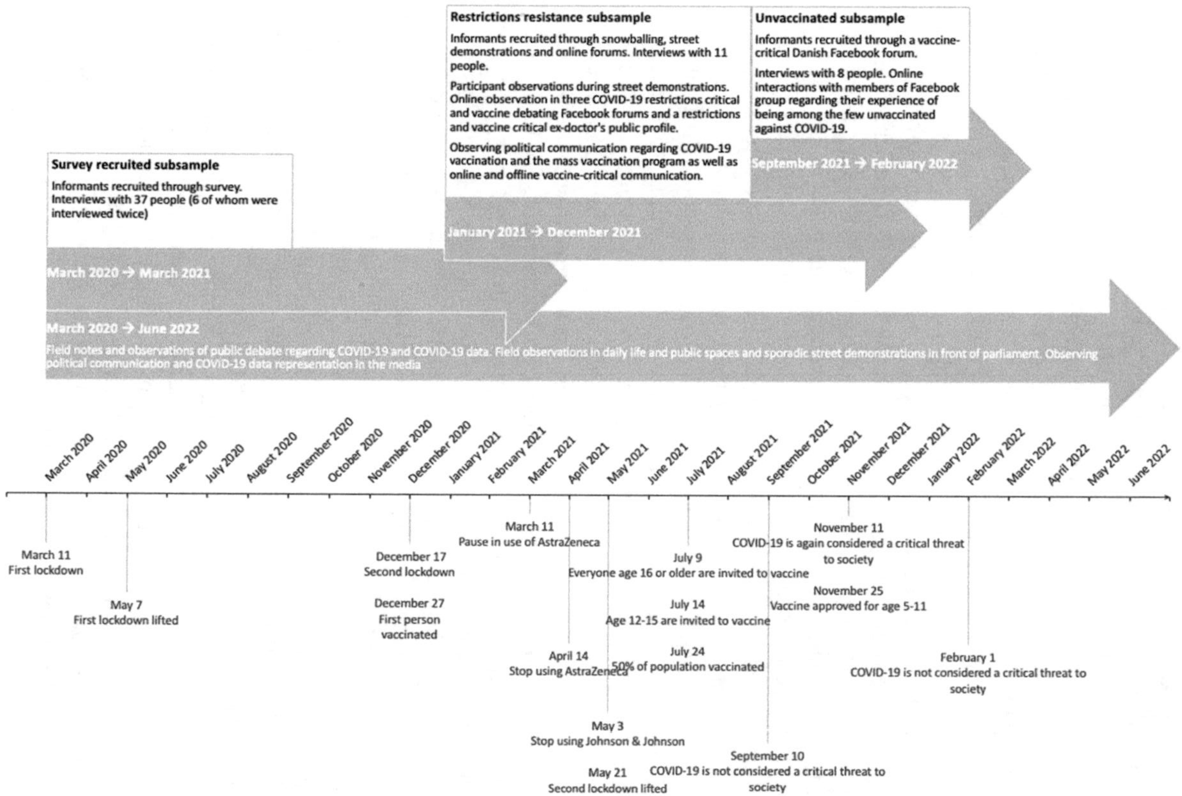

Figure 6.1 Timeline of pandemic response and fieldwork activities.

therefore became a sense-making activity with political connotations. Even though many vaccine-hesitant and restrictions-critical informants generally mistrusted institutions and sometimes science (or, rather, scientific institutions), they agreed to participate in our scientific study and shared with us their – sometimes controversial – views on restrictions and vaccines. They trusted us with their narratives. Even when we might not agree with their perception, we became obliged to respect it.

Introducing the Danish case

To understand the high level of support of vaccines within the general population in Denmark, we first provide some context. Denmark is a welfare state with a predominantly tax-financed healthcare system offering universal access (Olejaz et al. 2012). Denmark has a free child vaccination programme and offers seasonal flu vaccination free of charge to people over the age of 65, pregnant women, and certain risk groups. Uptake of child vaccines is generally high in Denmark – though uptake of vaccines against Human Papillomavirus (HPV) is lagging behind the other vaccines in the programme (Voss et al. 2021).

The Danish mass vaccination programme against COVID-19 included free mRNA vaccines from Pfizer/BioNTech and Moderna, and until March 2021, also Astra Zeneca's Vaxzevria. The digital infrastructures and integrated data pathways facilitated a relatively smooth and quick roll-out (Danske Regioner [Danish Regions] 2021). Data were also used to distribute vaccines based on medical criteria. In March 2021, the Danish Health Authority decided to pause the use of Astra Zeneca's Vaxzevria, due to the suspicion that the vaccine caused the severe side effects Vaccine-induced Immune Thrombosis and Thrombocytopenia (VITT), and in April 2021, it was permanently removed from the mass vaccination programme. The risk assessment was enabled by the existence of comprehensive Danish registers (Danmarks Radio 2021; Pottegård et al. 2021; Sundhedsstyrelsen [Danish Health Authority] 2021a). Vaccine uptake and support did not fall after Vaxzevria was paused (Sønderskov et al. 2021); rather, due to the global shortage of vaccines, the decision was criticised by many citizens for delaying the vaccination efforts. Parliament then decided to offer even these vaccines known to have side effects, but outside the official programme and on a voluntary basis, to accommodate the people who were not willing to wait. It became a very expensive solution (Heissel 2021a, 2021b). This battle to ensure *access* to vaccines suggests that Danes, overall, had a high level of willingness to be vaccinated against COVID-19, and by February 2022, 80% of all citizens had received COVID-19 vaccination (Petersen & Roepstorff 2021; Statens Serum Institut 2022). One study specifically related this to high levels of trust in the health sector (Sønderskov et al. 2021).

In August 2021, when everybody over the age of 15 had received an invitation to be vaccinated, the strategy shifted from rationing scarce vaccines to promoting vaccine uptake. Danish Health authorities established pop-up vaccination centres in supermarkets and in specific areas with low vaccine uptake, to make vaccination as easy and convenient as possible (Jørgensen 2021; Sundhedsstyrelsen [Danish Health Authority] 2021b, 2021c). The health authorities also targeted communication towards different ethnic groups, youth, and smaller children and their parents, to encourage them to vaccinate. Soon after the first Danes were vaccinated, dashboards in national media, which hitherto had been presenting COVID-19 infection data, started including daily numbers on vaccinations. Geographic coverage of vaccination down to parish level was presented as heat maps (Prakash & Keldorff 2021; Statens Serum Institut [State Serum Institute] 2021). In this way, data came to have a daily presence and inform people's sense-making strategies, including those related to COVID-19 vaccines.

As we now turn to the temporal dimensions of embodied and biographical ways of relating to vaccines – present, past, and future – we begin with how data were communicated in the media as a way of positioning and categorising people in the present at a time when many felt an extraordinary pressure.

The pandemic present

Between 6 March 2020 and 26 January 2022, Prime Minister Mette Frederiksen held 30 press conferences with other ministers and representatives from the authorities. They were live-streamed on national media and became a form of central arena for official narratives about the pandemic. The conferences were occasions for the current moment to be interpreted by those in power. As people were coping with pandemic-related distress, these events became important conveyors of narratives about groups and categories of people. As Frank points out, narratives both tie people together and divide them. From April 2020 onwards, vaccines began to be mentioned as the way out of the pandemic and to bring societal life back to normal (Statsministeriet [The Prime Minister's Office] 2020c). On 27 December 2020, when the very first Danes were vaccinated against COVID-19, Frederiksen said it was the "most hopeful day of 2020" (Statsministeriet [The Prime Minister's Office] 2020d). As vaccines were rolled out, they were called the "super weapon" by both the Prime Minister (Statsministeriet [The Prime Minister's Office] 2021b, 2021c) and the head of the Danish Health Authority, who said that this "super weapon should bring us safely through the winter" (Statsministeriet [The Prime Minister's Office] 2021e). The head of the Danish Medicines Agency also talked about vaccines as a "weapon arsenal" (Statsministeriet [The Prime Minister's Office] 2021a). In this narrative, the disease is the threat, and the vaccine the defence.

When in August 2021 the emphasis shifted from rationing vaccines to promoting them, the political communication also shifted. At one conference the Prime Minister, the Minister of Health, and the head of the Danish Health Authority all directly talked to the unvaccinated, appealing to their sense of responsibility for themselves, their family, and their community and to the aim of avoiding further lockdowns (Statsministeriet [The Prime Minister's Office] 2021c). Frederiksen appealed to the unvaccinated, saying: "So to you, who for one reason or another have not been vaccinated: Shouldn't you go do it now? … For your own sake, but also for the rest of us". Similarly, Søren Brostrøm, head of the Danish Health Authority, appealed to people in areas of low uptake, saying: "You should take the vaccine for your own sake. … You should also think about the rest of your neighbourhood. You should think of your family and friends" (Statsministeriet [The Prime Minister's Office] 2021c). On 8 November 2021, when the government reintroduced the COVID-19 passport necessitating a negative test or vaccination for entering restaurants, cultural institutions, and so on, the communication turned more to blaming, as when Prime Minister Frederiksen said: "I can't highlight enough the unfairness of the few [unvaccinated] potentially ruining it for the majority of us. So, in my eyes, there is no excuse – no moral excuse either – for not getting vaccinated" (Statsministeriet [The Prime Minister's Office] 2021d). Such moralising narratives served to categorise people, and can be seen as part of a sense-making strategy that gains strength when the present is full of confusion and distress.

Our interviews in all three subsamples contain a wide range of reactions to the political emphasis on vaccines being a "solution", as well as to the appeals to "responsibility". Many interviewees recruited through the survey directly mirrored the idea of vaccines being the means to overcome the pandemic. For example Torben (72, survey-recruited subsample) said in April 2020: "So I don't think we will get rid of COVID-19 infections before there's an effective vaccine". However, across the three samples there were people with more tempered hopes. In October 2020, 33-year-old Kasper (survey-recruited subsample) said: "Of course it's important to develop a vaccine. But I also know that the flu vaccines are guesswork. Because they [viruses] mutate … So I don't know if it is the solution, or when it may be the solution". So even among those who were supporters of the government and eager to have their vaccination, the science behind it was not seen as infallible. Data give rise to statistical probability, not ontological certainty. Doubt was part of the present even for some of those supporting vaccinations. For those more inclined to question the intentions of the authorities, however, such doubts inspired more fundamental reflections. In January 2021, 30-year-old Nanna (restrictions resistance subsample), imagined there would be a series of jabs as a result of virus mutations, calling this "a vicious circle". In the unvaccinated subsample, informants were generally very critical of the idea of vaccines as the solution. They requested "nuances" and recognition of side effects. They wanted a less "rosy" presentation. 45-year-old Niels (unvaccinated subsample, September 2021), who had himself been infected with COVID-19, commented that communication about natural immunity "just suddenly died, and now it's just vaccine, vaccine, vaccine".

Among the people under the age of 50 in the survey-recruited subsample, the idea of protecting others against infection rather than fear of getting severe COVID-19 mostly motivated their willingness to get vaccinated. It resonated with the political rhetoric of vaccinating for the sake of others, as described earlier. In contrast, many of the informants in the restrictions and unvaccinated subsamples reacted to idea of vaccination as a moral act, both as it appeared in the political communication and among fellow citizens. Nina, age 35 (unvaccinated subsample, October 2021), described how she felt: "We don't all feel like getting vaccinated, and that's not because we're egoistic. And the word *samfundssind* ['civic-mindedness'], it's implying that if you do as they say, you're a good citizen, and if you don't, you're a bad citizen". Mikkel, age 39 (restrictions resistance subsample), in February 2021, explained how he perceived the COVID-19 pass as unfair and as singling out some citizens as more worthy than others: "I think it's a very bad idea that a person is denounced as the black sheep". Vera, age 40 (unvaccinated subsample, September 2021), found the discourse patronising and thought those who were not vaccinated were hunted down as prey. She had recently lost her father. His health deteriorated immediately after he had a COVID-19 vaccination, and he died 35 days later. She blamed the vaccination. It made her uncomfortable when fellow citizens bragged about getting vaccinated:

> I don't know exactly why they do it [brag about getting vaccinated]. It's as if it's connected to being a good human. You share it on Facebook like that. … It's like a test of manhood to show that you're a good citizen, doing what is good for others. So, it hurts a bit every time you see it, because you feel like it gets connected with taking responsibility. And I'm not doing that, or what?

In this way, moral appeals to "civic-mindedness", referred to by Prime Minister Frederiksen several times from the first lockdown onwards (Statsministeriet [The Prime Minister's Office] 2020a; Villadsen 2021) can be experienced as a form of shaming. Health communication can thereby shape the experience of the pandemic in the present by categorising people. However, when people articulate their position towards vaccines, they do so not only through the categorisations of the present turmoil. They often build narratives based on past experiences.

Past

When comparing across the three subsamples, we see that informants use previous experiences to justify trust as well as mistrust. Interviewees from the survey-recruited subsample overall had positive experiences with vaccines and the institutions responsible. They did not request detailed evidence of the safety and benefits of COVID-19 vaccines. They trusted "the system" and its institutions' competence and procedures, and therefore did not need to know how the institutions had arrived at their conclusions. Anders, age 54 (survey-recruited subsample, second interview, November 2020), expressed his trust in the authorities' good intentions this way:

> I'm super naïve. If the health services and Søren Brostrøm [Head of the Danish Health Authority] say: "Just do it, God damn it", then I do it. No doubt. He doesn't tell me to do anything for his own sake. He's telling me for my own sake.

Anders specifically pointed out that it had worked for him in the past. Still, some – also from the population-recruited subsample – were uncomfortable with the economic interests related to vaccination development globally. No trust seems to be unconditional. Even those who personally have good experiences with the (healthcare) system have doubts, not least relating to big pharmaceutical companies with economic interests in vaccination. These concerns were shared by the restrictions resistance and unvaccinated subsamples, who sometimes also extended their mistrust to national and international institutions such as the World Health Organization. Some individuals from the restrictions resistance and unvaccinated subsamples also referred to Bill Gates and the conspiracy theories regarding his intentions for expanding vaccinations programmes worldwide (Fuchs 2021).

Besides this generalised mistrust in intentions and the interests of global vaccine actors, shared in varying degrees by those who support vaccines and those who become increasingly vaccine hesitant, interviewees from the restrictions resistance and unvaccinated subsamples invoked more specific past negative experience as formative for their vaccine hesitancy. We identify three kinds of negative experiences from the individual's past: those related to previous vaccination, previous experiences with the (health) system, and those related to one's own body.

A clear example of a negative vaccine experience was 40-year-old Vera (unvaccinated subsample, September 2021), who said her father had died from adverse reactions to the mRNA COVID-19 vaccination he received while ill. In her narrative, this explained her "boycott" of COVID-19 vaccination. Most often, however, informants drew on experiences with other vaccinations, such as those for flu or HPV. Overall, there are two ways in which HPV vaccination seems to have influenced COVID-19 vaccination attitudes among our informants: having seen people they care for experiencing side effects, or having experienced authorities not listening to those who want to talk about HPV vaccination side effects. Several informants in the unvaccinated subsample had relatives or people in their social network who had experienced some form of suffering in the period after an HPV vaccination. Lisa, age 51 (restrictions resistance, March 2021), recounts how this experience had fundamentally changed her approach to vaccination:

> It took me by surprise completely because I believed in the system. I've always supported all vaccines and believed a lot in vaccines, and for a time, I would even have supported forced vaccination, I think. So, I had an abrupt awakening when my daughter got seriously ill and had a high fever and a stiff neck the same night she got the HPV vaccine.

In Lisa's narrative, the experience of a seriously ill daughter fundamentally changed her approach to vaccination, and her trust in the system. Lisa explained how the experience with her ill daughter made her dig for information and browse vaccine research; she wanted to make sense of it. Her search on the internet, medical research databases, and social media bolstered her mistrust in vaccines, vaccine research, and their relation to big pharmaceutical companies with economic interests in vaccine programmes and uptake.

Other informants explained how their mistrust in vaccines was influenced by a lack of acknowledgement by the authorities of what informants perceive as vaccine side effects. Beate, age 24 (restrictions resistance, February 2021), for example, said:

> It was the HPV vaccine that put me off vaccines. Because there were so many girls who got ill. But now it's reported that it's only 25 girls who got ill. No doctors or health authorities will acknowledge that there was something in that vaccine which could make people ill.

We see in both Lisa's and Beate's narratives a sense of not being heard or respected by the Danish health system. Such a sense of not being heard or not receiving the help they need is further illustrated when people have negative experiences with the (health) system in general, and use this to explain their mistrust. For example, Niels, age 45 (unvaccinated, September 2021), mobilised the past in this way to explain his mistrust:

> I'm probably a bit more suspicious compared to the general public, because I've gone through this illness experience where I didn't get any help treating my disease in Denmark. So, I had to go abroad to get treatment [for a tick-borne borrelia infection]. So, it changed my perception of what and who you can trust.

Several informants in the unvaccinated subsample were, like Niels, also members of a Facebook group for people experiencing long-term effects of borrelia. In this group they found support from peers, and tips on how to alleviate symptoms that many of them felt were not handled appropriately in the Danish healthcare system. Such groups may also nourish a common narrative of reasons for mistrust and sustain identities of opposition. Yet others in the restrictions resistance and unvaccinated subsamples present negative experiences with the authorities or "the system" in general as reasons for mistrusting the communication about COVID-19 vaccines. Examples include (sexual) workplace harassment and conflicts with unemployment authorities. Common to these experiences is a narrative element of not being taken care of by "the system" – the welfare state – when needing it the most.

The third way vaccine-hesitant interviewees mobilise the past to explain mistrust related directly to their personal bodily biography, such as their experiences with illness. Returning to 45-year-old Niels (unvaccinated, September 2021), he for example stated:

> My problem is that I'm chronically ill and have a borrelia infection, that tick disease, and I've struggled to get rid of it and I've had it for many years. I have an immune system which goes crazy. Nobody really knows

> if it's overactive or underactive. So, I'm a bit in doubt [about] how I would react to vaccination, both against COVID-19 and other things. … I'm quite sick already so I wouldn't be able to forgive myself if I had really rough side effects after receiving a vaccination.

Having a body which cannot be trusted is an embodied experience of precariousness that potentially turns COVID-19 vaccines, *as well as* COVID-19 itself, into threats. Conversely, strong trust in one's own body and immune system also featured in the narratives of people in the restrictions resistance and unvaccinated subsamples.

Some informants saw vaccination against COVID-19 as an unwelcome intervention in a bodily system which would without intervention be able to successfully combat COVID-19. Such admiration for one's immune system is described by 51-year-old Tina (unvaccinated, September 2021):

> Think about how a flower can become a fruit, so full of nourishment. I mean that is so way beyond what humans can produce. And my body is likewise a divine creation. And therefore, I have an enormous trust that my immune system can do all sorts of things, especially if I don't load it with all sorts of things which are bad for it.

Here we suggest that mobilising one's bodily experience can serve as a way of building authority, as well as being a sense-making strategy. It does not preclude data or science. However, it inspires people to search for data in other ways, from other sources, with different conclusions. Many vaccine-hesitant people therefore engage with data and research studies with much more dedication than those declaring their trust. An example of this is 35-year-old Nina (unvaccinated, October 2021) who had just finished university and who stated:

> I don't trust the safety of the vaccines based on what I've read about the trials. For example, the vaccines have not been tested against true placebos like saline, and already after four months they ruined the control group by vaccinating them. … I wouldn't call it good science.

Her past experience with several health conditions for which she had not found mainstream medical relief, and her academic inclination to question had stimulated a search for reasons to question vaccines. While the past was invoked in ample ways in explanations of (mis)trust, the future also plays a role in the formation of (mis)trust.

Future

"To show trust is to anticipate the future", Luhmann (1979: 10) wrote. The various different narratives of trust and mistrust in COVID-19 vaccines involve very different imaginations of the future and of what kinds of future people hope for and/or fear. For interviewees in the survey-recruited subsample, a future without trust in the authorities is one of great uncertainty. Some supporters of vaccination express concern about the ongoing polarisation related to COVID-19 policies, and they consider that trusting the authorities in relation to restrictions and vaccination is an investment in the future. Vaccine hesitancy similarly relates to visions for the future and the type of society being built with pandemic measures. Among the vaccine hesitant, the future was mobilised in very fearful ways in some of their narratives. For example, 24-year-old Beate (restrictions resistance, February 2021) concluded, "If they can force us to vaccinate, what can't they force us to do?" Several informants in the unvaccinated subsample explained how they would migrate or defend themselves in case of forced vaccination. Tina, age 51 (unvaccinated, September 2021), expressed her fear of forced vaccination in the following way:

> I get very afraid when I see what happens in some other countries. I can't imagine that someone would force vaccinate me. I would rather be raped, to put it bluntly. You can come to terms with that and then it's over. But injecting something into the body that you didn't choose to [have], and which [you] can't get out again. That is such an assault, that even just considering it is a major landslide in human rights.

This quotation illustrates just how devastating and anxiety-provoking forced vaccination can be for the interviewees who do not wish to get vaccinated – and the kind of future they fear the most.

Some informants in the restrictions resistance and unvaccinated subsamples mentioned narratives that are labelled "conspiracy theories" by the authorities, for example of vaccines acting as a "bioweapon" (Olga, 60, unvaccinated, October 2021) or as part of a depopulation plan. Interestingly, the idea of vaccines as a weapon used in the political rhetoric described earlier is here turned around. For people mistrusting intentions, this weapon is directed not at a dangerous virus, but at people. The forecast they believe is driving the interventions is not prevention of disease, but dissemination of disease in order to depopulate the planet either via less reproduction (vaccine-induced infertility) or population thinning (killing through vaccination). As such, the imagined future interacts with fears and ideas about the intentions of those in power. Trust as well as mistrust involve caring about and for the future.

Conclusion

During the pandemic, data were omnipresent and figured in political communication, everyday conversation, online and offline resistance, and the media. With this chapter we have illustrated how trust and mistrust influence the navigation of these data, and how embodied experience shapes narratives of trust and mistrust. Moreover, for people to trust the data used to argue preventive measures such as restrictions and vaccinations, they need to trust the people presenting them and their intentions. Trust is rarely, if ever, unconditional. It takes a leap of faith. Not everyone will make this leap. Data do not deliver the necessary faith in and by themselves. Whether or not they do so will reflect how people make sense of the world around them. Rather than thinking that vaccine mistrust grows out of a propensity to listen to conspiracy theories (Rutjens et al. 2021), we have shown that both supporters of vaccines and the vaccine hesitant share general doubts about the incentives and intentions driving pharmaceutical industry and global vaccine actors. The vaccine hesitant, however, also tend to have more specific experiences informing their mistrust and how they make sense of the pandemic. They are unlikely to neglect these concrete experiences with generalised appeals to "science".

Sense-making is a bodily act embedded in biographical experience. We have taken insights into trust in general presented at the beginning of this chapter and developed them further by situating the mechanisms of trust and mistrust *phenomenologically* in a temporal play of past, present, and future. With our focus on embodied experience, we substantiate the claim referenced in the introduction: that more, and correct, information will not by itself diminish either vaccine hesitancy or the conspiracy theories that some people mistrusting vaccines refer to (Lazić & Žeželj 2021).

Experience and trust formation are always social. People narrate to an audience, and narratives can both tie people together and tell them apart. Narratives of COVID-19 vaccines are thus part of a process of group formation for both vaccine supporters and hesitators, a process which may contribute to group polarisation and negative attitudes towards the other. Recent research has shown that people vaccinated against COVID-19 hold discriminatory attitudes towards the unvaccinated, much more so than the other way around (Bor et al. 2022). Political rhetoric probably influences people's perceptions of both vaccines and vaccine behaviour. At least, we see how vaccine-hesitant people have felt shamed and marginalised by the rhetoric used by politicians and authorities in Denmark. People mobilise in relation to different communities. When exploring how people are building communities, we have suggested paying attention to how talk *about* trust is performative. It shapes the way people build group membership. Trust should therefore not only serve as analytical lens or a term we as scholars discuss and theoretically refine. It is an emic concept that people – vaccine supporters and hesitators, lay people and politicians – talked about, used, and altered as they made sense of the pandemic. When authorities or individuals shame people who hesitate to vaccinate, or scold them for lack of trust, it will probably only make them seek those that accept them. Listening carefully to people's narratives – symmetrically – may help to avoid both re-inventing the deficit-model and pushing vaccine-hesitant people toward those who will only confirm their doubts. Scholars as well as authorities might have to learn to think of mutual respect as the fertile soil from which a more fruitful dialogue can grow.

Note

1 We recognise that *distrust* and *mistrust* may not be completely interchangeable terms. We use the term "mistrust" as it may embrace more nuances and degrees of COVID-vaccine-related hesitancy than "distrust", which we understand as more certain lack of trust in something particular.

References

Asad, Talal. 1994. Ethnographic representation, statistics, and modern power. *Social Research* 61(1): 55–88.

Bjørnskov, Christian. 2007. Determinants of generalized trust: A cross-country comparison. *Public Choice* 130(1–2): 1–21. https://doi.org/10.1007/s11127-006-9069-1

Bor, A., F. Jørgensen & M. B. Petersen. 2022. Discriminatory attitudes against the unvaccinated during a global pandemic. *Nature*. https://doi.org/10.1038/s41586-022-05607-y

Bruner, Edward M. 1986. Experience and its expressions. In Victor W. Turner & Edward M. Bruner (eds.), *The Anthropology of Experience*, 3–32. Urbana and Chicago: University of Illinois Press.

Clotworthy, Amy, Agnete Skovlund Dissing, Tri Long Nguyen, Andreas Kryger Jensen, Thea Otte Andersen, Josephine Funck Bilsteen, Leonie K. Elsenburg et al. 2021. "Standing together – At a distance": Documenting changes in mental-health indicators in Denmark during the COVID-19 pandemic. *Scandinavian Journal of Public Health* 49(1): 79–87. https://doi.org/10.1177/1403494820956445

Danmarks Radio. 2021. LIVE: Pressemøde om AstraZeneca-vaccinen [LIVE: Press conference about the AstraZeneca vaccine], 14 April 2021. https://www.dr.dk/nyheder/indland/live-pressemoede-om-astrazeneca-vaccinen

Danske Regioner [Danish Regions]. 2021. International medieinteresse for dansk vaccinationsindsats [International media interested in Danish vaccination efforts], 20 January 2021. https://www.regioner.dk/services/nyheder/2021/januar/international-medieinteresse-for-dansk-vaccinationsindsats

Devlin, Kat & Aidan Connaughton. 2020. Most approve of national response to COVID-19 in 14 advanced economies. https://www.pewresearch.org/global/2020/08/27/most-approve-of-national-response-to-covid-19-in-14-advanced-economies/

Egher, C. 2020. Online expert mediators: The rise of a new "bipolar" stakeholder or going beyond interactional expertise in the blogosphere. *Science and Technology Studies* 33(2): 10–31. https://doi.org/10.23987/sts.60782

Frank, Arthur W. 2010. *Letting stories breathe: A socio-narratology*. Chicago and London: University of Chicago Press.

Fuchs, Christian. 2021. *Communicating COVID-19: Everyday life, digital capitalism, and conspiracy theories in pandemic times*. United Kingdom – North America – Japan – India – Malaysia – China: Emerald Publishing.

Goldenberg, Maya J. 2021. *Vaccine hesitancy: Public trust, expertise, and the war on science*. Pittsburgh: University of Pittsburgh Press.

Hausman, Bernice L. 2019. *ANTI/VAX: Reframing the vaccination controversy*. Ithaca and London: Cornell University Press.

Heissel, Anders. 2021a. Mange gange dyrere: Privat firma får kvart milliard for at tilbyde skrottede vacciner [Many fold more expensive: Private firm gets a quarter of a billion to offer tossed vaccines], 25 August 2021. https://www.dr.dk/nyheder/indland/mange-gange-dyrere-privat-firma-faar-kvart-milliard-tilbyde-skrottede-vacciner

Heissel, Anders. 2021b. Vaccinefirma fik 16 millioner kroner for at vaccinere 60 danskere på en uge [Vaccine firm received 16 million crowns to vaccinate 60 Danes in a week], 31 August 2021. https://www.dr.dk/nyheder/indland/vaccinefirma-fik-16-millioner-kroner-vaccinere-60-danskere-paa-en-uge

Hu, Ben, Hua Guo, Peng Zhou & Zheng Li Shi. 2021. Characteristics of SARS-CoV-2 and COVID-19. *Nature Reviews Microbiology* 19(3): 141–154. https://doi.org/10.1038/s41579-020-00459-7

Statens Serum Institut. 2022. Antal og andel siden 27. december 2020 (1. vaccinationsforløb). 16 February 2022. https://experience.arcgis.com/experience/9824b03b114244348ef0b10f69f490b4/page/page_3/

Jackson, Michael. 1996. Introduction: Phenomenology, radical empiricism, and anthropological critique. In Jackson, Michael (ed.) *Things as they are: New directions in phenomenological anthropology*. Bloomington: Indiana University Press.

Jackson, Michael. 2002. *The politics of storytelling: Violence, transgression and intersubjectivity*. København: Museum Tusculanum Press.

Jørgensen, Lars Bach. 2021. Vaccineret i amme-rummet i Bilka: Det har været en kamp at komme her [Vaccinated in the breast-feeding room in Bilka: It has been a struggle to come here], 11 September 2021.

Kreps, S. E. & D. L. Kriner. 2020. Model uncertainty, political contestation, and public trust in science: Evidence from the COVID-19 pandemic. *Science Advances* 6. https://doi.org/10.1126/sciadv.abd4563

Lazić, Aleksandra & Iris Žeželj. 2021. A systematic review of narrative interventions: Lessons for countering anti-vaccination conspiracy theories and misinformation. *Public understanding of science*. SAGE Publications Ltd. https://doi.org/10.1177/09636625211011881

Leach, Melissa & James Fairhead. 2007. *Vaccine anxieties: Global science, child health & society*. London: Earthscan from Routledge.

Lewis, J. D. & A. Weigart. 1985. Trust as a social reality. *Social Forces* 63(4): 967–985.

Lindholt M. F., F. Jørgensen, A. Bor & M. B. Petersen. 2021. Public acceptance of COVID-19 vaccines: Cross-national evidence on levels and individual-level predictors using observational data. *BMJ Open* 11: e048172. https://doi.org/10.1136/bmjopen-2020-048172

Luhmann, Niklas. 1979. *Trust and power*. Chichester, New York, Brisbane, Toronto: John Wiley & Sons.

Lynch, Michael. 2017. STS, symmetry and post-truth. *Social Studies of Science* 47(4): 593–599.

Martin, Emily. 2021. *Experiments of the mind: From the cognitive psychology lab to the world of Facebook and Twitter*. New Jersey: Princeton University Press.

Möllering, Guido. 2001. The nature of trust: From Georg Simmel to a theory of expectation, interpretation and suspension. *Sociology* 35(2): 403–420.

Mordecai, Mara. 2020. How people around the world see the World Health Organization's initial coronavirus response. https://www.pewresearch.org/fact-tank/2020/11/12/how-people-around-the-world-see-the-world-health-organizations-initial-coronavirus-response/

Nielsen, Julie Hassing & Johannes Lindvall. 2021. Trust in government in Sweden and Denmark during the COVID-19 epidemic. *West European Politics* 44(5–6): 1180–1204. https://doi.org/10.1080/01402382.2021.1909964

Nooteboom, B. 2002. *Trust: Forms, foundations, functions, failures and figures*. Cheltenham and Northampton: Edward Edgar Publishing.

Olejaz, Maria, Annegrete Juul Nielsen, Andreas Rudkjøbing, Hans Okkels Birk, Allan Krasnik & Christina Hernández-Quevedo. 2012. Denmark health system review. *Health Systems in Transition* 14(2): i-xxii, 1-192. PMID: 22575801

Petersen, Alan, Allegra Schermuly & Alison Anderson. 2022. "A platform for goodness, not for badness": The heuristics of hope in patients' evaluations of online health information. *Social Science & Medicine* 306: 115115. https://doi.org/10.1016/j.socscimed.2022.115115

Petersen, Michael Bang. 2021. COVID lesson: Trust the public hard truths. *Nature* 580: 237. http://ci.nii.ac.jp/naid/40007256857/

Petersen, Michael Bang & Andreas Roepstorff. 2021. Danskerne adfærd og holdning til corona-epidemien. Aarhus: School of Business and Social Sciences, Aarhus University. https://hope-project.dk/#/reports/danskernes_adfaerd_og_holdninger/versions/06-08-2021

Pottegård, Anton, Lars Christian Lund, Øystein Karlstad, Jesper Dahl, Morten Andersen, Jesper Hallas, Øjvind Lidegaard et al. 2021. Arterial events, venous thromboembolism, thrombocytopenia, and bleeding after vaccination with Oxford-AstraZeneca ChAdOx1-S in Denmark and Norway: Population based cohort study. *The BMJ* 373 (May). https://doi.org/10.1136/bmj.n1114

Prakash, Thomas & Peter Keldorff. 2021. Tingbjerg Og Gellerup topper liste over sogne med den laveste tilslutning til vaccine [Tingbjerg and Gellerup are on the top of the list of parishes with the lowest vaccine uptake], 14 June 2021. https://www.dr.dk/nyheder/indland/tingbjerg-og-gellerup-topper-liste-over-sogne-med-den-laveste-tilslutning-til#!/

Quinn, Sandra, Amelia Jamison, Donald Musa, Karen Hilyard & Vicki Freimuth. 2017. Exploring the continuum of vaccine hesitancy between African American and White adults: Results of a qualitative study. *PLOS Currents* 8.

Rutjens, Bastiaan T., Sander van der Linden & Romy van der Lee. 2021. Science skepticism in times of COVID-19. *Group Processes & Intergroup Relations* 24(2): 276–283.

Sheikh, Zainab & Klaus Hoeyer. 2018. "That is why I have trust": Unpacking what "trust" means to participants in international genetic research in Pakistan and Denmark. *Medical Health Care and Philosophy* 21: 169–179.

Sønderskov, Kim Mannemar & Peter Thisted Dinesen. 2014. Danish exceptionalism: Explaining the unique increase in social trust over the past 30 years. *European Sociological Review* 30(6): 782–795. https://doi.org/10.1093/esr/jcu073

Sønderskov, Kim Mannemar, Peter Thisted Dinesen & Søren Dinesen Østergaard. 2021. Sustained COVID-19 vaccine willingness after safety concerns over the Oxford-AstraZeneca vaccine. *Danish Medical Journal* 68(5).

Statens Serum Institut [State Serum Institute]. 2021. Statens Serum Institut deler nu opgørelser over vaccinationstilslutningen i sogne [The State Serum Institute now share inventories of vaccination uptake in parishes]. 14 June 2021. https://www.ssi.dk/aktuelt/nyheder/2021/statens-serum-institut-deler-nu-opgorelser-over-vaccinationstilslutningen-i-sogne

Statsministeriet [The Prime Minister's Office]. 2020a. Pressemøde om COVID-19 den 11. marts 2020 [Press conference about COVID-19, 11 March 2020]. 11 March 2020. https://www.stm.dk/presse/pressemoedearkiv/pressemoede-om-covid-19-den-11-marts-2020/

Statsministeriet [The Prime Minister's Office]. 2020b. Pressemøde den 30. marts 2020 [Press conference, 30 March 2020]. 30 March 2020. https://www.stm.dk/presse/pressemoedearkiv/pressemoede-den-30-marts-2020/

Statsministeriet [The Prime Minister's Office]. 2020c. Pressemøde den 6. april 2020 [Press conference, 6 April 2020]. https://www.stm.dk/presse/pressemoedearkiv/pressemoede-den-6-april-2020/

Statsministeriet [The Prime Minister's Office]. 2020d. Pressemøde den 29. december 2020 [Press conference, 29 December 2020]. https://www.stm.dk/presse/pressemoedearkiv/pressemoede-den-29-december-2020/

Statsministeriet [The Prime Minister's Office]. 2021a. Pressemøde den 5. januar 2021 [Press conference 5 January 2021]. https://www.stm.dk/presse/pressemoedearkiv/pressemoede-den-5-januar-2021/

Statsministeriet [The Prime Minister's Office]. 2021b. Pressemøde den 24. februar 2021 [Press conference 24 February 2021]. https://www.stm.dk/presse/pressemoedearkiv/pressemoede-den-24-februar-2021/

Statsministeriet [The Prime Minister's Office]. 2021c. Pressemøde mandag den 23. august [Press conference, 23 August 2021]. https://www.stm.dk/presse/pressemoedearkiv/pressemoede-mandag-den-23-august/

Statsministeriet [The Prime Minister's Office]. 2021d. Pressemøde den 8. november 2021 [Press conference, 8 November 2021]. https://www.stm.dk/presse/pressemoedearkiv/pressemoede-den-8-november-2021/

Statsministeriet [The Prime Minister's Office]. 2021e. Pressemøde den 1. december 2021 [Press conference, 1 December 2021]. https://www.stm.dk/presse/pressemoedearkiv/pressemoede-den-1-december-2001/

Sundheds- og Ældreministeriet. 2021. Skærpet forsamlingsforbud og øvrige tiltag for at imødegå Cluster B.1.1.7 [Stricter assembly ban and other measures to address Clusters B.1.1.7]. 5 January 2021. https://www.regeringen.dk/nyheder/2021/skaerpet-forsamlingsforbud-og-oevrige-tiltag-for-at-imoedegaa-cluster-b117/

Sundhedsstyrelsen [Danish Health Authority]. 2021a. Dansk-norsk studie om sjældne bivirkninger efter COVID-19 vaccinen fra AstraZeneca er offentliggjort [Danish-Norwegian study about rare side effects of the COVID-19 vaccine from AstraZeneca is published]. 6 May 2021. https://www.sst.dk/da/Nyheder/2021/Dansk-Norsk-studie-om-sjaeldne-bivirkninger-efter-COVID-19-vaccinen-fra-AstraZeneca-er-offentliggjort

Sundhedsstyrelsen [Danish Health Authority]. 2021b. Virksomheder Og organisationer bidrager til vaccinationsslutspurten [Companies and organizations contribute to the final vaccination sprint], September. https://www.sst.dk/da/Nyheder/2021/Virksomheder-og-organisationer-bidrager-til-vaccinationsslutspurten

Sundhedsstyrelsen [Danish Health Authority]. 2021c. Fremover kan du selv vælge, hvilken type vaccine du vil have ved 1. stik [From now on you can decide which type of vaccine you want at 1st jab]. 16 September 2021. https://www.sst.dk/da/Nyheder/2021/Fremover-kan-du-selv-vaelge_-hvilken-type-vaccine-du-vil-have-ved-1_-stik

Svendsen, Gert Thinggaard. 2020. Forsker: Danmarks verdensrekord i tillid hjælper os i kampen mod corona [Researcher: Denmark's world record in trust helps us in the fight against COVID]. 20 March 2020. https://videnskab.dk/forskerzonen/kultur-samfund/forsker-danmarks-verdensrekord-i-tillid-hjaelper-os-i-kampen-mod-corona

Vandendriessche, Joris. 2020. Cholera, corona and trust in numbers. *Journal for the History of Environment and Society* 5: 47–52.

Villadsen, L. S. 2021, One word to rule them all: "Civic-mindedness" and Danish prime minister Frederiksen's nationalist Covid-19 rhetoric. *Punctum. International Journal of Semiotics* 6(2): 229–248. https://doi.org/10.18680/hss.2020.0030

Voss, Sissel Skou, Sarah Kristine Nørgaard, Manon Chaine & Palle Valentiner-Branth. 2021. *Hvilke grupper af børn har behov for en målrettet vaccinationsindsats* [Which groups of kids need a targeted vaccination intervention]. Copenhagen: Infektionsepidemiologi og Forebyggelse, Statens Serum Institut. https://apps.who.int/immunization_monitoring/globalsummary/schedules

Warren, Rueben C., Lachlan Forrow, David Augustin Hodge & Robert D. Truog. 2020. Trustworthiness before trust: Covid-19 vaccine trials and the Black community. *New England Journal of Medicine* 383(22): e121. https://doi.org/10.1056/nejmp2030033

7 Trust and the public vaccine debate in Finland before and during the COVID-19 pandemic

Aapo Kuusipalo, Johanna Nurmi, Katri-Maria Järvinen, and Pia Vuolanto

Introduction

Societal discussions consist of and incorporate a large spectrum of vaccine-related attitudes, ranging from anti- to pro-vaccination standpoints endorsed by supporters and opponents of immunisation programmes and related public health campaigns. Citizens are affected by these public discourses, which can shape their views about vaccines. The COVID-19 pandemic and the vaccines developed to fight the disease have brought vaccination to the forefront of societal discussions all over the world. This is true even in contexts like Finland, where vaccines have historically sparked little controversy and vaccine-critical sentiments have been marginal. This chapter analyses vaccine-related discourses presented in both mainstream media and in a campaign promoting an alternative view, i.e., the *Let's Save the Children of Finland* campaign.

Finland is a Nordic country characterised by high levels of trust in national institutions and high vaccine uptake (Finnish Science Barometer 2019): only 0.7% of school-aged children have not received the basic vaccinations included in the national vaccination programme (THL 2022), despite all vaccines being voluntary for the general public. During the COVID-19 pandemic in Finland, as in many high-income countries (Esaiasson et al. 2021; Goldfinch et al. 2021), strong or even increasing levels of trust in scientific institutions and the government were witnessed, along with a simultaneous increase in the challenging of expert advice and public measures (e.g., mask recommendations, restrictions on events and gatherings, vaccination) related to the pandemic (Jallinoja & Väliverronen 2021; Jallinoja et al. 2021; Väliverronen & Jallinoja 2021).

Suspicions regarding COVID-19 vaccines in Finland were prominently voiced by the *Let's Save the Children of Finland* campaign, a movement started by doctors and other healthcare professionals who sought to prevent and end COVID-19 vaccinations for children. The campaign started its operation with the publication of a petition signed by the founding professionals in June 2021, at which time the expansion of COVID-19 vaccinations to children was being publicly discussed. While this campaign was mainly national, movements started by medical professionals critical of COVID-19 vaccinations are both a

DOI: 10.4324/9781003305859-9

Nordic and a global phenomenon (e.g., Läkaruppropet in Sweden, NZDSOS in New Zealand, Doctors for COVID Ethics internationally).

In research on vaccine refusal and hesitancy, lack of trust is one of the key reasons identified to explain criticism and questioning of expert advice on vaccination. However, these explanations often presume a simplistic dichotomy of trust vs. lack of trust and tend to frame lack of trust as a problem of hesitant individuals (see Leach & Fairhead 2007: 21) and compliance with vaccination systems as morally right (Heller 2008: 22–23). An alternative perspective is to see vaccine hesitancy as a sign of poor public trust in scientific and governmental institutions, as an institutional failure to engender and maintain public trust (e.g., Goldenberg 2021: 136). Trust in vaccination and in the actors implementing vaccination policies can thus be understood as a part of generalised trust, or trust in abstract systems (Leach & Fairhead 2007: 18; see also Giddens 1990; Luhmann 1988). When examining trust in relation to vaccination, it is important to clarify conceptually the different types of attitudes towards and engagements with health systems, institutions, and vaccine technologies that are expressed or promoted in public discussion. Relevant concepts for the analysis of publics' relationship with health systems such as vaccination include trust, confidence, mistrust, and distrust.

Smith (2005) has emphasised an analytical distinction between confidence and trust (see Table 7.1) in health and social care, with confidence centring on rational choice and risk calculation and trust centring on morals and uncertainty. Trust, in fact, can be understood as an alternative to rational prediction (Luhmann 1979: 4). While confidence relies on technical or ethical competence, trust is more reliant on moral and affective competence (Smith 2005). Both concepts have been central in research on vaccine attitudes and vaccine hesitancy, and they are sometimes used interchangeably (e.g., Goldenberg 2021: 114; Karafillakis et al. 2021). Smith (2005) argues that trust and confidence both contribute to different areas of healthcare, but that health systems have been emphasising confidence over trust. Health systems have thus been developing "confidence in systems rather than trust in the moral capacities of

Table 7.1 Differentiating between theoretical concepts

Confidence	*Trust*	*Mistrust*	*Distrust*
Predictability, rational choice, risk calculation	Uncertainty, morals	Caution, scepticism, doubt, questioning	Suspicion, cynicism,
Technical competence and ethical codes of conduct	Moral and affective competence	Sensitivity to new information	Settled belief of untrustworthiness
In the functioning of systems	In the moral capabilities of individuals	Hesitation, updating, assessment	Avoiding, distancing

individuals who are responsible for delivering health and social care" (Smith 2005: 310). This has promoted predictability and risk analysis, but offered fewer tools in developing trust.

Situations where trust is not present can be described with concepts of distrust and mistrust (see Table 7.1) and, again, these concepts are often used interchangeably. Lenard (2008) has outlined a useful distinction between mistrust and distrust by characterising mistrust as more ambivalent and precarious than distrust, which is more of a fixed position. Mistrust is a cautious, doubtful, questioning, and sceptic mindset (Jennings et al. 2021; Lenard 2008). It is an attitude marked by hesitation and a "lack of clear expectations" (Sztompka 1999: 26) characterised by a "continuous process of feedback and updating" (Jennings et al. 2021: 1178) as the possible (un)trustworthiness of a person or an institution is constantly assessed. Distrust, on the other hand, refers to an established belief of untrustworthiness (Lenard 2008). Sztompka (1999: 26) described distrust as "the negative mirror-image of trust" that may lead to avoiding social commitment, or distancing.

Our focus is particularly on discourses relating to hesitant and critical views and the concept of trust. Firstly, we utilise the theoretical delineation between trust and confidence as we ask: (1) How do Finnish discourses on vaccines, both mainstream and alternative, use elements of trust and confidence when seeking to build trust towards their message? Secondly, we employ the concepts of mistrust and distrust in asking: (2) How do these discourses express mistrust and distrust in situations where trust is not present?

This analysis will offer insight into the interplay between a vaccine-critical discourse originating amongst medical and scientific experts and a mainstream discourse deeply rooted in the Finnish context, characterised by high vaccination coverage and strong public trust in science, healthcare organisations, and healthcare professionals (Finnish Science Barometer 2019). The alternative discourse we analyse is critical only of COVID-19 vaccines, not all vaccination. The people presented in said discourse, while on the alternative side on this issue, thus share the views of the mainstream medical establishment with regard to all other vaccines, making the interplay, relations, and differences between discourses even more interesting. This analytical context could be considered as something of an "ideal case" for studying the appearance and discursive use of the conceptualisations of trust discussed earlier: the presumably small distance between mainstream and alternative positions can enable an analysis to focus on minute differentiations and thus shed light on processes which can, in many contexts, be shrouded by more pronounced difference.

Research design

This study utilised a qualitative approach in analysing both mainstream and alternative Finnish discourses relating to vaccine hesitancy and criticism. Our focus was on how trust and confidence were built in the research materials and on orientations of mistrust and distrust expressed in situations where trust was lacking. As we examine discourses that seek to affect the opinions of others, our analysis falls into the realm of rhetorical analysis in its broad definitions (see Perelman 1982). Our focus was further framed by the conceptual delineations between trust/confidence and mistrust/distrust discussed in the previous section.

The analysis was based on the Finnish media analysis for the EU-Horizon-funded research project *VAX-TRUST, Addressing Vaccine Hesitancy in Europe*, which incorporated semantic, rhetorical, and discourse analyses. The mainstream media data was coded using a codebook compiled for this project, while a separate coding scheme was designed and used for the alternative discourse data. For coding, we used the qualitative analysis software NVivo and ATLAS.ti. The analyses of both discourses were expanded and refocused on vaccine hesitancy and the concepts of trust, confidence, mistrust, and distrust. All presented quotations have been translated from the original Finnish by the authors of this chapter.

The data representing Finnish mainstream media discourse consisted of 607 articles from the time between 1 April 2019 and 10 April 2021 and were collected from three news portals: YLE, *Helsingin Sanomat*, and *Iltalehti*. The selection of news outlets was based on popularity and diversity, with the chosen portals representing the national public broadcasting company (YLE), the largest politically independent daily newspaper (*Helsingin Sanomat*), and one of the largest tabloid journals in Finland (*Iltalehti*). The data featured news articles and columns, but excluded materials like opinion pieces and comment sections. Quotations are marked with the news portal domain (yle.fi, hs.fi, or iltalehti.fi) and date of publication.

The alternative discourse was represented in this study by one of the more visible vaccine-critical movements active in Finland in recent years: the *Let's Save the Children of Finland* campaign. Data was collected between 1 November 2021 and 31 January 2022 from the campaign website, where the campaign published its materials, which included compilations of scientific information, open letters to policymakers and scientists, and reactions to current events. The analysed data consisted of all 55 pages viewable on the website at any given point during data collection. Quotations from these materials are marked in the analysis by a number arbitrarily assigned by the analysis software, which serves only to distinguish between materials.

Mainstream media discourse before and during COVID-19

The Finnish mainstream discourses we analysed relating to vaccines and vaccine hesitancy featured a wide variety of actors, viewpoints, and discursive threads. Vaccines were framed in an overwhelmingly positive way, with argumentation highlighting the benefits and necessity of vaccines and seeking to dispel any presumed fears or hesitations. This reporting was most commonly linked to COVID-19 vaccines, where statements from healthcare experts and officials regularly accentuated the seriousness of the pandemic and presented vaccines as the only way back to normal.

> According to him [interviewed intensive care physician], the amount of intensive care required to treat the most serious forms of the disease speaks to the severity of corona. [The physician] emphasises that it is only through vaccination that we can get back to normal everyday life.
>
> (yle.fi 2021-01-15)

As seen earlier, vaccines were often construed as the solution to the threatening pandemic situation, but this conceptualisation also had a larger framing. Vaccine reporting before the onset of the pandemic had a similar tendency to represent vaccines as the solution to a host of ailments and often reported on vaccine development against a host of serious diseases, like HIV, Alzheimer's, and malaria. Reporting linked to vaccine side effects had a corresponding proclivity to emphasise the positive overall effects of vaccinations, despite acknowledging the seriousness of some adverse effects. This discourse theme was often linked to the cases of narcolepsy caused by the swine-flu vaccine Pandemrix in Finland in 2009–2010, but was also utilised in the COVID-19 context to dispel fears of emerging side effects, like the blood clots resulting from the AstraZeneca COVID-19 vaccine.

> Concern [about blood clotting as a side effect] is understandable, but so far, all the data suggests that the risk of having a serious reaction from AstraZeneca, or any other vaccine, is very small compared to the benefits that this vaccine provides. I [interviewed chief physician of a regional public healthcare organisation] urge everyone to get the vaccine when it's their turn.
>
> (yle.fi 2021-03-18)

Mainstream discourses strongly associated vaccines with biomedical knowledge and research, and vaccine-related reporting was often accompanied by technical medical language and terminology with detailed descriptions of the workings of RNA, DNA, adjuvant substances, and adenoviral vectors.

> [This vaccine] utilises a gene vector, which imitates the early stages of the adenovirus, but transfers a gene producing the spike protein of the coronavirus to the cells of the vaccinated person.
>
> (iltalehti.fi 2020-05-06)

Along similar lines, the research, development, and testing of vaccines was meticulously covered, and numbers such as the efficacy percentages of COVID-19 vaccines were thoroughly reported on. These threads of reporting focused on building confidence as opposed to trust, with argumentation seeking to downplay the risks associated with vaccines, enhance confidence in the predictability of vaccination outcomes, and highlight the benefits of vaccines on a population-wide level (see Smith 2005). Thus trust, which becomes active and is necessary precisely in conditions of uncertainty (Harrison & Smith 2004: 376), was all but ignored by this focus on rendering the inherent indeterminacy of the pandemic calculable, predictable, and manageable by vaccines.

The appearance of voices critical of vaccinations was generally uncommon in Finnish mainstream media discourses. Where mentioned, reporting covering vaccine hesitancy had a tendency to focus on extreme forms of opposition – many articles addressing hesitant or critical viewpoints towards vaccination presented views and claims which were, in all likelihood, very marginal even amongst those most hesitant to take vaccines. These reports included conspiratorial descriptions of vaccines as means of population control with the aim of killing people and views linked to extreme religious interpretations:

> [the COVID-19 vaccine] contains a microchip or the mark of the beast … This microchip enables mind control. A kind man can be made into a man-beast controlled from the outside, not by the Holy Ghost.
>
> (hs.fi 2020-06-23)

The excerpt just shown is from a media report. It quotes a host from a national Christian TV network voicing views linking COVID-19 vaccines to mind control and the mark of the beast (see Fjell, chapter 12, this volume). This vein of reporting could be seen to function in a marginalising way in that it represented a view of vaccine criticism not easily amenable to logic and commonly held perceptions. It thus worked to create distance between the idea of (any) hesitancy or opposition towards vaccines and normal behaviour in society. The rarity with which vaccine-critical or hesitant views were mentioned further underscored this effect, as there were not a lot of news articles which would give context to the phenomenon of vaccine hesitancy to make it more comprehensive or relatable. Rather, media reporting was more likely to present any hesitancy regarding vaccines as anti-vaccination, leaving little room for a more encompassing view of vaccine hesitancy or any distinction between these concepts.

> The number of anti-vaxxers has remained very stable over time since the smallpox vaccine. About 1 per cent of the population does not want any vaccines. Anti-vaxxers are a loud but small group.
>
> (yle.fi 2019-06-16)

In the previous excerpt, a leading vaccination expert from the Finnish Institute for Health and Welfare emphasises the marginality of anti-vaccination attitudes when commenting on the effects on vaccine uptake caused by the vaccine-induced narcolepsy cases of 2009–2010. Thus, an equivalency was drawn between an effect on vaccination willingness and marginal anti-vax stances. Along the same lines, some reporting on vaccine-hesitant views contained labelling or mocking rhetoric using colourful expressions such as "the pro-epidemics", which tended to further marginalise these views and call into question the morality of people choosing not to vaccinate. This line of argumentation was especially noticeable during the COVID-19 pandemic, and it commonly insinuated that those not willing to vaccinate themselves against COVID-19 were selfish and did not care about other people in society.

In many of the rare cases where critical views and/or actors were presented, they tended to become objects of discussion, rather than active participants in discussions. Critical viewpoints were often reported as third-hand accounts, after which biomedical experts were brought in to comment and reject these claims with statistical and research data, while those expressing hesitant or critical views were left without a direct voice in discussions. The following excerpt from a news article exemplifies this tendency and features a Twitter message expressing an unwillingness to take COVID-19 vaccines, after which the leader of the Finnish Vaccine Research Centre is brought in to comment:

> [The Twitter message] Will I risk my healthy life on an experimental vaccine for a non-lethal disease? Of course not … [The expert] The death rate is not zero even in younger age groups, and even young people can suffer from serious long-term effects of the disease. On the other hand, no serious side-effects have been found to result from vaccinations in extensive testing on humans … Vaccines with sales permits are no longer experimental.
>
> (hs.fi 2020-12-03)

Many of the previous quotations exemplify the general proclivity of mainstream media reporting to serve as a direct communication channel for experts representing relevant healthcare organisations. The inherent credibility of these actors was exemplified by the tendency to leave their views unchallenged and by the publishing of their views as the facts to end discussion. These experts further served as direct conduits from which the scientific view was derived and were imbued with the authority to proclaim what the data, research and science indicated. From a trust/confidence standpoint (Smith 2005: 309), these actors, who constituted the dominant discourse on vaccines, mostly argued within a confidence framework, as the knowledge deemed relevant and published in news reports was almost exclusively linked to risk calculations and cost-benefit analyses performed on a population-wide level.

Trust, incorporating a moral component and relating to the particularities of concrete situations (Smith 2005), while seemingly overridden by the reliance on expert knowledge and risk calculations inherent to confidence, was not entirely missing in the observed mainstream discourse. In particular, some of the labelling and mocking lines of reporting related to vaccine-critical actors tended not to focus on the erroneousness of their arguments, but rather on their lack of social responsibility and morals. It could thus be said that while the building of trust, i.e., argumentation seeking to increase belief in the good intentions and moral competencies of officials in charge of vaccination programmes (see Smith 2005), was minimal to non-existent in mainstream discourses, the undermining of trust in vaccine-critical or hesitant actors was not.

The articles analysed in this chapter covered time periods both before and during the COVID-19 pandemic and thus reflect a shift in which vaccines, as topics of reporting, changed from a rather marginal issue to one on the forefront of societal discussion. There were some differences in how vaccines were reported on between the data from different times: vaccine-related reports after the onset of the COVID-19 pandemic were often closer to the immediate national context and more laden with emotions. Despite these differences, and relevant to the context of this analysis, the distinct positive undertone of vaccine-related reporting persevered, as did the focus on risk calculation and scientific rationale. If anything, these foci were more pronounced in media discourse following the onset of the pandemic. Mainstream vaccination discussion was likewise equally dismissive of critical voices both before and after the pandemic, while the host of official and trusted sources was even expanded after the onset of COVID-19 to include actors such as chief physicians of regional healthcare organisations.

Overall, the voices present in vaccine-related Finnish mainstream media reports were overwhelmingly those of organisations and experts working in biomedical fields. Biomedical knowledge formed the basis of argumentation and imbued actors with credibility, as did formal positions in relevant healthcare organisations. The hegemonic positions occupied by these actors were constructed most prominently by the omission of critical voices from discussions: even where critical viewpoints were reported on, they could be mocked and/or presented as objects of, rather than participants in, discussions. The mainstream media discourse could thus be seen to reflect a certain presumption of trust, or rather, confidence, in vaccines, and presented hesitancy as a marginal and extreme phenomenon which should be immediately corrected and dismissed where encountered.

Alternative discourse during the pandemic

In this analysis, alternative discourses were exemplified by the *Let's Save the Children of Finland* campaign, which was a vaccine-critical campaign started in Finland during the COVID-19 pandemic. Although mentions of the campaign in mainstream media were marginal, even the relatively small amount of publicity it received can be seen as exceptional for a vaccine-critical movement in the Finnish context. The campaign originated in June 2021 with the publication of a petition to prevent COVID-19 vaccinations from being given to children. At the time, Finnish public discussion revolved around the possibility of expanding COVID-19 vaccinations to the 12- to 15-year age group.

In its materials, the *Let's Save the Children of Finland* campaign sought to question and dispute the safety and effectiveness of (as well as the need for) COVID-19 vaccinations, while being careful to stress the campaign's acceptance of other vaccines as critically important tools of preventive healthcare. The most prominent themes in the campaign's argumentation were very reminiscent of the mainstream discourse: scientific studies, expert statements, and statistical information formed the basis of discourse. For example, the campaign used scientific referencing in much of its correspondence with health officials and regularly presented their argumentation as backed by studies and scientific evidence. Campaign materials featured a myriad of scientific sources ranging from highly reputable journals, such as *Vaccines* and *Nature*, to references to redacted studies and websites with little scientific credibility. The outspoken attachment to scientific reasoning was regularly reinforced by the exhaustive use of technical medical terminology in describing the processes causing alarm in those running the campaign:

> The mRNA encoding the S protein is stabilised and humanised (N-methyl-pseudo uridine, extra prolines at positions 986 and 987, which weaken the adhesion of S proteins to ACE2 receptors; humanised triplets that encode the viral S protein). This construction makes the mRNA stable, and it can remain inside and outside the cell for a long time.
>
> (D6)

The calculations and estimates of the safety, efficacy, and need of COVID-19 vaccinations were often packaged together in and crystallised by a medical cost-benefit analysis.

> The cost-benefit ratio of COVID-19 vaccines is abnormal for children and young people. Children and young people have generally had COVID-19 in a milder form. They don't seem to spread corona either.
>
> (D19)

These cost-benefit analyses were argued to show that administering COVID-19 vaccines was not in the best interest of children especially, though these reservations were expanded to the whole population in later campaign materials. These analyses, as forms of risk calculation characteristic of confidence (Smith 2005: 309), underscore the tendency of the campaign to focus large parts of its argumentation on the building of confidence instead of trust. This scientifically framed argumentation regularly had a distinctly questioning and inquisitive tone indicative of a mistrusting orientation (Lenard 2008: 313), with campaign materials and correspondence using wording such as "it seems likely" and "we would like your opinion on".

Despite the clear and oft-outspoken allegiance to scientific truth, the campaign's relation to scientific knowledge was ambiguous and without qualifications. Campaign materials demonstrated varying degrees of scepticism towards research and organisations funded by the pharmaceutical industry, with some materials being devoted to the dissecting of specific studies relating to the efficacy and safety of COVID-19 vaccines published by vaccine manufacturers. At times, an evaluation of scientific reliability was made based solely on the perceived motivations of the actors producing said research.

> We are against these vaccinations, or experimental and unfinished GMO injections, especially for children, until THL and FIMEA show with scientific investigations that they are safe. We cannot consider the research conducted by vaccine manufacturers to be scientifically reliable.
>
> (D31)

This position is an example of a distrusting orientation, as the belief in the untrustworthiness of these actors was settled (Citrin & Stoker 2018: 50), and actors as well as the science they produced were deemed unreliable due to perceived conflicts of interest. These suspicious dispositions were somewhat variable, as actors like the Finnish Institute for Health and Welfare (THL) and the Finnish Medicines Agency (FIMEA) who, in the previous excerpt, were called upon to produce scientific inquiries into the safety of COVID-19 vaccines, were, in other instances, seen as compromised since they had received funding from vaccine developers – they were thus considered just as untrustworthy as the vaccine developers.

> Doubts have arisen regarding insurmountable conflicts of interest and even corruption, as e.g. THL and the Vaccine Research Centre take millions of euros from vaccine manufacturers. Experts of theirs who have made public appearances have also been silent about the extensive and serious adverse effects and mainly spread the good news of these "vaccines" contrary to scientific evidence.
>
> (D41)

The perceived conflicts of interest exemplified by the previous excerpts were used by the campaign as a means of moral positioning of actors. The implication was that the financial dependence of publicly visible experts on vaccine developers made them unwilling or unable to act in morally responsible ways or in the public's interest (Goldenberg 2021: 125) and thus be worthy of trust. Here, the campaign's argumentation was directed not towards the system of vaccination or its risk calculations, but rather towards the actions and morality of the individuals working within this system. This form of argumentation is characteristic of trust as opposed to confidence (Harrison & Smith 2004: 377).

Along with scientific studies and journals, statistical data was frequently used in the alternative discourse. The statistics referenced by the campaign were almost exclusively materials used, and indeed published, by healthcare authorities, but the interpretations of such materials could be markedly different from the official ones. The campaign thus offered an alternative version of the reality of the pandemic situation based on its own estimation, which was a common theme in the campaign's rhetoric. For example, the campaign considered the number of cases and severity of side effects to be on a scale unprecedented in vaccine history. They described them as the greatest health catastrophe of the century, even while using official side effect statistics from around the world.

> We represent physicians from many different specialities, doctors, docents, other health care professionals and natural scientists, who have followed with great concern the international literature and information found on official websites, both here and elsewhere in the world, about the hundreds of thousands of cases of serious harm and incidents leading to death.
>
> (D8)

Here, as in many cases, the argument was buttressed by references to the high academic and/or professional statuses of those involved in the campaign. Generally, expertise and credibility in vaccine-related issues was constructed along lines following achievement in formal educational and professional settings, and the campaign presented itself as a voice for marginalised and even censored scientists, doctors, and other concerned parties seeking to generate an open scientific debate on COVID-19 vaccines. The selflessness of this endeavour was often emphasised: doctors involved in the campaign were described as willingly using their own free time and personal savings to save children and people in general from harm. The possible consequences for individuals' careers were also invoked and were seen as the reason why many like-minded doctors and other professionals chose to stay silent or participate anonymously.

> We now urge you to consider why hundreds of thousands of medical experts, doctors and researchers, including several Nobel laureates, take a huge personal risk and endanger their reputations and careers by rising up against the vaccine industry worldwide, by questioning the existence of the corona pandemic and by opposing vaccinations and the corona passport.
>
> (D14)

This underscoring of the costs associated with participation in the campaign functioned as a way to link ideas of trustworthiness and moral virtue to the people participating in the campaign and generate an image of the campaign as a just cause any moral individual would gladly participate in. Here, the campaign's claim was thus not only that they have the expertise and biomedical knowledge to participate in public discussion and challenge other expert opinions, but also that they have the moral high ground and are indeed unbiased and trustworthy on a personal and moral level. This view was accentuated by frequent references to the campaign members' immunity to external influences, which contrasted favourably with the compromised image created around experts working within official organisational contexts. This theme of alternative discourse was perhaps the clearest example of the building of trust rather than confidence; i.e., a trust in the moral capabilities, trustworthiness, and righteous motivation of the actors in question rather than a confidence in the accuracy of their risk calculations (Smith 2005: 309).

The perceived censorship and marginalisation of any views critical of COVID-19 vaccines, including and most notably of the campaign itself, was a key part of the campaign's argumentation. These practices attributed to the mainstream media and the forces controlling it were seen to exemplify the hold pharmaceutical companies and their interests had on public discussion and the experts visible in it. The public reactions of the media and representatives of key national organisations were closely reported on in campaign materials, which featured ample criticism towards the practices of the media and statements made by some notable figures in public discourse. As an example of the campaign's perceived marginalisation, the campaign references an article published in a newspaper in Helsinki, where a representative of the campaign was asked to elaborate on the campaign's concerns regarding COVID-19 vaccines.

> [M]ainstream media and media representing the official view completely censor health professionals such as professors, doctors, docents and specialist physicians with differing views based on independent science, or at least distort and twist their message. Essential points are left unsaid, and the representatives of official organisations are always given the upper hand and an opportunity to repeat the same false mantras they have repeated since the beginning of the corona crisis.
>
> (D10)

Criticism of this perceived deception and dishonesty was directed at the fact that the newspaper had published a simplified version of the scientific issues provided by the campaign's representative. Also, unbeknownst to the campaign representative, the newspaper had subsequently asked the chief physician of the Finnish Institute for Health and Welfare to comment on these claims without giving the campaign a chance to respond. As previously discussed, the practice of presenting vaccine-critical views as objects to be analysed and rejected by experts was not atypical for Finnish mainstream vaccine discourse. In this case, it served to provoke the campaign into providing answers marked by strong institutional suspicions and created a general distrusting orientation amongst those in the *Let's Save the Children of Finland* campaign. Along similar lines, other campaign materials took issue with and responded to derogatory statements made by the executive director of the Finnish Medical Association, which is the largest labour union for doctors in Finland:

> – Paranoia is a mental illness. I [the executive director referring to campaign members] wonder why a paid official of the union publicly insults the honour of members who independently – without pursuing the

> interests of any third party – draw attention to the risks of corona spike-protein-mRNA-injections based on scientific findings and the professional expertise of an experienced doctor. Bringing these risks to the fore is disadvantageous for pharmaceutical companies, and therefore these views are silenced.
>
> (D15)

Here, as in other cases, these mocking, marginalising, and discrediting ways of reporting on vaccine criticism in the mainstream discourse were mirrored in campaign materials by further suspicions towards the motivations of such attacks. From campaign materials, it seems clear that the effect of these reporting practices was a refocusing of the campaign's argumentation from raising questions regarding the rationale and justification of COVID-19 vaccinations to a more generalised suspicion and distrust towards a host of actors, most notably the media and national healthcare officials. Conceptually this shift was twofold: firstly, from confidence to trust as the basis for argumentation; and secondly, from an orientation of mistrust to distrust, marked by increased suspicions and even cynicism (Lenard 2008: 313).

The alternative discourse exhibited an interesting temporal component that becomes clear when looking at the development of the campaign's argumentation from the publication of the initial petition in June 2021 to the end of data gathering in February 2022. In many of the materials published during or soon after the campaign's initial debut, the language of the campaign was prone to pose questions, call attention to identified issues, and generally exhibit a questioning and investigative – mistrusting – orientation, whereas later materials tended to feature increased certainty and accusative tones, or distrust. This shift was perhaps best exemplified by the broadening of reservations held related to COVID-19 vaccinations. Whereas the original petition and early materials expressed concern only towards children's vaccinations, later materials adopted a position in which COVID-19 vaccinations were seen as harmful and unnecessary for everyone.

To summarise, the alternative discourse sought to question and dispute the effectiveness, safety, and need for COVID-19 vaccines and regularly utilised argumentation referencing scientific evidence, statistics, and expert statements. This construction of confidence was accompanied or superseded at times by argumentation tied to the moral motivations and trustworthiness of actors, which reflected the trust side of the trust-confidence continuum. Perceived marginalisation and mistreatment of vaccine-critical voices in mainstream media, particularly of the campaign itself, were salient themes of the alternative discourse and provoked increased suspicions.

Discussion

This chapter has analysed mainstream and alternative vaccine-related discourses with a focus on expressions of vaccine criticism and conceptualisations of trust, confidence, mistrust, and distrust. Confidence-based argumentation was the most prevalent in both discourses, although the alternative discourse also exhibited pronounced threads of discourse based on the trust side of the trust-confidence duality. From a mistrust/distrust perspective, the former was generally more descriptive of the alternative discourse's orientation. While distrust was visible especially towards mainstream media and the actors most visible in it, much of the campaign's argumentation assumed a questioning and inquisitive attitude, although there was a distinct temporal shift in focus from a predominantly mistrusting tone in the campaign's earlier materials to an increasingly distrusting orientation in the later ones.

Vaccine hesitancy and criticism were generally not very visible themes in mainstream media discourse, and reports covering these phenomena often featured marginalising, mocking, and dismissive tones. These practices left little room for expression of critical views and pushed those wishing to express such views to form alternative channels of communication, like the *Let's Save the Children of Finland* campaign. In all, much of the alternative channel's argumentation was notably similar to the mainstream discourse – the use of scientific references, statistics, and expert statements was commonplace in the building of confidence in both sets of materials. Central points of contention between official and alternative views of vaccine use and the pandemic situation were the selection of publications, studies, and experts which were deemed valid and credible, as well as their interpretations. Viewed as a whole, this interplay between discourses was a disagreement regarding confidence. The two parties generally sought to convince audiences of the accuracy and credibility of their data, estimates, and expertise. In other words, the technocratic framing generated by representatives of public health organisations – the prevalent actors in mainstream media – through the usage of scientific and biomedical research data (see Hausman 2019: 212) did not, in this particular case, form a barrier to understanding, but was responded to in kind in the alternative discourse.

The reactions exhibited by the *Let's Save the Children of Finland* campaign to the marginalising and dismissive reporting practices of the mainstream discourse are especially interesting when viewed through the conceptual lens applied in this chapter. As discussed earlier, the original orientation of the campaign was characterised most prominently by mistrust, an investigative attitude manifesting in a desire to assess the performance of the object of mistrust relative to expectations (Jennings et al. 2021: 1178). It seems that the campaign's responses to the marginalising reporting of mainstream media reflect the outcome of precisely this type of assessment. The corresponding deepening of reservations and hesitations can be further understood as "the negative effects of trust" (Smith 2005: 309), i.e., the results of an agent's reaction to untrustworthy behaviour. Thus, the campaign's original mistrusting orientation, a precarious attitude sensitive to available information (Lenard 2008: 318), was shifted, perhaps partly by these media practices, to the more settled attitude of distrust towards the mainstream media and the actors most prominent in its discourse.

Broadly speaking, a hegemonic discourse not responsive to dissident or critical voices can be inimical to the establishment of open discussion and the building of trust. The treatment of critical actors and their messages as objects to be rejected by experts might be beneficial from a confidence standpoint (these practices can indeed work to reduce uncertainty), thus improving confidence in the predictability of vaccination outcomes (see Smith 2005), but they also neglect trust and leave critical actors ignored and without recourse. When a mistrusting agent, typically wavering between trust and distrust (Lenard 2008: 318), is met with these responses, they cannot be expected to feel much of the respect and understanding presupposed by trust (Harrison & Smith 2004: 376). Unfulfilled trust leads to feelings of betrayal, as well as avoidance of social engagement and co-operation (Smith 2005: 309), which further distances mistrusting and critical agents from trusting behaviour. Thus, an attitude of mistrust manifesting as criticism can develop into distrust when this criticism is rejected and ignored. This is especially concerning when taking into account that a questioning, careful, and cautious attitude is not necessarily a negative thing in and of itself. A mistrusting attitude has been seen as vital to democracy (Lenard 2008) and linked to a higher likelihood of behavioural adjustments with regard to COVID-19 responses (Jennings et al. 2021: 1192).

While inflammatory reporting practices regarding vaccine hesitancy and criticism are not necessarily novel phenomena (e.g., Hausman 2019: 39), our analysis, and its specific focus on mainstream and alternative discourses (which are not necessarily all that dissimilar), underscores the somewhat arbitrary nature of the delineations of trustworthiness made by the mainstream media. The academic qualifications or medical expertise of the actors behind the *Let's Save the Children of Finland* campaign did not seem to affect reporting practices, nor did the fact that the campaign's argumentation was often based on the same types of sources, risk calculations, and biomedical language used by representatives of official healthcare organisations in the mainstream discourse. Mainstream media thus reported on vaccine-critical views and actors with a certain inherent assumption of untrustworthiness, or distrust. One possible explanation for these reporting practices is the dominance of the cultural narrative of vaccination, which can lead to vaccine hesitancy being portrayed as ignorance and a threat to public health (Goldenberg 2021; Heller 2008). Whatever the causes, a discourse seeking to generate trust must necessarily account for the vulnerability inherent in any trusting relationship (Harrison & Smith 2004: 377), be ready to accept actors with differing viewpoints into the discussion, and be careful not to break trust where it is once, however tentatively, extended.

References

Citrin, Jack & Laura Stoker. 2018. Political trust in a cynical age. *Annual Review of Political Science* 21(1): 49–70.

Esaiasson, Peter, Jacob Sohlberg, Marina Ghersetti & Bengt Johansson. 2021. How the coronavirus crisis affects citizen trust in institutions and in unknown others: Evidence from "the Swedish experiment". *European Journal of Political Research* 60(3): 748–760.

Finnish Science Barometer. 2019. *A study of the Finns' attitudes towards science and their opinions on scientific and technological progress*. Helsinki: Tieteen Tiedotus ry.

Fjell, Tove Ingebjørg. 2024. COVID-19, the mark of the beast, and the last days: A study on vaccine hesitancy in Norwegian Christian charismatic movements. In Lars Borin, Mia-Marie Hammarlin, Dimitrios Kokkinakis & Fredrik Miegel (eds.), *Vaccine hesitancy in the Nordic countries: Trust and distrust during the COVID-19 pandemic*. London: Routledge.

Giddens, Anthony. 1990. *The consequences of modernity*. Cambridge: Polity Press.

Goldenberg, Maya. 2021. *Vaccine hesitancy: Public trust, expertise, and the war on science*. Pittsburgh: University of Pittsburgh Press.

Goldfinch, Shaun, Ross Taplin & Robin Gauld. 2021. Trust in government increased during the COVID-19 pandemic in Australia and New Zealand. *Australian Journal of Public Administration* 80(1): 3–11.

Harrison, Stephen & Carole Smith. 2004. Trust and moral motivation: Redundant resources in health and social care? *Policy & Politics* 32(3): 371–386.

Hausman, Bernice L. 2019. *Anti/Vax: Reframing the vaccination controversy*. Ithaca: Cornell University Press.

Heller, Jacob. 2008. *The vaccine narrative*. Nashville: Vanderbilt University Press.

Jallinoja, Piia, Jonas Sivelä & Esa Väliverronen. 2021. Valtavirtaa ja vastavirtaa – koronanäkemykset yhteydessä halukkuuteen ottaa koronarokotus [Mainstream and the counter current – corona views connected with the willingness to take a corona vaccination], *Lääketieteellinen aikakausikirja Duodecim* 137(19): 2061–2068.

Jallinoja, Piia & Esa Väliverronen. 2021. Suomalaisten luottamus instituutioihin ja asiantuntijoihin COVID19-pandemiassa [Finns' trust in institutions and experts during the COVID-19 pandemic]. *Media & Viestintä* 44(1): 1–24.

Jennings, Will, Gerry Stoker, Victor Valgarðsson, Daniel Devine & Jennifer Gaskell. 2021. How trust, mistrust and distrust shape the governance of the COVID-19 crisis. *Journal of European Public Policy* 28(8): 1174–1196.

Karafillakis, Emilie, Mark R. Francis, Pauline Paterson & Heidi J. Larson. 2021. Trust, emotions and risks: Pregnant women's perceptions, confidence and decision-making practices around maternal vaccination in France. *Vaccine* 39(30): 4117–4125.

Leach, Melissa & James Fairhead. 2007. *Vaccine anxieties: Global science, child health and society*. London: Earthscan.

Lenard, Patti Tamara. 2008. Trust your compatriots, but count your change: The roles of trust, mistrust and distrust in democracy. *Political Studies* 56(2): 312–332.

Luhmann, Niklas. 1979. *Trust and power: Two works*. Chichester: John Wiley.

Luhmann, Niklas. 1988. Familiarity, confidence, trust: Problems and alternatives. In Diego Gambetta (ed.), *Trust: Making and breaking cooperative relations*, 94–107. New York: Basil Blackwell.

Perelman, Chaïm. 1982. *The realm of rhetoric*. Notre Dame: University of Notre Dame Press.

Smith, Carole. 2005. Understanding trust and confidence: Two paradigms and their significance for health and social care. *Journal of Applied Philosophy* 22(3): 299–316.

Sztompka, Piotr. 1999. *Trust: A sociological theory*. Cambridge: Cambridge University Press.

THL – Finnish Institute for Health and Welfare. 2022. *Lasten rokotuskattavuus* [Children's vaccine coverage] [Online]. Available at: https://thl.fi/fi/web/infektiotaudit-ja-rokotukset/tietoa-rokotuksista/kansallinen-rokotusohjelma/rokotuskattavuus/lasten-rokotuskattavuus (Accessed 27 September 2022)

Väliverronen, Esa & Piia Jallinoja. 2021. Suomalaisten näkemykset asiantuntijoista ja rokotuksista. Havaintoja muutoksista ensimmäiseltä koronavuodelta [Finns' views on experts and vaccinations. Observations on changes from the first corona year]. *Yhteiskuntapolitiikka* 86(3): 323–333.

8 Uncertainty at the needle point

Vaccine hesitancy, trust, and public health communication in Norway during swine flu and COVID-19

Karine Aasgaard Jansen

Introduction

> Anti-vaxxers are just a small group of crazy idiots. So in Norway there is … there is no vaccine reluctance in Norway.
>
> (interview with N1, the Norwegian Medicines Agency [NoMA], 12 December 2014)

This statement made by a key person within the Norwegian public health authorities following Norway's mass vaccination during the 2009–2010 A(H1N1) or swine flu pandemic, may appear controversial given raising global concerns over anti-vaccination movements throughout the COVID-19 or corona pandemic. Nevertheless, it also illustrates how vaccine hesitancy is not a status quo phenomenon, but rather has diverging meanings to different people and varies across time and contexts. To increase our knowledge about vaccine hesitancy and trust in Norway during COVID-19, in this chapter I argue that we need to look back at how the swine flu pandemic was handled, and its consequences thereafter. By comparing Norwegian public health communication during swine flu to that of COVID-19, my objective is to discuss whether transparency in public health communication may increase or decrease trust in public (mass) vaccination programme. How did Norwegian public health authorities communicate risk of infection during the two pandemics? Did they adopt similar or different rhetorical strategies? In what ways may public health messages influence laypeople's decisions to vaccinate or not?

While vaccination is the main preventive measure in a pandemic in Norway (The Norwegian Directorate of Health [DOH] 2014: 76), contrary to what has been the case with COVID-19, the influenza vaccine Pandemrix by GlaxoSmithKline (GSK) was already available for use during swine flu. From late October 2009, 2.2 million Norwegians – approximately 45% of the total population – were therefore vaccinated at schools, city halls, gyms, etc., across the whole country (DOH 2010: 46). This number also includes 600,000 children from the age of 6 months to 20 years (Aavitsland & Nøkleby 2011: 5). Among these were 121 minors who were later diagnosed with the chronic sleep

DOI: 10.4324/9781003305859-10

disorder narcolepsy as a serious side effect of the Pandemrix vaccine (The Norwegian System of Patient Injury Compensation; NPE 2020).[1] Have these Pandemrix-induced cases of narcolepsy affected laypeople's trust in the Norwegian public health authorities? Did they influence public health communication or vaccine uptake during the ongoing COVID-19 pandemic?

This chapter is primarily based on data collection conducted in 2014–2015 for the ethnological research project "Epidemics, Vaccination and the Power of Narratives" at Umeå University in Sweden, funded by the Marcus and Amalia Wallenberg Foundation. The study investigated perceptions of and experiences with the swine flu pandemic and subsequent mass vaccinations in Sweden and Norway. For the purpose of this chapter, I also draw upon online news sources and secondary literature to compare public health communication during COVID-19 to the swine flu. My use of research methods and empirical material will be further discussed in the first part of the chapter. This section also includes an overview of the Norwegian public health authorities' roles and responsibilities in a pandemic. Second, I will provide a brief historical analysis of vaccine hesitancy in Norway with a focus on swine flu. This will be followed by a discussion of trust in relation to side effects of vaccines. Lastly, I will compare transparency in Norwegian public health communication during swine flu and COVID-19. All translations from Norwegian or Swedish into English are mine.

Research methods and empirical material

The main methods and empirical material that inform the chapter are 196 responses to qualitative questionnaire no. 251 entitled *Cold and Flu*. In addition, I draw upon 17 semi-structured interviews with central Norwegian public health stakeholders about their decision to mass vaccinate during the swine flu pandemic.

The use of use of qualitative questionnaires for data collection is a well-established method within ethnological research in Sweden and Norway. Nevertheless, it has traditionally been little known outside of the discipline (Jansen 2018a; Klein 2003). Given the social restrictions during COVID-19, however, the method has also recently been discovered and adapted as a replacement for qualitative interviews in other related research fields such as media studies (Ytre-Arna 2022).

Qualitative questionnaires cover a wide range of everyday topics of concern to many of us and ask open-ended questions to retrieve respondents' reflections on the topics that are being investigated (Kjus 2013). The respondents are made up of a fixed group of regular contributors and one-time repliers who are recruited via social media channels such as Facebook. The respondents answer in writing, and replies can vary from single words or a few sentences to longer coherent narratives over several pages. This combination of regular contributors and one-time repliers makes thus for a rather heterogeneous group of respondents with various world views, experiences, and practices. For example, the youngest respondents to the *Cold and Flu* questionnaire were born in the 1990s, and the oldest in the 1920s. Of the 196 respondents, 43 were men and 153 were women.

The objective of using qualitative questionnaires is to learn about various social phenomena as understood and expressed by the respondents themselves (Hagström & Marander-Eklund 2005: 12). Rather than comparing qualitative questionnaires to quantitative surveys, it is therefore more useful to think of them as "an interview in letter form" (Kjus & Grønstad 2014: 383). In this regard, qualitative questionnaires offer unique insights into lived experience. As ethnologist Alf Arvidsson (2003: 101) puts it: "Responses to qualitative questionnaires, and other ethnological source materials, are attributed their distinctive scientific character due to their self-experienced quality". Since the responses are self-biographical, they can also provide rare and unexpected empirical material which may be harder to come by in a more formalised interview (Waldetoft 2003).

Qualitative questionnaire no. 251, which the research project's principal investigator Britta Lundgren and I developed in collaboration with the Norwegian Ethnological Research (NEG), was divided into a total of five sub-themes. These were "Being infected by cold or flu", "Protection against contagion", "Treatment", "The 2009–2010 swine flu", and "The risk of future pandemics". Each of the sub-themes consisted of five to ten questions. For this chapter, I will primarily focus on the questions related to the subsection on swine flu and vaccination. These include: *Did you vaccinate against swine flu? Why, or why not? What do you think about vaccines? Do you know anyone who's developed any side effects? If so, which ones and how serious are they?*

Like other qualitative methods, a qualitative questionnaire is not based on a representative sample. This means that the response rate is unknown, and that the replies cannot be generalised (Jansen 2018a). As a result, data analysis of qualitative questionnaires is inductive and involves careful, thorough, and repeated readings, which makes it possible to identify and extract recurrent themes across respondents' replies (Waldetoft 2003). Categorisation of the material has thus consisted of identifying and subtracting such overarching themes. This includes themes that may be described as typical on one hand, and untypical on the other. As implied by the chapter's title, so-called typical replies represent, for example, uncertainty and concerns about side effects of (new) vaccines. So-called untypical quotes are those that represent outright vaccine refusal. For this chapter, I have selected quotes that illustrate the various points made in the analysis.

Data analysis of the 17 semi-structured, recorded, and transcribed interviews with public health experts were conducted with the same inductive analytical approach. The research participants were recruited through purposive sampling on the basis of their involvement in pandemic preparedness, decision-making, evaluation, and care. Since some of the participants were very visible in the media during the swine flu pandemic, and continued to be so during COVID-19, most subjective information, such as their positions as spokespersons, age, gender, and so on, has been removed according to agreement, and in line with Norwegian research ethical guidelines (Norway's National Committee for Research Ethics in the Social Sciences and the Humanities [NESH] 2021). This was also a strategy to ensure that they would be able to talk freely even if their personal views were contradictory to official governmental lines. Contrary to respondents' replies to qualitative questionnaire no. 251, however, most answers resembled each other. This may be because the interviews took place at a time when official consensus had already been reached with regard to the Norwegian public health authorities' handling of the swine flu pandemic. As a result, the selection of quotes represents to a large extent a unified discourse wherein the discovery of Pandemrix was described as a very unfortunate, but unexpected occurrence (Jansen 2018b).

Although most of the interviewees represent the strategic level of so-called crisis management – that is, the political and administrative command level within the public health sector – some also belonged to the operational level, such as emergency medical personnel and district GPs (McConnell et al. 2008, in Byrkjedal-Bendiksen 2012: 34). The participants represented the Ministry of Health and Care Services (HOD) at the very top of the strategic level, followed by the DOH, the Norwegian Institute of Public Health (NIPH), the Norwegian Medicines Agency (NoMA), and the Directorate of Civil Protection and Emergency Planning (DSB), which was responsible for the evaluation of the Norwegian public health authorities' handling of the swine flu pandemic. While HOD has the supreme responsibility for all matters of concern to national public health, in a pandemic it is DOH, on the authority of HOD, which oversees crisis management (Byrkjedal-Bendiksen 2012: 35). During both swine flu and COVID-19, the DOH worked closely together with the NIPH, which is the national public health competence institution. The NIPH is responsible for the national surveillance and prevention of communicable diseases, and for Norway's public vaccination programme (Jansen 2018b). While the role of the NIPH is primarily oriented towards research, and the DOH is an executive agency, both institutions are active in pandemic preparedness and public health communication (Brekke et al. 2017; Offerdal et al. 2021).

Vaccine hesitancy in Norway

Vaccine scepticism is not a new phenomenon in either Norway or elsewhere. In Norway, vaccine scepticism first became first visible with the introduction of the smallpox vaccine in the mid-1800s (Fjell 2005: 42). It increased around the 1930s, and then again in the 1950s with the implementation of mandatory vaccination in 1954 (Harthug 2014: 33; Schiøtz 2003: 420). Today, all vaccination in Norway is voluntary. This remained the case during both swine flu and COVID-19. While vaccine scepticism has most likely been around for as long as vaccines themselves, people's motives to abstain from vaccination have changed over the course of history. Early examples of vaccine scepticism were based primarily on religious convictions and concerns about animal welfare due to the cross-pollination used to develop the cowpox vaccine (Fjell 2005). In more recent times, vaccine scepticism has largely targeted the MMR-vaccine Priorix against measles, mumps, and rubella, which was first introduced in 1983 (Fjell 2005; Jansen 2018c). A reason for this is a study published in the renowned medical journal *The Lancet* by the physician Andrew Wakefield, who claimed that there was a link between Priorix and autism among children. While the findings were later discredited and the article (Wakefield et al. 1998) was retracted, the study still appears to have taken on a life of its own, especially among some groups of vaccine sceptics, including in Norway (Fjell 2005: 49, 2021: 70).

Vaccine scepticism is currently a rapidly growing phenomenon worldwide (Greenhough & Blume 2017). In 2019 the World Health Organization (WHO) identified vaccine hesitancy as one of ten threats to global health. As seen during both swine flu and COVID-19, the vaccines that people are mostly concerned about, and critical against, are usually new vaccines (Fjell 2021; Jansen 2018c). This could also be seen in several respondents' replies to qualitative questionnaire no. 251 as illustrated here by respondent 44893:

> No, I did not vaccinate against swine flu. I was, and I still am, sceptical against new vaccines. I want it [the vaccine] to be tried out for a long time on other people before I get it myself. I am generally in favour of taking the good old ones for children, and those [vaccines] that keep the most serious diseases at bay. Those vaccines have been thoroughly tried out and are some of the best things that has ever happened in the fight against diseases.
>
> (44893, F1980, disabled)

Although respondent 44893 is positive towards the vaccines that are offered in the Norwegian childhood immunisation programme, she is more sceptical towards recently introduced ones. Since new vaccines have been available for a shorter time period than established ones, they are often considered to be riskier, especially when it comes to side effects:

> We chose not to vaccinate [against swine flu] since we felt that the vaccine had not been sufficiently tested. In addition, none of us belonged to a risk group. Afterwards we have been very happy about this [decision] since we have heard about all of those who suffered from side effects … In general, I am sceptical against new vaccines, and I did not let my children get vaccinated against meningitis, and my eldest daughter was also not vaccinated against cervicitis.[2] The reason is that I think we always hear about unanticipated side effects for years afterwards; either because they were not foreseen when vaccination first started, or because they [the side effects] only show up after several years.
>
> (44858, F1970, student)

In addition to being perceived as risky, new vaccines are also prone to more rumour spreading (Larson 2020; Hammarlin et al. 2024, chapter 10, this volume). Over the last decades wide access to internet and social media has also radically increased both the reach and speed in which misinformation about vaccines can spread (Fjell 2021). This includes conspiracy theories (Færseth 2013). According to Fjell (2021: 63) these conspiracies closely resemble those voiced in the United States. There are, for example, COVID-19 vaccine rumours concerning 5G magnetic tracking chips, sterilisation, and the New World Order of a secretly emerging global totalitarian regime (Bodner et al. 2021).

Despite the increasing impact of populist knowledge on social media, none of the respondents based their decision to vaccinate or not against swine flu on conspiracy reasoning. Instead, such beliefs were rather described as far-fetched and ridiculous (44947, M1983, academic), echoing the statement made by N1 from the Norwegian Medicines Agency (NoMa; interview 12 December 2014). Nevertheless, as illustrated by the aforementioned quotes from 44893 and 44858, many respondents were still hesitant about vaccination. But do raising concerns over side effects, or having doubt about certain vaccines, necessarily entail vaccine scepticism? In contrast to public health and medical understandings of vaccine scepticism as conviction (Goldenberg 2021), my argument is that hesitation is rather relational and situational. Vaccine hesitancy is not the same as refusal (Goldenberg 2021; Jansen 2018c). Instead, those who are uncertain at the needle point often ask for more information about the contents and potential side effects of the vaccine that is recommended (Biss 2015). As previous studies show, the ones who are most critical of vaccines are often highly educated (Fjell 2005: 42; Greenhough & Blume 2017: 6). When their requests are ignored, or even written off as ignorant by public health experts, Goldenberg (2021) therefore argues that their views are more likely to harden rather than to persuade them about the benefits of vaccination.

Vaccine side effects and trust in public health authorities

The decision to vaccinate or not depends on several factors, but as argued throughout this anthology, the issue of trust appears to be key to all of them. While trust is a somewhat elusive concept with a multitude of definitions, it becomes important when there is a power imbalance between two parties due to information asymmetry (Larson et al. 2018: 1559). Trust refers thus to someone acting under uncertain circumstances, but who still choose to rely on the other party to have their best interests at heart (Smith 2005). Vaccine compliance relies, for example, on having trust in the safety and efficacy of vaccination, the respective vaccine and its producer, the health care personnel who administer the vaccine, and the wider public health system that recommends it (Larson et al. 2018).

As raised in the Introduction to this anthology, trust in authorities is overall exceptionally high in and across the Nordic countries (Borin et al. n.d.). Norway is no exception. Then again, trust, like vaccine hesitancy, can fluctuate in time. Pandemics such as the swine flu and COVID-19, and not the least the implementation of invasive public health measures during the latter, can put people's trust in authorities to the test (Borin et al. 2024). Following swine flu, the main cause for such increased mistrust was the discovery of the Pandemrix-induced cases of narcolepsy among children and young adults:

> It quieted down after the storm. Few people died and people breathed out. But the quiet did not last for long because then all the reports came out about side effects and the [vaccination] price of 700 million NOK. The last part was not a problem since the Norwegian Oil Fund have such huge stocks in the pharmaceutical industry that we got the full amount back, or even more so. But the first part is serious. Dozens of children and young people had their lives ruined because of the vaccine. Those responsible were confronted, but our trust in the white coats is so big that when they stand looking serious and a bit regretful while saying "it is sad that some have gotten side effects but think about how many people we saved from dying from the swine flu". Without blinking. Without the journalist asking for evidence for the incredible claim that we were saved from dying. Without the Minister of Health having to resign from having instigated a scandalous hysteria. After the scandal it just went quiet … That is why me and my two children stopped taking vaccines. My trust is completely diminished.
>
> (44949, M1966, museum employee)

To assess whether respondent 44939's accusations against the Norwegian government and public health authorities are accurate or not is beyond the scope of this chapter. Nevertheless, the statement clearly illustrates how the way the Norwegian public health authorities handled the narcolepsy cases have turned respondent 44939's "dial" from hesitancy to refusal as argued by Goldenberg (2021). Lundgren (2015) also shows how Swedish parents of children with narcolepsy often blamed the public health authorities for recommending mass vaccination which, in turn, led their children to fall ill. The primary critical narrative among these parents revolved around a sense of having been pushed into a normative decision of vaccination as the right thing to do in the face of pandemic threat (Lundgren 2015: 153). While vaccination against swine flu was, as already mentioned, voluntary, this was not necessarily how it was experienced at the time:

> No-one I know caught swine flu. The whole thing seemed exaggerated. My sister was pregnant, and the doctor gave her the vaccine without her consent, just grabbed her arm and injected. We chose not to vaccinate. The school nurse vaccinated both at school and in the nursery, something we experienced as a major imposition. We got scolded for "not understanding that we put everyone else in danger if we fall ill".
>
> (respondent 44860, F1969, teacher)

The school nurse's argument plays into the issue of solidarity, in which vaccination is considered a collective responsibility so that those who for various reasons cannot vaccinate are still protected against infection. In medical terms, this is known as herd immunity, and requires 80%–95% vaccine coverage depending on how contagious the disease in question is (Jansen 2018c: 78). Lundgren (2015: 162) shows for example that while none of the Swedish parents opposed vaccination in general, their doubts about vaccination had still been strengthened.

Did any of these negative experiences with Pandemrix affect vaccine uptake in Norway during COVID-19? It was known from early on, for example, that although the swine flu could have severe consequences for a small number of people, the outbreak would overall be mild (Jansen 2018b: 82). Yet, like Sweden, the Norwegian public health authorities still recommended vaccination. Respondent 45023 (F1969, student and self-employed) fears, therefore, that a new pandemic will not be taken seriously "because the reactions against swine flu were so exaggerated. Like the boy who yelled 'wolf, wolf' in the fairy tale". With a total COVID-19 vaccine coverage of 93.2% among 18 years and older with two doses as of 23 September 2022 (The Norwegian Institute of Public Health; NIPH 2021), it seems safe to say that that is not the case. There may be several reasons for this. In the wake of COVID-19, many seem to have forgotten about the swine flu or do simply not think of it as a pandemic anymore (Jansen 2021). Since Norway had an agreement with the vaccine producer GlaxoSmithKline, which would release two doses of Pandemrix as soon as the WHO declared a pandemic, mass vaccination against swine flu could commence quite rapidly. As a result, there was no need for the implementation of highly restrictive public health measures such as lockdowns, social distancing, use of face masks, and travel quarantines as seen during COVID-19 while awaiting vaccination. In addition, contrary to the swine flu, COVID-19 is a much more severe disease. Of 900,000 cases, there were 32 confirmed deaths from swine flu in Norway in 2009 and 2010 (The Norwegian Directorate of Health [DOH] 2010: 3). In comparison, there were 943 confirmed deaths due to COVID-19 as of 9 June 2022 (NIPH 2022a).

Transparency in public health communication

Solidarity as an argument for vaccination against swine flu appears to have been more outspoken among public health authorities in Sweden than in Norway (Lundgren 2016). According to N3 (NPHI, interview 18 December 2014), to avoid referring to solidarity was a conscious rhetorical move due to the seeming unpredictability and uncertainty of swine flu (Jansen 2018c: 79). This uncertainty concerned the evolvement of the disease, those who were at risk of developing severe symptoms, and side effects of the Pandemrix vaccine. Based on this, for example, N4 (NIPH, interview 15 December 2014) described the swine flu as "Doctor Jekyll and Mr. Hyde". Dealing with this uncertainty also appears to have influenced public health communication (Brekke et al.

2017; Jansen 2018c: 87). For example, part of the criticism against Norwegian public health authorities following the swine flu mass vaccination was a lack of transparent communication with regards to potential side effects of vaccination (Brekke et al. 2017: 75).

Was this still the case during the COVID-19 pandemic? In its function to negotiate between medical and lay knowledge, public health communication plays a particularly important role in increasing either vaccine compliance or resistance. In the following discussion, I will refer to transparency in its broader meaning of honesty and openness, as this is how the concept is usually understood among the general public (Löfstedt & Way 2016: 1082). Transparency is not merely about disclosure of information, however (Ihlen et al. 2022: 2). As argued by Ihlen et al. (2022), it concerns several dimensions simultaneously. These include substantiality; that is, that information must be "relevant, complete, reliable and understandable" (Bachmann et al. 2015 in Ihlen et al. 2022: 3). Transparency also concerns accountability, which entails willingness to admit mistakes and tolerate criticism. It also requires public participation, meaning that authorities must be open to feedback through engaging actively with their audience (Ihlen et al. 2022).

During the swine flu pandemic, risk of infection was communicated to the general audience through the adoption of two rhetorical strategies simultaneously: that is, concern and reassurance (Briggs & Nichter 2009: 191). The aim was to communicate that swine flu appeared to be less severe than what was initially feared, and not least that the responsible authorities had the situation under control. The ambiguity of the swine flu pandemic itself became a communicative problem in Norway, however (Brekke et al. 2017: 75). This was exacerbated by the mere frequency in which information was given which would normally indicate a much more serious risk situation than what was in fact the case (Brekke et al. 2017).

Contrary to what was the case during swine flu, Norwegian public COVID-19 communication remained open about what was unknown and uncertain (Kjeldsen et al. 2022; Pileberg 2021). This relates both to the general uncertainty of the evolvement of the pandemic itself and admitted uncertainty in lack of knowledge (Kjeldsen et al. 2022). While vaccination was strongly recommended, Norway was for example among the first countries in the world after Denmark to discontinue vaccination with AstraZeneca's Vaxzevria after two reported deaths in Denmark and Austria caused by vaccine-induced blood clots (Vestreng 2021). Shortly thereafter, five cases also occurred in Norway, including three deaths (NIPH 2022b).[3]

Would the discontinuation of vaccination with Vaxzevria have occurred had it not been for Pandemrix? In being so quick to change their vaccine recommendations and put the use of Vaxzevria on hold, one may argue that the public health authorities displayed transparency through accountability. This was arguably not the case during the swine flu pandemic. Instead, the leading narrative among Norwegian public health authorities during swine flu remained one of saving lives (Jansen 2018b). In this highly uncertain situation, the Pandemrix vaccine thus became the magical medical bullet which could control the spreading of the disease (Singer 2009: 202). This was also alluded to by N1 (NoMA, interview 12 December 2014):

> I am myself a vaccine supporter, but I have also worked with side effects throughout most of my professional life at NoMA ... So it makes you wonder whether there are these "do not want to see attitudes", that is if you talk to true vaccine supporters they do not see side effects of vaccines at all. Because the [public health] authorities actually tend to downplay problems concerning vaccination.

While Brekke et al. (2017) have shown how both DOH and particularly NIPH aimed towards transparent communication, based on respondents' views on how Norwegian public health authorities handled the pandemic and subsequent mass vaccination, it does not appear as if they were entirely successful in achieving this goal. In addition, despite disagreements backstage, Norwegian public health authorities also appeared to be primarily concerned with displaying a united front in engagement with the general audience (Brekke et al. 2017).

During COVID-19, however, differences in opinion between NIPH and DOH, and between public health authorities and the government, have been openly acknowledged to the general public. Approximately one month after then Norwegian Prime Minister Erna Solberg declared on 12 March 2020 that "today the Norwegian government will implement the strongest and most invasive measures we have had in Norway in times of peace" (Røed-Johansen & Torgersen 2020), the DOH and the NIPH were, for example, about to hold a press conference to announce the first easing of restrictions since the onset of COVID-19. These included the opening of nurseries and the lifting of the controversial ban on visits to secondary property such as cabins. While feedback from the government indicated that their opinions would be overruled, they still chose to communicate their recommendations (Offerdal et al. 2021: 261).

While publicly expressing conflicting opinions may cause confusion among the general audience, according to Offerdal et al. (2021: 262), it rather functioned "as a demonstration of virtue, in this case professional integrity, honesty and the courage of conviction".

Displaying transparency about disagreements contributed thus to increase the public health authorities' trustworthiness among the Norwegian population. According to respondents, Norwegian public health communication during swine flu appears instead to have been lacking in all three domains regarding transparency. Not only did they not feel adequately informed about the necessity of vaccination (sustainability), but as raised by respondent 44949, the public health authorities also did not admit to their mistakes when it was discovered that Pandemrix could have an unexpected, but a severe, side effect (accountability). In doing so, they also appeared less open to feedback (public participation). In terms of public participation during COVID-19, both the DOH and NIPH actively displayed empathy and identification with their audience in their communication (Offerdal et al. 2021: 263). This was achieved by the implementation of simple, informal, and personalised rhetorical moves such as the use of "you" and "those close to you" (Offerdal et al. 2021). In addition to press conferences and interviews, they also engaged actively in televised debates and online discussions informed by a more dialogical approach than what can be achieved when merely answering questions (Ihlen et al. 2022: 8). This was also a method to transparently communicate uncertainty, but on their own terms. While admitting to uncertainty, it was one of conditionality (Kjeldsen et al. 2022: 100). While communicating that they were uncertain about a situation, they would simultaneously reassure their audience that they were seeking more information, that they had access to exclusive information shared with other experts around the world, and that they still knew what was possible to know in the current situation. Admitting to this kind of conditional uncertainty thus placed them in the position of competent experts since it illustrated how they, despite all this openly acknowledged uncertainty, still knew best how to act (Kjeldsen et al. 2022: 100).

Conclusion: transparency and trust

Uncertainty at the needle point and otherwise was characteristic of both swine flu and COVID-19. While Norwegian public health authorities were quick to stop the use of Vaxzevria, narcolepsy was an unexpected side effect of Pandemrix which was discovered only after mass vaccination. The irony perhaps, is that this side effect would not have occurred had it not been for the highly efficient pandemic preparedness exhibited through mass vaccination (Lundgren 2015: 162). A public health measure that could potentially have been a medical success story, and contributed towards building trust in public health authorities, contributed thus to mistrust among some of the Norwegian respondents. This was not only because of the narcolepsy cases, but also because public health communication during swine flu appeared to be lacking in transparency.

Taking these factors into account, the swine flu and COVID-19 appear as two very different pandemics. As such, one may also argue that they are not comparable, because they happened at two different points in time. In terms of Norwegian public health communication, there appears to have been a rhetorical shift from one pandemic to the next, however (Offerdal et al. 2021). While public health has traditionally framed vaccine hesitancy as a problem to be overcome by persuasion instead of transparent communication and information, I agree with Goldenberg (2021) that this can ultimately increase rather than decrease mistrust in health authorities and public vaccination programs. Then again, transparency is not unproblematic and may in some cases weaken rather than strengthen trust in health care (Licht 2011: 183). In terms of COVID-19 communication, for example, Petersen et al. (2021) show how disclosing negative information about vaccines decreased acceptance among a large, representative sample of Americans and Danes. Nevertheless, they also argue that while negative transparent COVID-19 vaccine communication may indeed harm vaccine uptake here and now, it simultaneously increases trust in public health authorities which is essential for vaccine compliance in the long run. Moreover, it hinders the spread of conspiracy beliefs (Petersen et al. 2021).

In contrast to the swine flu, the conditional transparency which characterised the Norwegian public health communication during COVID-19 proved to be successful (Offerdal et al. 2021). In communicating uncertainty at the needle point, Norwegian public health authorities also appear to have recognised and reflected lay people's concerns, rather than rejecting them. This rhetorical strategy may not have been possible if trust in public institutions was not already as high as it is in Norway (Offerdal et al. 2021: 265). Rather than rebuilding trust as argued by Goldenberg (2021), in the case of Norway, transparent public health communication was rather key to sustaining it (Offerdal et al. 2021: 265). As argued by Petersen et al. (2021), this is essential in preparation for future pandemics and other health emergencies. In the case of COVID-19 communication in Norway, it appears thus as if the Norwegian public health authorities have learnt from previous shortcomings during the swine flu pandemic. I will even claim that they may have something to teach others about the importance of transparency to establish trust in the wake of growing vaccine hesitancy worldwide.

Notes

1 Narcolepsy is characterised by excessive daytime sleepiness causing the affected person to suddenly fall asleep at inappropriate times. Other symptoms are cataplexy, which is the temporary loss of muscle control in response to emotions or efforts; sleep paralysis when falling asleep or waking up; and hallucinations (Lundgren 2015).

2 While the meningitis vaccine is recommended to all young adults between the ages of 17 and 19, it is not part of the Norwegian childhood immunisation programme. The HPV (human papillomavirus) vaccine became part of the programme for girls in 2009–2010, and for boys in 2018–2019 (NIPH 2008).

3 From 2021, a total of 19 deaths from COVID-19 vaccination have been registered in Norway (NIPH 2022a).

References

Aavitsland, Preben & Hanne Nøkleby. 2011. *Foreløpig rapport om narkolepsi etter Pandemrix, 2. august* [Preliminary report on narcolepsy after Pandemrix, 2 August]. Oslo: The Norwegian Public Health Institute.

Arvidsson, Alf. 2003. Självbiografiska positioner och berättar-röster. En typologisk skiss [Self-biographical positions and voices of narration. A typological draft]. In Bo G. Nilsson, Dan Waldetoft & Christina Westergren (eds.), *Frågelist och berättarglädje: Om frågelistor som forskningsmetod och folklig genre* [Qualitative questionnaires and narration joy. On qualitative questionnaires as research method and popular genre], 89–101. Stockholm: Nordiska Museets Förlag.

Biss, Eula. 2015. *On immunity: An inoculation*. London: Fitzcarraldo Editions.

Bodner, John, Wendy Welch, Ian Brodie, Anna Muldoon, Donald Leach & Ashley Marshall. 2021. *Covid-19 conspiracy theories: Qanon, 5G, the New World Order and other viral ideas*. North Carolina: McFarland & Company.

Borin, Lars, Mia-Marie Hammarlin, Fredrik Miegel & Dimitrios Kokkinakis. 2024. Vaccine hesitancy and the COVID-19 crisis in the Nordic countries. In Lars Borin, Mia-Marie Hammarlin, Dimitrios Kokkinakis & Fredrik Miegel (eds.), *Vaccine hesitancy in the Nordic countries: Trust and distrust during the COVID-19 pandemic*. London: Routledge.

Brekke, Ole A. Kari Ludvigsen & Kristian Bjørkdahl. 2017. Handling og usikkerhet. Norske myndigheters kommunikasjon om svineinfluensapandemien i 2009 [Action and uncertainty. Norwegian authorities' communication about the swine flu pandemic in 2009]. *Norsk statsvitenskapelig tidsskrift* 33(1): 54–77.

Briggs, Charles S. & Mark Nichter. 2009. Biocommunicability and the biopolitics of pandemic threats. *Medical Anthropology* 28(3): 189–198.

Byrkjedal-Bendiksen, Øyvind. 2012. *Svineinfluensaen – en varslet krise* [The swine flu – a warned crisis]. Master's thesis, Department of Administration and Organization Theory, University of Bergen.

Færseth, John. 2013. *KonspiraNorge* [ConspiraNorway]. Oslo: Humanist Forlag.

Fjell, Tove I. 2005. Fri tvang eller tvingende frihet – eller begge deler? Om vaksineringspraksikser i samtids-Norge [Free force or forced freedom – or both? On vaccination practices in contemporary Norway]. *Tidsskrift for kulturforskning* 4(3): 41–54.

Fjell, Tove I. 2021. Covid–1984: En studie av motnarrativ om koronatiltak [Covid-1984: A study of counter narratives about corona measures]. *Tidsskrift for kulturforskning* 1: 61–81.

Goldenberg, Maya J. 2021. *Vaccine hesitancy: Public trust, expertise and the war on science*. Pittsburgh: University of Pittsburgh Press.

Greenhough, Paul & Stuart Blume. 2017. Introduction. In Christine Holmberg, Stuart Blume & Paul Greenhough (eds.), *The politics of vaccination: A global history*, 1–17. Manchester: Manchester University Press.

Hagström, Charlotte & Lena Marander-Eklund. 2005. Att arbeta med frågelistor: En introduktion [To work with qualitative questionnaires: An introduction]. In Charlotte Hagström & Lena Marander-Eklund (eds.), *Frågelistan som källa och metod* [*Qualitative questionnaires as source and method*], 9–31. Lund: Studentlitteratur.

Hammarlin, Mia-Marie, Fredrik Miegel, Dimitrios Kokkinakis & Jullietta Stoencheva. 2024. Fearing mRNA: A mixed methods study of vaccine rumours. In Lars Borin, Mia-Marie Hammarlin, Dimitrios Kokkinakis & Fredrik Miegel (eds.), *Vaccine hesitancy in the Nordic countries: Trust and distrust during the COVID-19 pandemic* (Chapter 10, this volume). London: Routledge.

Harthug, Henrik. 2014. *Mellom påbud og frivillighet: Strategier i det norske vaksinasjonsprogrammene 1940–1980* [*Between injunction and voluntariness: Strategies in the Norwegian vaccination programs from 1940–1980*]. Master's thesis, Department of Archaeology, History, Cultural Studies and Religion, University of Bergen.

Helsedirektoratet (The Norwegian Directorate of Health [DOH]) 2010. *Håndtering av pandemisk influensa 2009–10* [*Handling of pandemic influenza 2009–10*].

Helsedirektoratet (The Norwegian Directorate of Health [DOH]) 2014. *Nasjonal beredskapsplan for pandemisk influensa* [*National preparedness plan for pandemic influenza*].

Ihlen, Øyvind, Sine N. Just, Jens E. Kjeldsen, Ragnhild Mølster, Truls S. Offerdal, Joel Rasmussen & Elin Skogerbø. 2022. Transparency beyond information disclosure: Strategies of the Scandinavian public health authorities during the COVID-19 pandemic. *Journal of Risk Research*. DOI: 10.1080/13669877.2022.2077416

Jansen, Karine A. 2018a. Etnografi og (kon)tekst: En metodologisk komparasjon av deltagende observasjon og spørrelister [Ethnography and [con]text: A methodological comparison of participant observation and qualitative questionnaires]. *Kulturella perspektiv* 27(1–2): 49–58.

Jansen, Karine A. 2018b. What to expect when you're expecting a pandemic: Public health and lay perceptions of the 2009–2010 swine flu outbreak and mass vaccination in Norway. *Ethnologia Scandinavica* 48: 82–98.

Jansen, Karine A. 2018c. Å vaksinere, eller ikke å vaksinere, er det (det eneste) spørsmålet? Norske holdninger til vaksinasjon og svineinfluensapandemien i 2009 til 2010 [To vaccinate, or not to vaccinate, is that [the only] question? Norwegian perceptions of vaccination and the 2009 to 2010 swine flu pandemic]. *Tidsskrift for kulturforskning* 17 (1): 73–89.

Jansen, Karine A. 2021. Forestillinger om pandemier. Svineinfluensa i lys av korona [Imagined pandemics: Corona in light of swine flu]. *Kulturella perspektiv* 30(2–3): 1–8.

Kjeldsen, Jens E., Ragnhild Mølster & Øyvind Ihlen. 2022. Expert uncertainty: Arguments bolstering the ethos of expertise in situations of uncertainty. In Steve Oswald, Marcin Lewinski, Sara Greco & Serena Villata (eds.), *The pandemic of argumentation*, 85–104. Berlin: Springer.

Kjus, Audun. 2013. Hvorfor spørre? Norsk etnologisk gransking og spørrelistas framtid [Why ask? Norwegian Ethnological Research and the future of the qualitative questionnaire]. *Tidsskrift for kulturforskning* 12(1): 41–57.

Kjus, Audun & Line Grønstad. 2014. Skriv fritt og selvstendig: Skriftlige, kvalitative spørreundersøkelser [Write freely and independently: Written, qualitative questionnaires]. *Sosiologisk tidsskrift*, 22(4): 383–393.

Klein, Barbro. 2003. Nm. 223 Personlig hygien: Reflektioner kring frågelistor, meddelarsvar och vetenskap [No. 223 Personal hygiene: Reflections about qualitative questionnaires, respondents' replies and science]. In Bo G. Nilsson, Dan Waldetoft & Christina Westergren (eds.), *Frågelist och berättarglädje: Om frågelistor som forskningsmetod och folklig genre* [Qualitative questionnaires and narration joy: On qualitative questionnaires as research method and popular genre], 69–89. Stockholm: Nordiska Museets Förlag.

Larson, Heidi J. 2020. *Stuck: How vaccine rumors start – and why they don't go away*. New York: Oxford University Press.

Larson, Heidi J., Richard M. Clarke, Caitlinn Jarett, Elisabeth Eckersberger, Zachary Levine, Will S. Schultz & Pauline Paterson. 2018. Measuring trust in vaccination: A systematic review. *Human Vaccines & Immunotherapeutics* 14(7): 1599–1609.

Licht, Jenny de F. 2011. Do we really want to know? The potentially negative effect of transparency in decision making on perceived legitimacy. *Scandinavian Political Studies* 34(3): 183–202.

Löfstedt, Ragnar & Dominic Way. 2016. Transparency and trust in the European pharmaceutical sector: Outcomes from an experimental study. *Journal of Risk Research* 19(9): 1082–1103.

Lundgren, Britta. 2015. *Narrating narcolepsy: Centering a side effect. Medical Anthropology* 34(2): 150–165.

Lundgren, Britta. 2016. Solidarity at the needle point: The intersection of compassion and containment during the A(H1N1) pandemic in Sweden. *Sociology and Anthropology* 4 (12): 1108–1116.

National Committee for Research Ethics in the Social Sciences and the Humanities (NESH). 2021. *Guidelines for research ethics in the social sciences, the humanities, law and theology*.

NIPH. 2008. https://www.fhi.no/nettpub/vaksinasjonsveilederen-for-helsepersonell/vaksinasjon/barnevaksinasjonsprogrammet/ (reading date 2022-08-19).

NIPH. 2021. https://www.fhi.no/en/id/vaccines/coronavirus-immunisation-programme/coronavirus-vaccination---statistic/ (reading date 2022-09-23).

NIPH. 2022a. https://www.fhi.no/hn/helseregistre-og-registre/dodsarsaksregisteret/tall-for-covid-19-assosierte-dodsfall-i-dodsarsaksregisteret-i-2021/ (reading date 2022-09-23).

NIPH. 2022b. https://www.fhi.no/nettpub/koronavaksinasjonsveilederen-for-kommuner-og-helseforetak/bakgrunn-og-overordnede-foringer/om-bruken-av-vaxzevria-astrazeneca-i-norge/ (reading date 2022-09-29).

NPE. 2020. https://www.npe.no/no/Erstatningssoker/utvalgte_skadeomraader/pandemrix/ti-ar-med-erstatninger-etter-vaksine-mot-svineinfluensa/ (reading date 2022-09-26).

Offerdal, Truls S., Sine N. Just & Øyvind Ihlen. 2021. Public ethos in the pandemic rhetorical situation: Strategies for building trust in authorities' risk communication. *Journal of International Crisis and Risk Communication Research* 4(2): 247–270.

Petersen, Michael B., Alexander Bor, Fredrik Jørgensen & Marie F. Lindholt. 2021. Transparent communication about negative features of COVID-19 vaccine decreases acceptance but increases trust. *Proceedings of the National Academy of Sciences (PNAS)* 118(29): 1–8.

Pileberg, Silje. 2021. Norske styresmakter har vore meir opne om det uvisse i pandemien enn Sverige og Danmark: Klar tale om covid-19 kan ha redda liv [Norwegian authorities have been more open about uncertainties in the pandemic than Sweden and Denmark: Clear communication about Covid-19 may have saved lives]. *Forskning.no*. Published article, 12 December, https://forskning.no/kommunikasjon-media-partner/norske-styresmakter-har-vore-meir-opne-om-det-uvisse-i-pandemien-enn-sverige-og-danmark/1948233 (reading date 2022-05-27).

Røed-Johansen, Daniel & Hans O. Torgersen. 2020. Regjeringen setter inn "de sterkeste tiltakene vi har hatt i fredstid" [The government is implementing "the strongest restrictions we have ever had in times of peace"]. *Aftenposten*, published article, 12 March, https://www.aftenposten.no/norge/i/mR4pRL/regjeringen-setter-inn-de-sterkeste-tiltakene-vi-har-hatt-i-fredstid (reading date 2022-09-27).

Schiøtz, Aina. 2003. *Folkets helse – landets styrke: 1850–2003* [*Citizens' health – the country's strength: 1850–2003*]. Oslo: Universitetsforlaget.

Singer, Merill. 2009. Pathogens gone wild? Medical anthropology and the "swine flu" pandemic. *Medical Anthropology* 28(3): 199–206.

Smith, Carole. 2005. Understanding trust and confidence: Two paradigms and the significance for health and social care. *Journal of Applied Philosophy* 22(3): 299–317.

Vestreng, Tom. 2021. AstraZeneca-vaksinen: Dette skjer med de som har fått første dose. Og dette skjer med vaksinene på vent [The AstraZeneca vaccine: This happens to those who have received the first shot. And this happens to the vaccines on hold]. *Dagsavisen*. Published article, 15 March, https://www.dagsavisen.no/oslo/2021/03/15/astrazeneca-vaksinen-dette-skjer-med-de-som-har-fatt-forste-dose-og-dette-skjer-med-vaksinene-pa-vent/ (reading date 2022-05-12).

Wakefield, Andrew J. et al. 1998. Ileal-lymphoid-nodular hyperplasia, non-specific colitis, and pervasive developmental disorder in children. *Lancet* (RETRACTED) 358: 637–641.

Waldetoft, Dan. 2003. Vad vill vi med våra frågelistor? [What do we want from our qualitative questionnaires?]. In Bo G. Nilsson, Dan Waldetoft & Christina Westergren (eds.), *Frågelist och berättarglädje: Om frågelistor som forskningsmetod och folklig genre* [*Qualitative questionnaires and narration joy: On qualitative questionnaires as research method and popular genre*], 89–101. Stockholm: Nordiska Museets Förlag.

Ytre-Arna, Brita. 2022. Tre spørsmål om metodeutvikling [Three questions about the development of methods]. *Norsk medietidsskrift* 29(1): 1–4.

9 Where the fringe and mainstream meet

Discussions on vaccine hesitancy among public radio listeners on Facebook

Emma Ricknell

Introduction

Some of the unprecedented amount of information that washed over the internet as the COVID-19 pandemic unfolded was generated by journalists, government officials, and others who worked hard to maintain accuracy in an extremely uncertain situation. However, the "infodemic" the World Health Organization (WHO) as early as February 2020 began to warn about is primarily associated not with such information, but instead with false and misleading information (United Nations 2020). When it comes to vaccines, misleading and false information online is not a new phenomenon, particularly when it comes to prevalence on social media, but has been explicitly linked to COVID-19 vaccine hesitancy in a number of studies (e.g. Pierri et al. 2022).

The WHO's warning specified that infodemics create confusion and distrust in a population, and are ultimately harmful to people's health (United Nations 2020). The term "infodemic" has at the same time received criticism for oversimplifying a highly complex phenomenon and potentially painting an exaggerated, threatening picture of a problem that is not entirely unfamiliar (Simon & Camargo 2021). Indeed, any attempt to illustrate a parallel between exposure to and subsequent infection of a new virus to how people receive and manage information online may in fact obfuscate aspects of resilience among citizens. In this chapter I aim to highlight these aspects at risk of being obscured. I do so by analysing online discussions regarding the COVID-19 vaccine among Swedish public local radio listeners.

A number of circumstances surrounding such discussions create a foundation for analysis. Scepticism towards the COVID-19 vaccine was at the time of the vaccine roll-out towards the end of 2020 very low (see Rönnerstrand 2024), a pattern in line with the generally high level of trust in both public authorities and other people among Swedes (Holmberg & Rothstein 2017). Swedes furthermore relied on local media when navigating the intense spread of information regarding the crisis (Ytre-Arne & Moe 2023), meaning interaction via social media in reaction to such news reporting was likely. Taken together, the expectation would therefore be that casual interactions via social media

DOI: 10.4324/9781003305859-11

concerning the COVID-19 vaccine would not be characterised by rampant disinformation. Nevertheless, all discussions via social media platforms exist in a comprehensive network of information exchange, one that during the COVID-19 pandemic included a significant spread of extreme, false, and conspiratorial content (e.g. Gruzd et al. 2021). Sweden is in this regard certainly not an isolated country impervious to false and misleading information generated either outside its borders or within. While thus not downplaying the existence of false and misleading information online during the pandemic and in relation to the COVID-19 vaccine, the aim here is to examine to which extent such content did in fact reach discussions in Swedish in the context of local news, and if so, how participants handled such content. The primary question is, how do citizens in a high-trust society respond to social media content that is possibly fuelled by false and misleading information, in this case concerning a vaccine?

In the next section I explain how high levels of trust can be theoretically explained in the Swedish context, followed by an overview of the role of local media and the COVID-19 vaccine roll-out. I then describe how the data was collected, coded, and analysed, and subsequently present the results. I end the chapter with a discussion of the results and what they tell us about how citizens act online while under significant stress.

Trust in Sweden

As has been well established in previous research (e.g. Holmberg & Rothstein 2017; Rothstein & Stolle 2003), Swedes tend to trust one another as well as the public institutions that manage their universal welfare state, which consistently ranks high on a number of global indices capturing, e.g., human development, democracy, freedom of the press, and gender equality (Strömbäck 2022). This high level of trust has remained fairly stable over time, challenging the argument presented by various thinkers regarding the decline in trust as a consequence of living in modern, highly individualistic, market-based economies where we no longer have a connection with others in our community (e.g. Putnam 2000).

It is, however, precisely the conditions of living in a modern society marked by an individualistic social order that have been argued to have contributed to the high levels of trust in Sweden. Drawing upon Cross (2005), Trägårdh (2013) argues that trust should be seen as varying in type between different types of societies. In modern societies, marked by individualism and the rule of law, trust is broad and "cooler", less emotional, and based on rationality, in contrast with more "hot", emotionally, and even irrationally based form of trust found in traditional societies where the tribe or clan comes first. A key aspect in the particular form of trust that has developed over time in Swedish society is a form of individualism Trägårdh (1997) calls "statist individualism", a solution applied by the modern Swedish welfare state that maximises individual freedom for citizens by guaranteeing services and support that free the individual from reliance on family, friends, churches, or various forms of charity. As described by Trägårdh (1997: 262), the Swedish welfare state "can be viewed as a gigantic deal whereby individuals have bought themselves collectively free from personal, individual responsibilities under the guise of state-run solidarity". Notably, however, this form of social contract or alliance between the state and the individual citizen does not challenge basic social order in society (Trägårdh 2013), and Swedes are generally very supportive of collectivistic solutions as part of a strong welfare state.

Trust during something as extreme, unpredictable, and serious of a threat to people's health and lives as a pandemic arguably puts both cooler and warmer variants to the test. Yet even during the COVID-19 pandemic, Swedes maintained their relatively high level of trust. A rally-around-the-flag effect was found during the early period of the pandemic (Esaiasson et al. 2020); a development that can often be found in times of crisis and emergencies that generates heightened levels of political trust and support for public institutions (Nielsen & Lindvall 2021). This effect may have dissipated slightly over time, and research carried out during the ongoing pandemic was able to show that there were significant differences in levels of trust among Swedes, for example among those of different ideological convictions (Andersson 2021; Nielsen & Lindvall 2021). This ideological polarisation was visible also in a survey on COVID-19 vaccine acceptance among Swedes, with right-leaning individuals expressing greater concern about the vaccine and its side effects compared to individuals voting for leftist parties. However, the proportion of Swedes that could count as being hesitant towards the vaccine was only 4% (Rönnerstrand 2021). When a COVID-19 vaccine finally became a reality by late 2020 in Sweden, most Swedes did decide to take it. By the end of 2021, 81.9% of the population had received at least two doses (Public Health Agency of Sweden (Fohm) Authority 2022).

Local media and vaccination roll-out

In what thus appears as a society that trusts authorities to administer a new vaccine, successful communication between government and citizens nevertheless remains an important factor. Media serves as the intermediary arena where this can occur, and is part of the greater system that allows for levels of trust to be maintained. It can not only convey messages from public authorities and other officials, but also serve to uphold important aspects such as transparency and openness by monitoring government. But this function depends on citizens seeing media as a trustful source of information in itself.

In Sweden, much like in many other countries, the media landscape is deeply fragmented, with digital media, including social media, creating individualised consumption patterns that can both facilitate new arenas for communication and create difficulty in maintaining cohesion (Nord & Grusell 2021). This constantly evolving media environment and subsequent highly divergent user patterns have been argued to have a negative effect on the view of traditional mainstream media as an institution that represents "the truth" (Dahlgren 2018a); truth being of utmost importance in the roll-out of a new vaccine to the entire public.

Despite considerable transformation of the media landscape, particularly with the introduction of social media platforms, Swedes nevertheless hold media in high regard. In particular, public service radio and television continue to attract significant audiences (Nord & Grusell 2021). About eight out of ten citizens consider public service media to be of high societal value, a level of appreciation that is present even among people with low usage of public service (Andersson 2022). In terms of trust in public service media and the COVID-19 crisis, levels rose during the early part of the pandemic only to decline somewhat by 2021, but over time public service retained its significant position in the Swedish media system (Andersson 2021, 2022).

Social media and the internet as a whole pose a challenge to more traditional conveyors of news and information such as public service broadcasting to reach audiences that have individualised their intake of information. While thus adapting to a new and evolving media landscape online, public service broadcast media at the same time constitute the only regional and local news providers when it comes to radio and television (Nord & von Krogh 2021). Central in this limited local media market when it comes to radio and television is P4, Swedish Public Radio's most popular radio channel. Its primary focus is local news, but it also broadcasts news at the national and international levels (Swedish Radio 2020). Like many other news media, P4 via its 26 different local radio stations has a presence on social media platforms, where listeners can interact with news stories and hold conversations among each other. Facebook is the most popular platform for keeping up to date with local matters in Sweden, such as via local Facebook groups, but is also important for citizens to take part of and engage with news stories produced by local media (Nygren 2018).

The function of P4's stations in terms of providing local news is a factor of considerable importance considering the pandemic and the COVID-19 vaccination campaign. Once a vaccine is ready for roll-out, vaccinations are after all a practical and ultimately local matter, setting the bar high for accurate, transparent information available to the public via all possible channels in order to ensure that people feel safe and confident in taking the vaccine. In the next section, I present the different considerations taken when collecting and analysing data from Facebook pages of P4 stations.

Methodological considerations

A number of choices have been made regarding the collection of Facebook comments that form the basis for analysis in this study. First, the study only comprises comments on news stories that in some way relate to the COVID-19 vaccine. Comments on stories that primarily deal with the pandemic from a wider perspective are thus not included. Second, as the first vaccine was administered by the end of December 2020 (Fohm 2022), the time period examined includes the month of December 2020 as well as November that same year in order to catch comments relating to stories about the implementation of the upcoming vaccination programme. The relevancy of the starting date is confirmed by a study of the overall news reporting in Sweden that indicates a significant rise in reporting on the vaccine by late fall 2020 (Dahlgren 2021). Vaccination roll-out continued over the course of 2021, whereby the entirety of the year 2021 is also included. Third, a selection of local radio stations was made. Out of Swedish Public Radio's 26 local stations, 25 were at the time of writing present on Facebook. Out of those 25, a random sample of five stations was selected. In addition to these, the Facebook pages of local stations in Sweden's three largest cities (Stockholm, Gothenburg, and Malmö) were included. The number of Facebook comments reacting to vaccine-related posts on these eight stations' Facebook pages November 2020 to December 2021 totalled 19,854 and were obtained via the online tool Export Comments.

I rely on a content analysis of the Facebook comments collected, involving a number of coding decisions. First of all, a determination was made regarding what would constitute comments that do not fall under vaccine acceptance. The Strategic Advisory Group of Experts on Immunization (SAGE), a working group of WHO, defines vaccine hesitancy as "the delay in acceptance or refusal of vaccines despite availability of vaccination services" (MacDonald 2015). In an attempt to break down this very broad definition, this study applies two main categories: *hesitant* and *opposed*. In practice, these main categories correspond to comments that differ from each other in a decisive way, namely that the first expresses hesitancy towards taking the vaccine, exemplified by comments like "I'm afraid to", or "I'm going to wait", typically in response to a question on whether to vaccinate or not, whereas a comment that belongs to the second category contains statements like "No" or "Never" in response to the same type of question.

Secondly, when a user provides a reason explaining a hesitant or oppositional position, such are also coded. A comment such as "There's no way I'm taking the vaccine" would be categorised as opposing the vaccine but lacking any explanation as to why. In contrast, a comment stating "I'm not taking it right now. No one knows about the side effects" explicitly refers to a reason as to why the person is hesitant. Comments that contain clear reasoning along these lines are subsequently divided into three categories: *side effects*, *big pharma*, and *conspiracy theories*, adapted from the Stanford Internet Observatory's Virality Project report on COVID-19 anti-vaccine narratives (The Virality Project 2022). The first category is used for comments that include fears about the vaccine's possible side effects, the second for those that instead misrepresent the vaccine production and roll-out and express mistrust in pharmaceutical companies with claims of the vaccine being about profitmaking. The last category is broad and may relate to the first two comments, but are separated from the first two as comments in this category contain references to the many conspiracy theories that have circulated regarding COVID-19 and the vaccine (see, e.g., The Virality Project 2022). These comments generally refer to deliberate and detrimental actions taken by known figures or institutions in order to harm, exploit, or deceive regular citizens (The Virality Project 2022).

Third, comments are coded for engagement, in this case meaning when someone replies to a comment that expresses vaccine hesitancy or opposition. Conditions for such responses are complex. On the one hand, users in the discussions under study are not members of a closed Facebook group comprised of people with common interests and similar opinions. Users can therefore expect both agreeing and disagreeing responses, or no responses whatsoever. On the other hand, users involved in a discussion may share geographic location and even know each other; conditions which may cause some to hesitate to comment in the first place, or try to correct someone else due to social consequences (Theocharis et al. 2021). However, based on the overwhelming supportive sentiment regarding the COVID-19 vaccine among Swedes (Rönnerstrand 2021), comments that stand out as extreme or outlandish can nevertheless be expected to generate some responses. Such replies are therefore counted and categorised. Adapted from the characterisation of replies to misinformation on social media by Tully et al. (2020), replies are coded as *supportive* (agreeing with the original comment), *questioning* (e.g., replying with a non-hostile question or expressing curiosity), *neutral* (e.g., with appeals to fact and reason, without judgement), and *uncivil* (e.g., mocking, angry, accusative, or hostile).

Lastly, while the comments analysed in this chapter are public, expressions relating to the vaccine regardless of content nevertheless constitute sensitive material. The analysis is therefore concentrated only on the content of the comments, the date when they were posted, and the news stories for which they were posted in reaction. No additional information about the commenter, such as user ID and other identifying pieces of information, is part of the downloaded dataset, nor the analysis. For integrity purposes, the analysis is furthermore presented at aggregate level, meaning no differentiation is made between the eight Facebook pages examined. Comments used to exemplify the content are also translated from Swedish to English by the author and presented in a way that reduces similarities with the original comment text in order to avoid identification to the furthest extent possible while maintaining original meaning.

A stable barrier faces pressure

The following analysis provides insight into how Facebook users reacted to and engaged with other users in the context of COVID-19 vaccine-related local public radio news stories posted from November 2020 to December 2021. The expectation is that comments reflect the overall very high level of vaccine acceptance among Swedes, seen in this study as a form of barrier, but the examination also aims to uncover patterns regarding vaccine hesitancy and opposition, and importantly also reactions to such less commonly expressed sentiments. The presentation of the results will start from a more general level of engagement when it comes to comments on news stories, to focus on the prevalence and content of expressions of vaccine hesitancy and opposition, ending with patterns regarding replies to comments that express such less common sentiments.

Beginning with the general level of engagement when it comes to the many news stories that appeared relating to the vaccine, Figure 9.1 displays the total number of comments each month (left-hand y-axis) as well as the average number of comments per news story (right-hand y-axis). In terms of the former, March 2021 is by far the most intense month when it comes to the total number of comments. At that point, the vaccination campaign was primarily aimed at seniors and certain medical care staff and had not expanded to include the entire population. Approximately 8.4% of the adult population had received at least one dose by 10 March (Fohm 2021a). Despite a rather modest start to the vaccine roll-out in the first couple of months, news reporting was nevertheless intense. For example, multiple stories related to AstraZeneca's COVID-19 vaccine, both due to the company's difficulty in delivering enough doses (12 March) and subsequently due to its being halted by the Public Health Agency pending the European Medicines Agency's review of possible adverse side effects (16 March) (Olofsson & Vilhelmsson 2022). Towards the end of the month (24 March), Swedish Radio also presented results of a major poll on vaccine acceptance among Swedes, with results from residents belonging to the geographical area of each individual public local

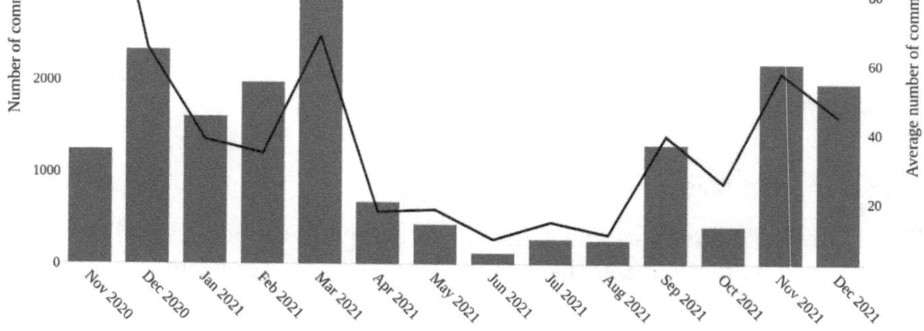

Figure 9.1 Comments over time (total number and average per news story).

radio station presented separately (Swedish Radio 2021). News stories on the poll, which showed overwhelming support for the vaccine, generated significant commentary.

While the average number of comments per news story in March 2021 is relatively high, it is not nearly as high as at the beginning of the examined time period, in November–December 2020 leading up to the start of the vaccination campaign. The fewer number of stories that were posted during those two months (45 in total compared to 75 in March 2021) were thus ones that users were very engaged with. The vaccine roll-out had not yet started, meaning the level of uncertainty was much higher compared to later months, in terms of both the efficiency and possible side effects of the vaccine as well as the actual practical matters of the upcoming campaign, from the national level down to the local authorities responsible. Some of the local radio stations engaged with their listeners and added questions to their vaccine-related stories, or in some cases simply posted questions on Facebook asking directly how people felt about the vaccine.

This somewhat uneven pattern relates to the proportion of the total number of comments that expressed vaccine hesitancy and opposition, and what those comments expressed as a primary concern. Figure 9.2 indicates that November and December 2020, along with being very comment-intense months, are also the two most intense months when it comes to the total number of comments indicating hesitancy and opposition. Sentiments indicating hesitancy represent

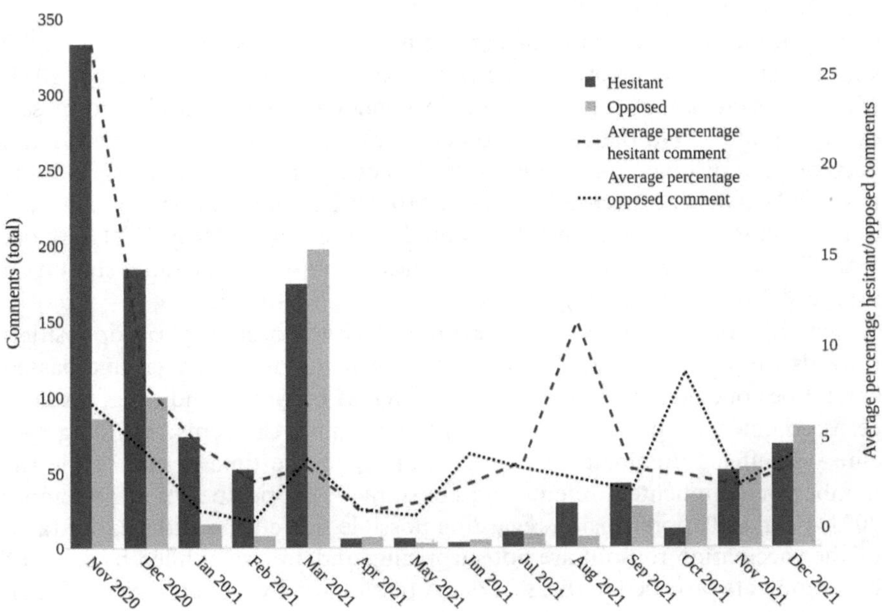

Figure 9.2 Comments indicating COVID-19 vaccine hesitancy and opposition (total number and average in percentage of total comments).

about 25% of all comments in November; a figure that drops drastically until the month of August 2021 when news reporting and overall engagement levels are otherwise generally low. During the month of August the number of Swedes that had received two doses of the vaccine increased from about 50% to 65% (Fohm 2022), but the temporary spike in hesitant comments can be explained by the occurrence of news stories about, on the one hand, the possibility of a third dose being necessary (Fohm 2021b) and, on the other hand, the vaccination roll-out to minors (Fohm 2021c). However, considering the low total number of comments during this month, as visible in Figure 9.1, this temporary spike is not indicative of a more significant pattern. Similarly, the proportion of comments expressing opposition to the vaccine is relatively high in October 2021, but that month is one of overall low activity.

The main result concerning the level of hesitancy is that it was prominent in comments in 2020, only to drop dramatically and remain at around 5% of all comments each month, August being an exception. Regarding the content of the comments posted in November and December 2020 that expressed hesitancy, some were elaborate, others very brief. Examples of more elaborate reasoning were, e.g., “I’m more afraid of the vaccine compared to the virus. But they’re good at convincing people like it’s a new type of religion”; “No, I’m going to wait a few months, they’ve rushed the vaccine. Plus it doesn’t give 100% protection”; and “What if diabetes type 1 is one of the side effects of the corona vaccine?” Brief comments posted in response to the local radio station engaging with its listeners and asking for their views on the vaccine were, e.g., “Doubtful” and “Sceptical”.

Regarding the proportion of comments opposing the vaccine, Figure 9.2 shows that it hovers below 5% except for November 2020 and October 2021. More elaborate comments were, e.g., “A confident no. I’ve vaccinated myself enough in life”; “No thank you! You can make it by washing your hands and keeping your distance”; and “Of course I’m not going to vaccinate. This is the first mRNA-vaccine given to humans”. More brief comments expressing clear opposition to the vaccine were, for example, those stating “Nope”, “No thank you:-)”, and “No way” in response to a question posed by the radio station on listeners’ thoughts on taking the vaccine.

Whether the individuals who expressed either hesitancy or opposition towards the vaccine in late 2020 changed their minds or not as time passed cannot be concluded from the data. However, as Figure 9.3 indicates, the concerns commenters provided shift slightly over time. Concerns regarding vaccine side effects dominate the earlier months of the time period, while the number of commenters referencing conspiracy theories peaks in December 2021. Fear and apprehension regarding possible side effects at the early stages of the vaccination roll-out are not surprising, and are exemplified by some of the comments provided in this section. A population living in a society of high political trust is thus not exempt from these types of fears and, in many ways, legitimate concerns amongst great uncertainty.

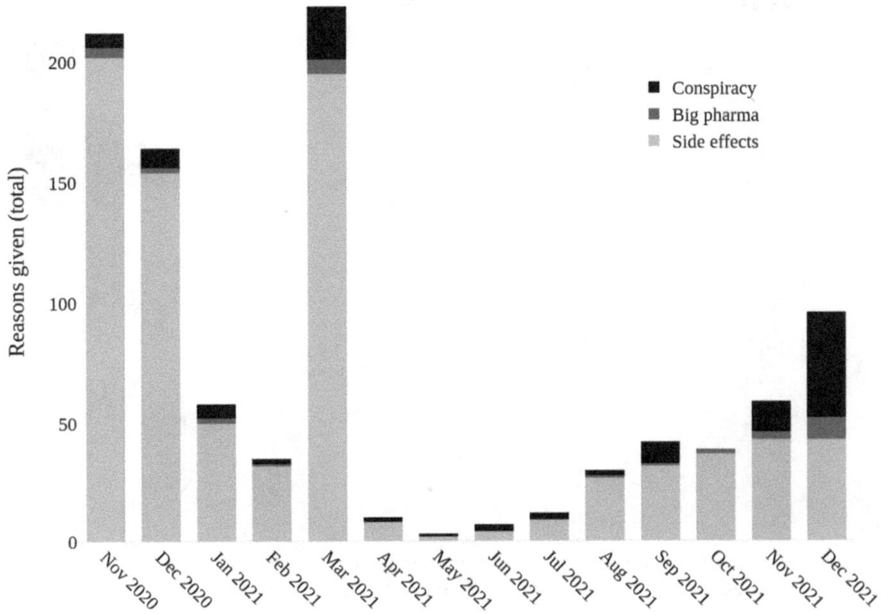

Figure 9.3 Reasons provided in comments expressing hesitancy and opposition (total number by month).

In contrast, the rise in comments referencing conspiracies is not entirely expected. Engagement levels had risen by November 2021 after a far less active summer (see Figure 9.1). Vaccine-related news stories during the latter part of year often centred on the increasing number of COVID-19 cases and the Public Health Agency of Sweden's subsequent and increasingly more strict infection control measures, including a COVID-19 vaccination certificate (Fohm 2021d). Comments posted towards the end of 2021 and that fall into this category referred to different aspects of conspiracy theories that developed over time concerning the virus itself, and eventually the vaccine. These aspects were sometimes referred to in more elaborate form and included links to various anti-vaccination websites, or commented on the new restrictions and the vaccination certificate by referring to a "mass psychosis" or "brainwashing", including by media, with calls to "wake up from this disgusting fraud/plandemic [*sic*] against humanity" and stating that various companies and well-known individuals, such as Bill Gates and George Soros, "own the world's governments now". Not all expressions of conspiracies referred to more globally circulating conspiratorial claims regarding the vaccine, but instead described well-known Swedish individuals such as the prime minister as personally benefiting from the vaccine, or claimed that Swedish politicians would benefit from a better-functioning health care system without so many old and frail people, as they were now dying from the vaccine.

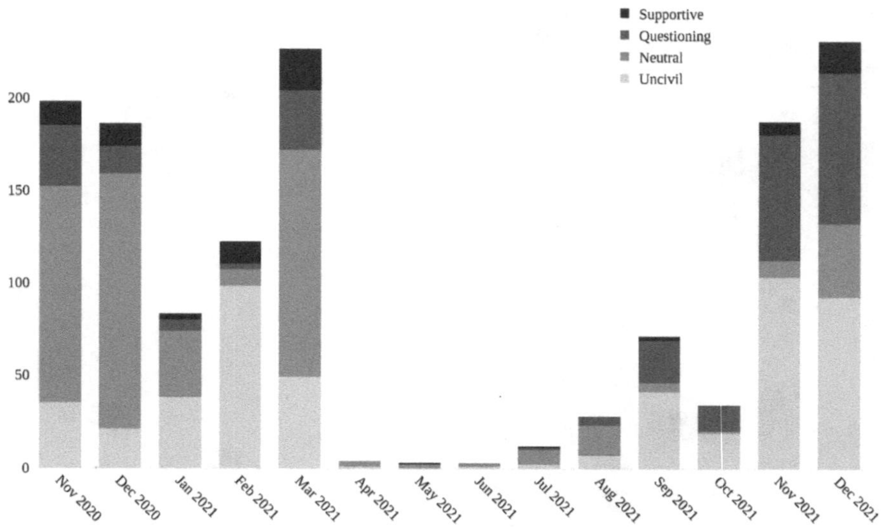

Figure 9.4 Categorisation of replies to comments expressing reason behind COVID-19 vaccine hesitancy and opposition (total number by month).

Finally, this study focuses not only on the presence of expressions of vaccine hesitancy and opposition, but also whether such expressions generated replies from other users and if so, what type of reply. From Figure 9.4, it is possible to see a similar pattern in terms of activity, i.e., that months when news stories generate a lot of comments, many of them are also replies. In some cases, a hesitant or oppositional comment can generate several replies, in other cases none. Over time, there is some variation in the proportion of uncivil replies to stated concerns, with such becoming proportionally more common towards the end of 2021. According to Figure 9.3, that is when conspiracy theories provided as reasons for hesitancy and opposition were more common in number than previously.

The results thus show that expressions of vaccine hesitancy and opposition did indeed generate further engagement in the form of replies, but that the tone during the studied time period went from one marked primarily by appeals to reason and fact, curiosity, and general, non-hostile questioning of such statements, to featuring also a generally more uncivil tone, that expressed, e.g., anger, hostility, or ridicule. Examples of replies that maintained a more civil tone during the beginning of the time period were e.g. "You have to check all that have received the vaccine. The US alone has vaccinated one million and all countries report side effects", "When it comes to excess mortality I recommend you google 'excess mortality Sweden'", and "The Pfizer vaccine was tested on 43,000 people and no one showed any serious complications. You also have to weigh possible side effects with what it means to catch covid". In contrast, the angrier, sarcastic, and/or accusatory replies that were slightly more common towards the end of 2021 were, e.g., "Does anyone think we will get rid of this shit unless everyone vaccinates. No, you go ahead and keep infecting old and frail people", "Your comment does not answer the question. So stop with your goddamn conspiracy theories!!!", and "That's what you think, but we're following the recommendations by authorities and take responsibility but you don't give a shit about it. You're really a responsible citizen". As noted earlier, this pattern mirrors the shift over time regarding reasons given as to why a person is hesitant towards or opposes the vaccine. Supportive comments were not common during any part of the studied time period.

Conclusions and discussion

This chapter has aimed to examine what happens when individuals interact with each other on a social media platform while under considerable pressure due to an ongoing health crisis and in the context of an intense spread of both accurate and inaccurate information. The COVID-19 vaccine roll-out is treated as a critical test, and the online context is one far removed from the more extreme corners of the internet. A number of conclusions regarding the results can be drawn, and inform us of how citizens in a society characterised by high trust respond to sentiments online that in varying ways deviate from the expected.

First, individuals who were hesitant towards the vaccine, particularly those who felt apprehensive regarding potential side effects, were willing to make their sentiments public and engage in conversation about their views with others who had taken part of the same local public radio news story, i.e., likely a person in the same geographical region of Sweden. They were willing to do so even though their opinion did not follow the general norm. After a period of such comments being relatively common while the vaccine was still in the process of being rolled out, they eventually declined in number, as did comments that were straightforward in their opposition to the vaccine. This is not a surprising result considering the level of uncertainty surrounding the COVID-19 vaccine as it was being made available to the public, and instead highlights the importance of open and constructive communication between the public and professionals during a stressful time period.

Second, it can also be concluded that users who saw hesitant comments responded to them, and when the vaccine was still very new, they did so primarily by appealing to rational thinking, logic, and facts. A cool, laid-back reaction, if you will, where one citizen is trying to help another to help themselves, with the efforts of government and public authorities there in the background. However, the results also show that the propensity to post such replies changes over time, and when more conspiratorial hesitant and oppositional comments appear towards the end of 2021, some of the patience may have run out. For context, it is important to remember that many people's patience was under considerable strain during that particular point of the COVID-19 pandemic, as the virus kept spreading not just in Sweden but globally. Even though the results cannot ascertain whether this development towards late 2021 was temporary or not, there are lessons to learn regarding what happens online as extreme conditions take a significant and long-term hold on people's lives.

Third, from a wider perspective, the results of this study indicate that as an arena where citizens can engage with others interested in keeping up with news about their local communities, Facebook has some potential for genuine engagement and public, primarily civil conversations, even in times of crisis and tremendous societal pressure. While capturing only a fraction of the online engagement in the context of the COVID-19 vaccine, the results relatedly show signs of a general level of resilience. They reveal signs of an active, constructive, and caring citizenry, rather than a passive one lacking the ability to withstand what some would liken to a form of informational virus. Considering all the issues involved with misinformation and disinformation as referenced in this chapter, along with a whole host of other issues of online participation on private, business-run spaces (see, e.g., Dahlgren 2018b), it is at the same time certainly not a flawless space. How to harness the potential among citizens who are able to maintain their cool online in extremely stressful times is nevertheless an avenue worth examining further.

References

Andersson, Ulrika. 2021. *Myndighetsförtroende under coronapandemin. SOM-undersökningen om coronaviruset 2021* [*Government trust during the corona pandemic. The SOM survey about the corona virus 2021*]. Gothenburg: SOM-institutet, University of Gothenburg.

Andersson, Ulrika. 2022. Användning och värdering av medier – om sociala mediers betydelse och public services starka stöd [Use and evaluation of media – on the importance of social media and strong support for public service broadcasting]. In Ulrika Andersson, Henrik Oscarsson, Björn Rönnerstrand & Nora Theorin (eds.), *Du sköra nya värld* [*You fragile new world*], 277–293. Gothenburg: SOM-institutet, University of Gothenburg.

Cross, Frank B. 2005. Law and trust. *Georgetown Law Journal* 93(5): 1457–1545.

Dahlgren, Peter. 2018a. Media, knowledge and trust: The deepening epistemic crisis of democracy. *Javnost – The Public* 25(1–2): 20–27. https://doi.org/10.1080/13183222.2018.1418819

Dahlgren, Peter. 2018b. Public sphere participation online: The ambiguities of affect. *Les Enjeux de l'information et de la communication* 19(1): 5–20. https://doi.org/10.3917/enic.024.0005

Dahlgren, Peter M. 2021. *Medieinnehåll och mediekonsumtion under coronapandemin: Datoriserade metoder för insamling och analys av stora mängder text- och mediedata* [*Media content and media consumption during the corona pandemic: Computerized methods for collection and analysis of large quantities of text- and media data*]. Gothenburg: The Department of Journalism, Media and Communication, University of Gothenburg. Available at: https://www.gu.se/sites/default/files/2021-09/Nr88-Dahlgren-Medieinnehall.pdf (Accessed 20 June 2022).

Esaiasson, Peter, Jacob Sohlberg, Marina Ghersetti & Bengt Johansson. 2020. How the coronavirus crisis affects citizens trust in institutions and in unknown others: Evidence from "the Swedish experiment". *European Journal of Political Research* 60(3): 748–760. https://doi.org/10.1111/1475-6765.12419

Gruzd, Anatoliy, Manilo De Domenico, Pier Luigi Sacco & Sylvie Briand. 2021. Studying the COVID-19 infodemic at scale. *Big Data & Society* 8(1): 1–6. https://doi.org/10.1177/20539517211021115

Holmberg, Sören & Bo Rothstein. 2017. Trusting other people. *Journal of Public Affairs* 17(1–2): e1645. https://doi.org/10.1002/pa.1645

MacDonald, Noni E. 2015. Vaccine hesitancy: definition, scope and determinants. *Vaccine* 33(34): 4161–4164. https://doi.org/10.1016/j.vaccine.2015.04.036

Nielsen, Julie H. & Johannes Lindvall. 2021. Trust in government in Sweden and Denmark during the COVID-19 epidemic. *West European Politics* 44(5–6): 1180–1204. https://doi.org/10.1080/01402382.2021.1909964

Nord, Lars & Marie Grusell. 2021. Media and politics in Sweden. In Eli Skogerbø, Øyvind Ihlen, Nete Nørgaard Kristensen & Lars Nord (eds.), *Power, communication, and politics in the Nordic countries*, 113–132. Gothenburg: Nordicom, University of Gothenburg. https://doi.org/10.48335/9789188855299-6

Nord, Lars & Torbjörn von Krogh. 2021. Sweden: Continuity and change in a more fragmented media landscape. In Josef Trappel & Tales Tomaz (eds.), *The Media for Democracy Monitor 2021: How leading news media survive digital transformation* (Vol. 1), 353–380. Gothenburg: Nordicom, University of Gothenburg. https://doi.org/10.48335/9789188855404-8

Nygren, Gunnar. 2018. En komplicerad lokal medieekologi: Facebook den nya lokala offentligheten? [A complicated local media ecology: Facebook the new local public sphere?]. In Ulrika Andersson, Anders Carlander, Elina Lindgren & Maria Oskarson (eds.), *Sprickor i fasaden: SOM-undersökningen 2017* [*Cracks in the facade: SOM survey 2017*], 195–212. Gothenburg: SOM-institutet, University of Gothenburg.

Olofsson, Tobias & Andreas Vilhelmsson. 2022. Dataset: COVID-19 epidemic policy and events timeline (Sweden). *Data in Brief* 40: 107698. https://doi.org/10.1016/j.dib.2021.107698

Pierri, Francesco, Brea L. Perry, Matthew R. DeVerna, Kai-Cheng Yang, Alessandro Flammini, Filippo Menczer & John Bryden. 2022. Online misinformation is linked to early COVID-19 vaccination hesitancy and refusal. *Scientific Reports* 12: 5966. https://doi.org/10.1038/s41598-022-10070-w

Public Health Agency of Sweden (Fohm). 2021a. Över en miljon vaccindoser inregistrerade [Over one million vaccination doses registered]. 10 March. Available at: https://www.folkhalsomyndigheten.se/nyheter-och-press/nyhetsarkiv/2021/mars/over-en-miljon-vaccindoser-inregistrerade/ (Accessed 3 August 2022).

Public Health Agency of Sweden (Fohm). 2021b. Tredje dos mot covid-19 troligen nästa år [Third dose against Covid-19 likely next year]. 3 August. Available at: https://www.folkhalsomyndigheten.se/nyheter-och-press/nyhetsarkiv/2021/augusti/tredje-dos-mot-covid-19-troligen-nasta-ar/ (Accessed 10 August 2022).

Public Health Agency of Sweden (Fohm). 2021c. Stort intresse för vaccination bland unga [Great interest in vaccinations among youth]. 19 August. Available at: https://www.folkhalsomyndigheten.se/nyheter-och-press/nyhetsarkiv/2021/augusti/stort-intresse-for-vaccination-bland-unga/ (Accessed 3 August 2022).

Public Health Agency of Sweden (Fohm). 2021d. Nya åtgärder för att begränsa spridning av covid-19 [New measures to limit spread of covid-19]. 7 December. Available at: https://www.folkhalsomyndigheten.se/nyheter-och-press/nyhetsarkiv/2021/december/nya-atgarder-for-att-begransa-spridning-av-covid-19/ (Accessed 16 August 2022).

Public Health Agency of Sweden (Fohm). 2022. Statistik för vaccination mot covid-19 [Statistics for Covid-19 vaccinations]. Available at: https://experience.arcgis.com/experience/6df5491d566a44368fc721726c274301 (Accessed 15 August 2022).

Putnam, Robert D. 2000. *Bowling alone: The collapse and revival of American community*. New York: Simon & Shuster.

Rönnerstrand, Björn. 2021. *Svenskarnas vaccinvilja och oro för vaccinets biverkningar. SOM-undersökningen om coronaviruset 2021* [*Swedish people's vaccination willingness and concerns about the vaccination side effects. The SOM survey about the corona virus 2021*]. Gothenburg: SOM-institutet, University of Gothenburg.

Rönnerstrand, Björn. 2024. Distrust and COVID-19 vaccine hesitancy in Sweden. In Lars Borin, Mia-Marie Hammarlin, Dimitrios Kokkinakis & Fredrik Miegel (eds.), *Vaccine hesitancy in the Nordic countries: Trust and distrust during the COVID-19 pandemic*. London: Routledge.

Rothstein, Bo & Dietlind Stolle. 2003. Introduction: Social capital in Scandinavia. *Scandinavian Political Studies* 26(1): 1–26.

Simon, Felix M. & Chico Q. Camargo. 2021. Autopsy of a metaphor: The origins, use and blind spots of the 'infodemic'. *New Media and Society*. Online First. https://doi.org/10.1177/14614448211031908

Strömbäck, Jesper. 2022. Beyond the political framing battles: Sweden in an international comparison. *Futurion*. Report no. 2022: 1. Available at: https://futurion.se/wp-content/uploads/2022/09/futurion-rapport-bortom-verklighetsbilden-2022-eng-rev-lowres.pdf (Accessed 9 September 2022).

Swedish Radio. 2020. Our channels. Available at: https://sverigesradio.se/artikel/733463 (Accessed 26 July 2022).

Swedish Radio. 2021. Nio av tio vill ta vaccin mot covid-19 [Nine out of ten want to take covid-19 vaccine]. 24 March. Available at: https://sverigesradio.se/artikel/bara-sex-personer-av-100-sager-nej-till-vaccin (Accessed 22 June 2022).

The Virality Project. 2022. *Memes, magnets and microchips: Narrative dynamics around COVID-19 vaccines*. Stanford Digital Repository v1.0.1. Available at https://purl.stanford.edu/mx395xj8490 (Accessed 3 August 2022).

Theocharis, Yannis, Ana Cardenal, Soyeon Jin, Toril Aalberg, David Nicholas Hopmann, Jesper Strömbäck, Laila Castro, Frank Esser, et al. 2021. Does the platform matter? Social media and COVID-19 conspiracy theory beliefs in 17 countries. *New Media & Society*: 1–26. https://doi.org/10.1177/14614448211045666

Trägårdh, Lars. 1997. Statist individualism: On the culturality of the Nordic welfare state. In Bo Stråth & Øystein Sørensen (eds.), *The cultural construction of Norden*, 253–285. Oslo: Scandinavian University Press.

Trägårdh, Lars. 2013. The historical incubators of trust in Sweden: From the rule of blood to the rule of law. In Marta Reuter, Filip Wijkström & Bengt Kristensson Uggla (eds.), *Trust and organizations: Confidence across borders*, 181–203. New York: Palgrave Macmillan.

Tully, Melissa, Leticia Bode & Emily K. Vraga. 2020. Mobilizing users: Does exposure to misinformation and its correction affect users' responses to a health misinformation post? *Social Media + Society* 6(4). https://doi.org/10.1177/2056305120978377

United Nations. 2020. UN tackles "infodemic" of misinformation and cybercrime in COVID-19crisis. Availableat: https://www.un.org/en/un-coronavirus-communications-team/un-tackling-'infodemic'-misinformation-and-cybercrime-covid-19 (Accessed 1 August 2022).

Ytre-Arne, Brita & Hallvard Moe. 2023. Citizens' news use during Covid-19: Concerns about misinformation and reliance on local news in Denmark, Finland, Norway, and Sweden. In Bengt Johansson, Øyvind Ihlen, Jenny Lindholm & Mark Blach-Ørsten (eds.), *Communicating a pandemic: Crisis management and Covid-19 in the Nordic countries*, 303–324. Gothenburg: Nordicom, University of Gothenburg. https://doi.org/10.48335/9789188855688-14

Part III

The growing chorus on the margin

10 Fearing mRNA

A mixed methods study of vaccine rumours

Mia-Marie Hammarlin, Dimitrios Kokkinakis, Fredrik Miegel, and Jullietta Stoencheva

Introduction

There are well-spread ideas among vaccine-critical individuals around the world that "new" vaccines might be more dangerous to health than other, "traditional" vaccines, which can lead to vaccine hesitancy; the "*delay in acceptance or refusal of vaccination despite availability of vaccination services*" (MacDonald 2015: 4163, emphasis in original). For example, a recurring remark made in social media is that mRNA technology resembles a chip that alters the human DNA, which might permanently and irreparably damage the immune system. These ideas sometimes take the shape of rumours and conspiracy theories (Loomba et al. 2021; Larson et al. 2022). Drawing on rumour theories and social cognitive perspectives, the aim of this chapter is to account for the purpose and the spreading of medical rumours that encircle mRNA COVID-19 vaccines. Our research questions are: How are rumours concerning mRNA expressed and established? In terms of trust and distrust, what function do the rumours have?

We rely upon DiFonzo and Bordia's definition of rumours as "unverified and instrumentally relevant information statements in circulation that arise in contexts of ambiguity, danger, or potential threat and that function to help people make sense and manage risk" (DiFonzo & Bordia 2007: 13). In relation to the present context, we develop this definition in the following manner: We analyse the fast circulation of a medical journal article concerning mRNA vaccines among members of the public that took place during the COVID-19 pandemic; a societal crisis characterised by danger, threat, and uncertainty.

The unfortunate bad reputation of vaccine rumours

Vaccines effectively protect ourselves, our children, and our fellow human beings from harmful infectious diseases, COVID-19 being one of them (Watson et al. 2022). Ultimately, vaccines protect people from risks of dying. Along these lines, the action of taking vaccines *and* the action of spreading vaccine refusal arguments encompass matters of illness, disease, and the fear of suffering. To stretch it even further, vaccine rumours could be seen as a phenomenon

DOI: 10.4324/9781003305859-13

that encompasses existential questions, of life and death and what it means to be living. This is not the case for all kinds of rumours. Therefore, we contend that vaccine rumours are a special category of rumours that need to be understood and studied on its own terms, where a compassionate approach is suitable (Pertwee et al. 2022; Hammarlin et al. 2023). However, this is not the most common way of dealing with the vaccine hesitancy problem in society. Actively debunking vaccine rumours may appear as a more constructive action, but this may lead to even stronger negative sentiments, especially if the refuting of the rumours is led by public authorities, as the sharp edge of the vaccine rumour sword often is pointed towards "experts" and "elites". Or as á Rogvi and Hoeyer (Chapter 6, this volume) put it: "for people to trust the [medical] data used to argue preventive measures such as restrictions and vaccinations, they need to trust the people presenting them and their intentions". So, instead of trying to reject the vaccine rumours, a better strategy would perhaps be to target the catalyst behind the rapid dispersion of these rumours (Larson et al. 2022: 1419). Therefore, we will contribute to an understanding of the function of mRNA vaccine rumours by analysing their actual content.

With Goldenberg (2021) and Hausman (2019), we argue that vaccine hesitancy is not primarily an expression of scientific ignorance or anti-scientific attitudes. Instead, we see it as an articulation of decreased trust in the scientific consensus regarding the conceivable risks of vaccines in favour of a more individualised and personal, rather than general and societal, approach. Hence, there is not necessarily a conflict between, on the one hand, being aware of the general safety and societal benefits of vaccines and, on the other hand, entertaining a personal scepticism of vaccinating oneself or one's children (Goldenberg 2021: 32–33). Viewing the expressions of vaccine hesitancy instead as a matter of *debating* how to interpret and evaluate the consensual comprehension of the vaccines' safety and effectiveness makes it an issue of negotiating knowledge and beliefs rather than one of scientific illiteracy. Similar to how Rosanvallon (2008) distinguishes between the concepts of anti-democracy and counter-democracy, we propose an understanding of the discussions regarding mRNA vaccines not as anti-scientific but rather *counter-scientific*, or, for that matter, *counter-epistemic*; ideas that will be developed further in the chapter.

Furthermore, Larson (2020) points out that rumours can be true or false or a mixture of the two. Rumours can save lives. They can also mislead people into making severely wrong decisions that might put them into dangerous situations. In a Swedish context, the medical historian Motzi Eklöf (2016) has shown how vaccine rumours became widely spread in 1932 in the city of Malmö, caused by an outburst of smallpox. The rumouring encompassed the evident risks at that time of severe adverse effects caused by the vaccine on the one hand, and the great fear of the disease itself on the other (Eklöf 2016). And rumours do have an influence on people's decisions. During the 1970s, false rumours were spread concerning a worry that the vaccine against whooping cough could cause severe brain damage in children, which resulted in a dramatic decline in the willingness to take the vaccine, especially in Sweden, Britain, and Japan (Blume &

Zanders 2006: 1828). One of the most well-known current vaccine rumours concerns a presumed connection between autism and the measles, mumps, and rubella (MMR) vaccination, a rumour that has been spread since the late 1990s. Albeit soundly refuted by the international research community, this story still causes parents to refrain from vaccinating their children against serious infectious diseases (Shevell & Fombonne 2006; Harrison 2010; Rao & Andrade 2011).

So, instead of seeing vaccine rumours as inherently bad, Larson underscores their complexity. She uses the word "resources" to describe them (Larson 2020: xxviii). Through negotiating reason and emotion, these communication resources clarify power relations in society – "who are the influencers and who are the followers" (Larson 2020: xxviii) – especially so in times of uncertainty. Vaccine rumours may unleash underlying sentiments about collective histories, relationships between people and governments, international organisations, and big business (Blume 2017: 216–242; Larson 2020). Larson takes the rumouring that led to a boycott of the polio vaccine in Nigeria in 2003–2004 as an example. The boycott was not caused by any evidence of problems with the vaccine. The resistance was triggered by what the vaccine represented, namely the global powers designing the campaign and the central Nigerian leadership, that people distrusted (Larson 2020: xxix).

Thus conceived, we find it appropriate to take as our empirical case the fast spreading of a medical scientific article, titled "Intracellular Reverse Transcription of Pfizer BioNTech COVID-19 mRNA Vaccine BNT162b2 in Vitro in Human Liver Cell Line" (Aldén et al. 2022), written by a group of infectious medicine researchers, that boosted an already-established vaccine rumour. Our analysis will show how mRNA rumours are not primarily based on anti-scientific sentiments, but rather on distrust regarding the officially sanctioned, positive narrative of new vaccine technologies.

mRNA scare (the case)

This is not the place to dive deeply into messenger RNA (mRNA) technology and its history, but it is worthwhile to note that it is not as new as it is sometimes described by sceptics. In fact, the first discovery that mRNA – molecules that carry the genetic information needed to make proteins – together with droplets of fat could make human cells absorb the mRNA and start to produce protein from it, was made in the 1980s (Dolgin 2021). In 2021, after four decades of research efforts, mRNA vaccines were mass distributed to people around the world as a protection against the virus SARS-Cov-2. This was the first time that mRNA vaccines were used on humans. Barely two years later, Katalin Karikó and Drew Weissman were awarded the Nobel Prize for their discoveries of the importance of base modifications in mRNA, which contributed to millions of lives being saved and allowed societies to return to normal conditions, the Nobel Assembly wrote in their motivation.[1]

So, how do these vaccines differ from others? To trigger an immune response, many vaccines put an inactivated germ or protein antigens from a germ into our bodies. This is not the case for mRNA vaccines; mRNA is a molecule that contains the instructions that directs the cells to make a protein, using its natural machinery. It travels within a protective bubble called a lipid nanoparticle, which helps it to enter cells smoothly. Once inside the body, our cells read the mRNA as a set of instructions, building proteins that match up with parts of the microorganism that causes the disease, called antigens. The immune system reacts by handling these foreign antigens as invaders, thus, training the immune system for potential future attacks by developing antibodies. So, after having received an mRNA vaccination against COVID-19, the body recognizes the SARS-Cov-2 virus, sounding the alarm to help defend against the infection.

It is also worth noting that the person who first made this groundbreaking finding is the physician Robert Malone, or so he claims. Malone also alleges that he has been written out of history (Dolgin 2021). During the COVID-19 pandemic, Malone became one of the medical doctors that anti-vaccination communities turned to in order to legitimise their opinions and arguments, especially concerning mRNA vaccines. While Malone has been celebrated in so-called alternative media, extensive critical journalism has been produced about him; the vaccine scientist that became a vaccine sceptic, as *The Atlantic* puts it (Bartlett 2021).

During the intense vaccination phases against COVID-19 between 2020 and 2021, numerous public health officials and authorities around the world strived to refute rumours related to mRNA vaccines. "No, COVID-19 vaccines do not alter your DNA", the Australian government's Health Department stated,[2] and approximately in the same wording also UNICEF,[3] the U.S. federal Centers for Disease Control and Prevention (CDC),[4] the South African government,[5] and the World Health Organization (WHO),[6] stating that "mRNA vaccines … do not interfere with human DNA". Sorted underneath "vaccine facts" on their official web page, the Washington State Department of Health writes: "No, the COVID-19 vaccines do not change or alter your DNA … The vaccine does not enter the part of the cell where our DNA is kept".[7] In sum, public authorities around the world seemed convinced that this particular mRNA scare was based on harmful rumours that might hinder people's willingness to take the vaccinations against COVID-19, notably the Pfizer BioNTech and the Moderna vaccine, and therefore needed to be rebutted; conceivably not very effective, but still a reasonable action as studies show that this particular rumour could have a negative effect on the willingness to take the jab (Pertwee et al. 2022).

Subsequently, the earlier-mentioned molecular biology mRNA study from Lund University, Sweden, was published. The title of the scientific paper is something of a riddle for people with scarce knowledge of biomedicine: "Intracellular Reverse Transcription of Pfizer BioNTech COVID-19 mRNA Vaccine BNT162b2 in Vitro in Human Liver Cell Line" (Aldén et al. 2022). Nonetheless, the specialist knowledge needed to interpret the results of the investigation did not prevent it from going viral. In August 2022, six months after it was published, it had been viewed in full-text more than 1.1 million times. At the time of writing this chapter in the autumn of 2023, 2.1 million people have viewed the article. With a so-called weighted attention score[8] of 28.780, the article quickly placed itself in the top 5% of all research outputs ever tracked by the data science metric tool.[9] It has been shared through social media at a fast speed, especially on the social media platform Twitter,[10] where 97% of the 89,400 tweets – from 57,600 tweeters, with upwards of 14 million followers in total – were written and spread by members of the public. So, what was this mRNA vaccine study about?

The question that the researchers set out to answer was the following: "Does the Pfizer-BioNTech mRNA vaccine get converted to DNA or not?" In a Q&A session, arranged by Lund University's press centre, Yang de Marinis, one of the authors, said:

> This study does not investigate whether the Pfizer vaccine alters our genome. Our publication is the first in vitro study on the conversion of mRNA vaccine into DNA, inside cells of human origin. We show that the vaccine enters liver cells as early as 6 hours after the vaccine has been administered. We saw that there was DNA converted from the vaccine's mRNA in the host cells we studied.
>
> (Lund University 2022)

Yang De Marinis's colleague, Magnus Rasmussen, added that the findings were observed under experimental conditions. He continued: "we do not yet know if the converted DNA is integrated into the cells' DNA in the genome – and if so, if it has any consequences". More studies need to be done, particularly on living human bodies, he concluded.

A counter-epistemic take on mRNA rumours

Why, then, did the Lund study get the amount of public attention it did? And why was it vigorously shared by laypeople? To answer these questions, we need to understand the driving forces behind people's engagement in controversial matters online. Asking how the information milieu on the internet affects people's cognitive processing, Sparrow and Chatman (2013: 279) investigate how people increasingly make consequential choices based on material they find on the internet which is not evaluated according to established scientific or other standards of accuracy, concluding that this has considerable effects on the process and content of how we socially negotiate reality (Sparrow & Chatman 2013: 288). In a similar vein, Rosanvallon (2021: 40–41) argues that, for instance, conspiracy theories could be seen as efforts to bring order in matters people experience as impenetrable, complex, and fearful. Paired with a psychological proneness to prefer simplified but comprehensible explanations over complex and complicated ones, he suggests that conspiracy theories comprise a cognitive mechanism allowing people to find and hold on to apparently more apprehensible, and less appalling reasons for problems they have to deal with in their lives.

In a similar vein, we take rumours to have functions corresponding to the ones Sparrow and Chatman and Rosanvallon, respectively, point out. A counter-epistemic approach to the mRNA rumours, thus, leads to an interest in the social dissemination and circulation of assumptions and propositions regarding the mRNA vaccines. We believe that this process can tell us something about how people process and evaluate online information and fit it into their perception of reality. A key social psychological concept regarding the cognitive functions of rumours on the internet is trust and trustworthiness. Rosanvallon (2008: 3) describes trust as an *invisible institution* that partly serves to reduce the need for other sources of proof. Similarly, Goldenberg (2021) argues for the importance of *building trust* rather than questioning the lacking faith in experts as intrinsically erratic and irrational. Both hold that we currently live in a society of mistrust, explained partly by an increased anger among parts of the public for having their views on matters important to them ignored and derided by "the elites". Goldenberg (2021: 17) describes this development as an unsuccessful science–public relation which makes people feel disrespected and silenced when they express their concerns.

Next, we turn to our empirical analysis of how rumours concerning mRNA vaccines are expressed and sustained, and how they, in this particular case, were reinforced by the complex medical article from Lund University. What do the tweets tell us about people's trust and distrust in mRNA vaccines and the "elite" discourses surrounding them? And what is the function of the Lund study for the vaccination-sceptical arguments?

Data collection and preprocessing

We collected Swedish tweets discussing mRNA vaccines, posted between 10 February and 10 November 2022, encompassing the initial and most intense phase of the popular dissemination of the Lund medical article. As mentioned earlier, during the studied time period Twitter was the most popular platform for spreading the Lund study globally. It is not, however, the most common social media for everyday use in Sweden; in comparison, Facebook and Instagram are much more popular.[11] When introduced in Sweden in 2006, Twitter was commonly referred to as the Swedish elite's platform, a view that might have changed with time.

The tweets were collected by searching with the keywords "m-RNA" or "mRNA", as well as all compounds beginning with these words, and setting the language to Swedish. The final tweet data set consisted of 2,028 unique tweets from 903 different users. Preprocessing is an important step in the data preparation stage that ensures that the topic model is identifying interesting and useful patterns instead of noise. Therefore, each tweet was pre-processed in various ways. First, we converted the tweets to lowercase. During a normalisation process, identified token variants such as "mrna vaccin," "mrna vax" and "mrnavaccin" were converted to a single uniform format; here, "mrna-vaccin". Furthermore, the dataset was further tokenized, separating punctuation and metadata from words, and then punctuation marks like ",.;:?!" were removed. Multiword expressions such as phrasal verbs and statistically significant collocations were also recognized, and their contiguous components were joined with an underscore prior to further processing (e.g., *big_pharma*; *in_vitro*, *nödgodkänt vaccin* 'emergency approved vaccine' or *spruta_in* 'to inject'). Stopwords, like *och* 'and', *på* 'on', *är* 'is', and *att* 'to', were also removed because those words are so common in any Swedish sentence that they tend to be over-represented in the results. Finally, posts with fewer than three words were removed as being too short, and the rest was used as input to the topic modelling software.

Topic modelling

Topic modelling is a method for the unsupervised classification of textual documents which allows people to get a bird's-eye view of large text collections. A popular topic model algorithm is *latent Dirichlet allocation* (LDA), proposed by Blei et al. (2003). LDA is a quantitative method based on a Bayesian probabilistic model that groups words with high co-occurrence probabilities into topics. Furthermore, we apply an extension to LDA, called *structural topic model* (STM),[12] that allows the integration of covariates, such as time and date of publication, into the prior distributions for document-topic compositions and topic-word proportions. Thereby, STM can be used to model how the content of a collection of documents changes as a function of document-level covariates, and to provide valuable insights and understanding on how topics evolve.

Since there is no "correct" solution for determining the optimal number of topics *k* that should be generated during the model selection process, several diagnostic aspects of the topic modelling were evaluated to decide the number of topics, *k*, to use. This parameter can be optimised by comparing the results of models run with different values of *k* (the number of topics), using several quantitative metrics such as the distribution of *exclusivity*, *held-out likelihood*, and *semantic coherence*, as well as other qualitative measures of interpretability. High semantic coherence implies that topics are semantically interpretable, while low-scoring topics are usually artefacts of statistical inference (Mimno et al. 2011). Exclusivity measures the extent to which the top words for each topic do not appear as top words in other topics (Bischof & Airoldi 2012). The held-out likelihood approach is based on document completion. The higher the held-out likelihood, the more predictive power the model has on average (Wallach et al. 2009). According to Roberts et al. (2019), such metrics capture what humans qualitatively perceive as good topics. We run multiple models with a varying number of *k* values, ranging from 2 to 40. Choosing the "best" *k* is a critical challenge, since a very small *k*-value divides the document collection into a few very general semantic contexts. However, if the *k*-value is too large, the document collection is divided into too many topics of which some may overlap and others are hardly interpretable. Figure 10.1 shows these three

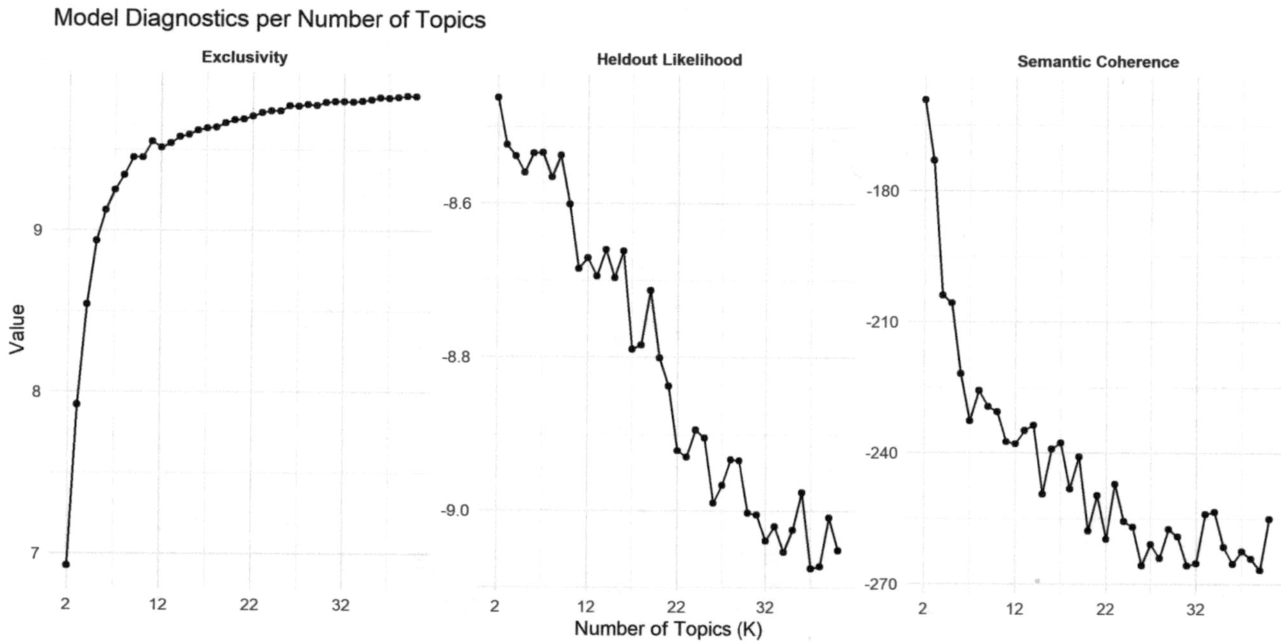

Figure 10.1 Model evaluation metrics for the number of topics *k*: exclusivity, held-out likelihood, and semantic coherence.

metrics for a grid of k between 2 and 40 with step size five. A number of topics k, between $k = 9$ and $k = 12$, seem to be good choices according to these important metrics, and we chose $k = 9$.

The Lund study seems to play an important role in the context of mRNA scepticism during the studied time period, and the analysis of the Swedish tweets provides some insights into people's limited trust and high distrust in the mRNA vaccine landscape. People clearly highlight their concerns on the efficacy and safety of the technology. Some common subjects that emerged include fear of vaccine side effects, perceptions of rushed development processes, mistrust in pharmaceutical companies such as Pfizer, and wealthy individuals such as Bill Gates, George Soros, and the Wallenberg family,[13] who wield their authoritarian power to promote their ultimate goal: the global and total control of humanity (see the discussion in the next section). The tweeter sceptics question the long-term effects of potential adverse reactions. Distrust in mRNA vaccines seems to also stem from concerns about personal freedom and autonomy. Tweets expressing this viewpoint emphasise the right to make individual health decisions without government or societal mandates. Tweets promoting distrust often make unsupported claims, such as vaccines being used for population control (*genpreparat ges för att kontrollera folket* 'genetic substances are given to control the people') or containing harmful ingredients (*mRNA-vaccinen innehåller metaller som bildar oorganiska "växter" i blodomloppet* 'the mRNA vaccines contain metals that form inorganic "plants" in the bloodstream'). Although one would have expected some Twitter users to express trust by referencing reputable health organisations such as the World Health Organization (WHO) to counteract the negative voices, the positive mRNA opinions are few and far between. When WHO is mentioned, it is in a negative tone of voice, sometimes paired with anti-Semitic imaginaries and conspiracy theories (*WHO agerar marionett för vaccinindustrin samt globalisterna* "the WHO acts as a puppet for the vaccine industry and the globalists").

A qualitative refinement of the quantitative selection

To refine our analysis, we took a closer look at the results of the STM, in which several general themes emerged based on the topics identified. Structural topic models are quantitative by nature and deal with the challenge of retrieving thematically similar documents (i.e., in our case tweets) from the textual collection. To achieve this objective, the document input to topic modelling is decontextualized with the aim of developing themes. Decontextualization, according to Eickhoff and Wieneke (2018), implies that (a) documents are pre-processed into a term-document matrix; and (b) the topic model itself further detaches words from their original context to arrive at topics suitable to model the entire document collection. Figure 10.2 shows the top ten probable words for each of the nine generated topics.

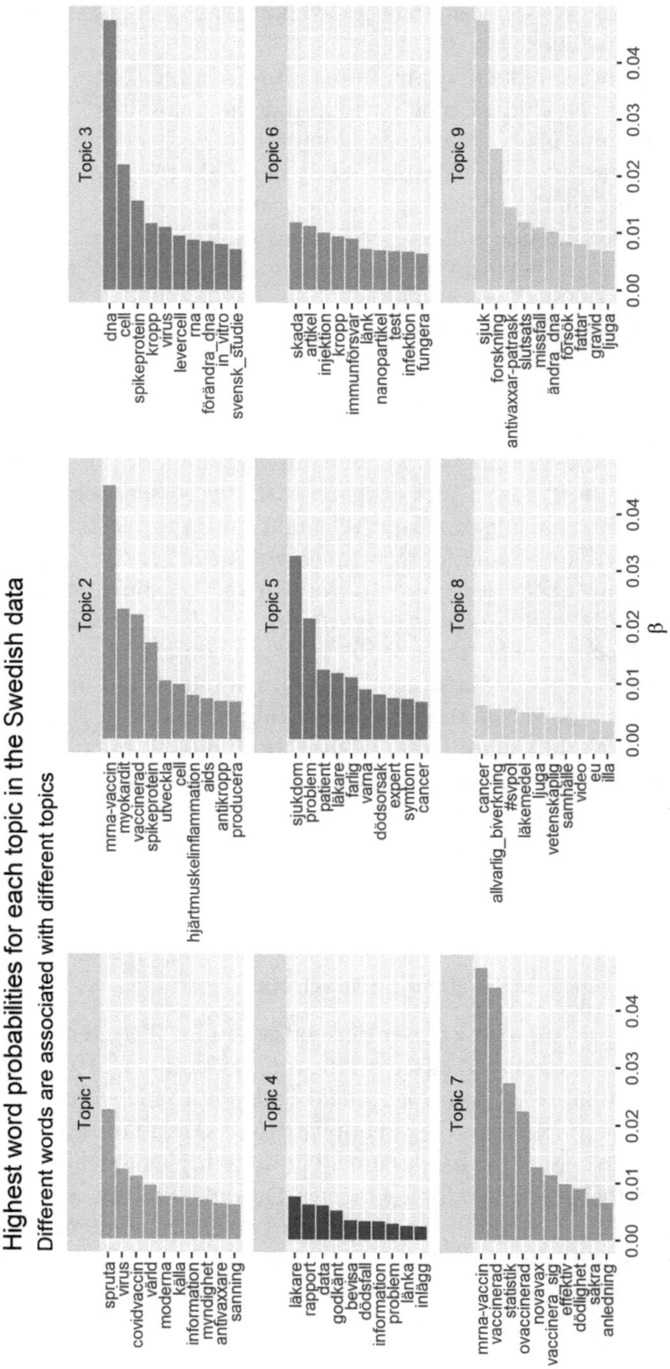

Figure 10.2 The top ten probable words for each of the nine generated topics in the text corpus.

In these graphs, topic 3 makes a clear reference to the Lund study, topic 9 in Figure 10.2 makes a reference to risks related to breast feeding and the traces of mRNA found in lactating mothers who received the vaccine, and topic 2 covers the risks related to myocarditis among young males.

In our research design, the combination of quantitative and qualitative elements is achieved by re-contextualising the previously decontextualised results, identifying and labelling the key themes that arose from the statistical analysis of the document collection. This mixed-methods research design offers several advantages for our study (Ivankova et al. 2006). It provides a more comprehensive and holistic understanding of the users' views and thoughts on mRNA vaccines. It also enables us to explore both the breadth and the depth of the mRNA discussions by leveraging the complementary strengths of the statistical quantitative method on the one side with the qualitative contextualisation and interpretation of the users' experiences, perceptions, and context, on the other; this complementarity enables a more comprehensive and nuanced understanding of the mRNA vaccine discussions.

For the qualitative thematic analysis, we used a data analysis software tool, manually categorising each tweet into one or several of the main themes it addressed. Table 10.1 showcases the three most distinct – and interrelated – themes that we identified in the material (for a complete overview of the themes and examples of each theme, see Appendix 10.1).

We notice that the way these mRNA rumours are communicated, they leave little space for doubt. In our data, shown here translated from Swedish to English, rumours were expressed with confidence regarding their validity. "A shocking new study conducted at Lund University in Sweden has *confirmed* that mRNA nanoparticles from Pfizer's Covid-19 vaccine enter human cells and are reverse-transcribed into DNA, causing a permanent change to the person's genetic code", writes one user, while another states that "it's gene therapy that has been *proven* to change the recipient's DNA. A Swedish study from Lund published in Current issues of Molecular Biology *shows* this". In times of uncertainty, when everyone is looking for answers, confidence is reassuring and convincing, and can help create trust.

The Lund study was centrally present in the dataset. The tweets mentioning the study were very rarely shared in a neutral manner, and (mis)interpretations were presented as facts. Strong language and emotive words were frequently invoked – a tweet, for example, stated that "mRNA becomes DNA, *vaxxed get genetically modified*, researchers believe". Some even referred to vaccinated people as "Human 2.0", meaning a genetically modified human, and the mRNA vaccines were referred to as "gene therapy" or a "genetic experiment". The Lund study served as a tool to cement and legitimise mRNA vaccine-related rumours, and it was mentioned in mRNA-related discussions even in cases where the topic at hand was not directly related to the study's findings, such as in a discussion about the fast-tracking of the vaccine containing the following tweet: "Anyone who hasn't understood that a fast-track vaccine … is risky is dumb. Read the following article from Lund University [link]".

Table 10.1 Most prominent themes among the tweets collected

Theme	*Top addressed issues*
Does mRNA alter our DNA?	Could mRNA vaccines change DNA; Lund study; mRNA vaccines "gene therapy"/"genetic experiment"; mRNA WHO/government/media conspiracy to change human DNA
Adverse side effects of mRNA vaccines	Transcribing of mRNA to DNA in the body = risk of autoimmune diseases, cancer and reproductive issues; Pfizer document submitted to the FDA reporting thousands of adverse side effects; mRNA Covid-19 vaccines and HIV; mRNA vaccines could lead to deaths; athletes and myocarditis
mRNA vaccine novelty	How well is mRNA tested, why hasn't mRNA been used for any publicly available vaccines before, and what its potential side effects could be; not safe, or possible, to release a mass use vaccine in such a short time frame; the vaccine approved in order to prevent the use of effective medicine; uncertainty about potential long-term side effects that wouldn't be possible to detect in the vaccine's short trial period; doctors warning against mRNA/Joe Rogan-Robert Malone interview

Ascribing mRNA-critical claims to Lund University solidified their veracity, as a reference to a reputable Swedish university offered credibility to statements that would otherwise be considered dubious and met with suspicion.

The perceived reluctance of experts to listen to public concerns has, according to Rosanvallon (2008), stimulated a willingness to engage in this type of discussions on the internet where one can find groups and fellowships willing to recognise and take seriously one's worries, experiences, and opinions. Such engagement also constitutes a counter-democratic civic watchdog function based on vigilance, denunciation, and evaluation, he argues (Rosanvallon 2008: 32). Analogously, we view the Twitter discussions generated by the mRNA study from Lund University (Aldén et al. 2022) as counter-epistemic or counter-scientific expressions, *questioning* and *challenging* rather than *denying* or *dismissing* science and established knowledge. The disclosure of the Lund article, we argue, is a result of the vigilant continuous attention and monitoring of what is published and posted regarding the mRNA vaccines; the exposing and displaying of what is regarded to be the findings and conclusions of the researchers constitute the denunciation element. The evaluative aspect is shown by the demands on the authorities to react and provide convincing and trustworthy answers to the questions, concerns, and fears inherent in the rumours building on the Lund study. Acknowledging the counter-epistemic function of vaccine rumours based on alternative or complementary interpretations and understandings of expert knowledge is essential in order to meet the sceptics on trustful common grounds.

Additionally, trust in the Lund study was contrasted to the distrust in media, government bodies, and the medical industry. A strain of tweets discussed the

Lund study's findings in the light of WHO and national governments' debunking of the myth that mRNA could alter the DNA, framing it as proof that this so-called false conspiracy theory was actually true. Some examples of this were: "Another conspiracy theory bites the dust. Swedish study: mRNA turns into DNA!"; "Suddenly it feels great to be 'another tinfoil hat' who refused to inject this 'vaxxine'!"; "Pfizer's vaccine enters liver cells – and transforms to DNA. The tinfoil hats were right, again". In that sense, the tweeters utilised their interpretation of the Lund study to engage in what we term *counter-debunking of an already-debunked rumour*, thus, challenging the established narrative around the rumour's correctness. That researchers from Lund University would "go against" what is considered an "epistemic truth" and publish such controversial findings was for the tweeters a solid proof of the counter-mRNA vaccine argument's correctness, and the lack of engagement with the study from the Swedish officials' side was framed as additional proof that the results of the study "debunked" the public narrative: "Media and government are quiet about this study from Lund".

The Lund study was not the only "source of truth" present in the data – referring to sources in order to legitimise claims was a frequent practice. Tweets addressing the potential risks and adverse side effects of mRNA vaccines contained a mix of personal stories and links to news and documents in (alternative) media, both frequently combined with a call-to-action to refuse taking the mRNA vaccines. Most commonly cited were (alternative) media websites (i.e., YouTube, *NewsVoice*, *Nya Dagbladet*), particular individuals (i.e., Robert Malone, John Campbell, Carrie Madej, Zev Zelenko, Mikolaj Raszek) and platforms (i.e., Telegram and Facebook groups). Notably, many supported their claims by pointing to studies – including the Lund study – and/or physicians. A large portion of the tweets referred to a viral interview between Joe Rogan and Robert Malone, in which Malone sowed doubts about the safety and efficiency of mRNA COVID-19 vaccines. Citing concrete numbers or statistics was also common practice that added legitimacy to statements, giving the impression that the user posting the claim was well-informed on the matter.

Humour also plays a significant part in the counter-narrative of mRNA distrust – rhetorical questions, irony, and sarcasm are centrally present. In contrast to communication techniques such as providing arguments or referring to sources to convince the audience of the legitimacy of a rumour, humour acts as an active demonstration of confidence. Using humour allows interlocutors to challenge established beliefs while avoiding accountability, and any expression of dissent becomes the subject of mockery. In our dataset, governments, experts, and public institutions were ridiculed as incompetent, and so were the few users that challenged mRNA distrust. One sharing of the Lund study, for example, was accompanied by the caption "The vaccine changes the DNA. Thank you, government and FHM! Fast-growing cancer, anyone?", and another tweet finding fault with the uncritical willingness of people to vaccinate stated, "mass quaxxination! Everyone is in!". Resorting to jokes was a way to express criticism or dissent, or to refute established narratives in a way that does not invite discussion, and that removes the burden of proof from the tweeters. In this respect, rhetorical questions were often posed to create or amplify rumours – some implying particularly serious dangers, such as "Does anyone know if it's routine to add HIV protein to vaccines, or is it something specific to the Covid vaccine? Grateful for answers". This points to the use of humour as a strategic means of disseminating rumours, as short, catchy messages have a stronger shareability potential. Comparable to meme communities on the internet (cf. Doona 2024, Chapter 5 of this volume), satirical irony among the tweeters here studied, points to the community aspects of Twitter; the tweeters who enjoy sharing this kind of uncertainty with others tacitly express "a form of solidarity built on the uncomfortable unstableness of ontological insecurity" (Doona 2024).

Conclusions

In this chapter, we have accounted for how rumours concerning mRNA vaccines are expressed and established in Swedish-language Twitter posts. Our point of departure was to create a suitable dataset for our experiments, which we then started to analyse with a computational distant reading approach based on structural topic modelling, and continued with the close reading analysis of the results. Further, the qualitative thematic analysis revealed seven overarching themes that drove the interlocutors' distrust in mRNA vaccines, the most prominent three among them being the worry that mRNA vaccines would alter human DNA, the technology's alleged experimental nature, and the potential adverse side effects from these vaccines. Our study subscribes to DiFonzo and Bordia's (2007) definition of rumours, but our findings differ from theirs in some substantial ways. Firstly, DiFonzo and Bordia discuss the sense making of information already acknowledged as rumours, whereas in our case the sense making concerns a piece of scientific information which *produces* the rumour. Secondly, while DiFonzo and Bordia argue that sense making is the main function of rumours in their studies, in our data people were *not* trying to deliberate whether mRNA technology was safe and effective, but instead treated it as integrally bad. Rumours about the dangers with mRNA vaccines were spread in order to challenge the public narrative about their reliability and efficacy. The goal of this spreading is, on the one hand, to delegitimize the trust in mRNA vaccines and discourage others from taking them, and, on the other hand, to handle fear, which aligns with Knapp's (1944: 31) definition of certain rumours as a "*defense* against anxiety" (emphasis in original).

The specific affordances of a platform like Twitter, with a character limit on messages and encouraging real-time discourse via hashtags, could also account for this difference. Similar to a message broadcast platform, Twitter is not designed in a way that encourages elaborate debate – it is rather a place to share current information in real time, such as revealing a discovery or starting a rumour. It is also worthy of notice that the negative sentiments towards mRNA vaccines, held by the vast majority of tweeters in our sample, are not representative of the general perception of the Swedish population, which has one of the highest COVID-19 vaccination rates in Europe. This points to distrust as a driver of rumour spreading on the platform. The fact that it was Twitter that stood for the fast spreading of the Lund study also aligns with the quick, real-time broadcasting nature of the platform. We found that the participants in the Twitter discussions about mRNA in Sweden exhibited a general sentiment of distrust in the capacity of governments, public actors, and institutions to adequately handle the COVID-19 pandemic. While media and public actors engaged in debunking rumours sowing doubts about mRNA, on Twitter, the Lund study became a tool for counter-debunking an already-debunked rumour.

A further in-depth analysis of the dynamics of rumour propagation on social media could also involve the study on how rumours originate, spread, and evolve within the digital ecosystem (cf. Zubiaga & Ji, 2014; Vosoughi et al. 2018; Sun et al. 2023). To conduct such an analysis, it would be necessary to focus more on examining how social media channels guide individuals toward specific content. This may include: content analysis, in the form of examining the language, tone, and visual elements used in the rumour to understand its appeal and emotional impact on users; network analysis, by mapping the propagation of a rumour across the social network, identifying key influencers or nodes that play a significant role in disseminating the information; algorithmic impact, that could investigate how social media algorithms affect the visibility and virality of rumours by requiring an understanding on how algorithms prioritise content, potentially amplifying or limiting the reach of rumours; and, geospatial analysis, which would look at the geographic spread of a rumour, revealing whether the rumour is localised to specific regions or has a global reach.

A concluding remark from a broader perspective is that the debate about the rightness or wrongness of people's ideas about vaccines with respect to scientific data will not take us very far. The frequent references to the Lund study and other acknowledged sources of knowledge challenge the mainstream narrative that vaccine-critical individuals deny or repudiate science. On the contrary, our findings show that vaccine sceptics rely heavily on scientific sources to strengthen the arguments for their stance. What is questioned is rather the authorities' interpretation of the scientific results and the measures taken based on them. Similarly, the Lund study is taken as proof that the pharmaceutical industry has not tested the vaccines enough to be scientifically satisfactory. The strategy is to question and oppose the authorities' recommendations by turning the very research they rely upon to motivate and legitimise their policies against them, thus, nurturing trust among the vaccine sceptics themselves and, ultimately, their individual decision-making, emphasising *their* capability to find and interpret scientific studies (Hausman 2019: 123–130; Goldenberg 2021: 30–33).

In line with Hausman (2019: 212), we believe that the things we do to our bodies, in the service of (public) health, could never solely be an effect of medical data and scientific considerations; a framing that helps us to see that vaccine controversy stages another conversation altogether that encompasses the promises and assumptions of modern medicine, and, by extension, modernity.

Appendix 10.1 Examples of theme content

Theme	*Top addressed issues*	*Examples*
Does mRNA alter our DNA?	Could mRNA vaccines change DNA; Lund study; mRNA vaccines "gene therapy"/"genetic experiment"; mRNA WHO/government/media conspiracy to change human DNA	*En chockerande ny studie genomförd vid Lunds universitet i Sverige har bekräftat att mRNA-nanopartiklar från Pfizers covid-19-vaccin går in i mänskliga celler och omvänt transkriberas till DNA, vilket ger en permanent förändring av personens genetiska kod.* A shocking new study conducted at Lund University in Sweden has confirmed that mRNA nanoparticles from Pfizer's covid-19 vaccine enter human cells and are reverse transcribed into DNA, causing a permanent change to the person's genetic code. *Men kalla det inte för ett vaccin, det är en genterapi som bevisats kunna förändra DNA hos mottagaren. En Svensk studie från Lund publicerad i Current Issues in Molecular Biology visar detta.* But don't call it a vaccine, it's gene therapy that has been proven to change the recipient's DNA. A Swedish study from Lund published in Current Issues in Molecular Biology shows this. *Media och Regering VÄGRAR DELA DENNA STUDY FRÅN LUND.* Media and Government REFUSE TO SHARE THIS STUDY FROM LUND. *För att det var en bluff allting. Rädsla för luft så att folk skulle låsa in sig. Maska blöja som en efterbliven chimpans för att avslutas med en Kosher desert bestående av DNA ändrade parasiter i nanopartiklar (av läkare kallat spikprotein) Vad visste du, Nisse?* Because it was all a scam. Fear of air so people would lock themselves up. Wear a mouth diaper like a backward chimpanzee to finish with a Kosher dessert consisting of DNA-altered parasites in nanoparticles (called by doctors spike protein). What did you know, Nisse?

Adverse side effects of mRNA vaccines	transcribing of mRNA to DNA in the body = risk of autoimmune diseases, cancer and reproductive issues; Pfizer document submitted to the FDA reporting thousands of adverse side effects; mRNA Covid-19 vaccines and HIV; mRNA vaccines could lead to deaths; athletes and myocarditis	https://mdpi.com/1467-3045/44/3/73/htm *Enligt studie från Lunds universitet omvandlas spikproteinet i Modernas och Pfizers covid19-vaccin i levern med genetiska förändringar till följd. Komplicerade samband för en lekman, men processen verkar kunna vålla autoimmuna sjukdomar.* https://mdpi.com/1467-3045/44/3/73/htm According to a study from Lund University, the spike protein in Moderna's and Pfizer's covid19 vaccine is converted in the liver with genetic changes as a result. Complicated connections for a layperson, but the process seems capable of causing autoimmune diseases. *Vaccinen ändrar DNA. Tack regeringen och FHM. Snabbväxande cancer någon?* The vaccine changes the DNA. Thank you, government and FHM. Fast-growing cancer anyone? … *att ha fått Pfizers covidvaccin. Om menstruationsrubbningarna också påverkar fertiliteten vet vi inte. Även mäns spermier påverkas av covidvaccinen. En studie har visat lägre koncentration och rörlighet av spermier i mannens sädesvätska upp till 5 mån …* https://obgyn.onlinelibrary.wiley.com/doi/epdf/10.1002/ijgo.14356 … to have received Pfizer's covid vaccine. We do not know whether the menstrual disturbances also affect fertility. Even men's sperms are affected by the covid vaccine. A study has shown a lower concentration and mobility of sperm in the man's seminal fluid up to 5 months … https://obgyn.onlinelibrary.wiley.com/doi/epdf/10.1002/ijgo.14356 *Covid viruset~vaccinet ~HIV Se ni deras plan? HIV har varit hos människor så många år, har forskare hittat vaccinet mot HIV? Nu kom plötsligt ett vaccin mot viruset, sedan leder det till HIV, Labyrint har de byggt men men var är utgången? CCP* The Covid virus ~ the vaccine ~ HIV Do you see their plan? HIV has been in humans for so many years, have scientists discovered a vaccine against HIV? Now suddenly there is a vaccine against the virus, then it leads to HIV. They have built the labyrinth, but where is the exit? CCP

(*Continued*)

Theme	*Top addressed issues*	*Examples*
		Tegnell kan ju kommentera den här nya studien från bland annat Lunds Universitet som visar att hans hyllade sprutor oavsiktligt kan ändra i vårt DNA. Vilka risker han utsatt folk för … helt sinnesrubbat. Jävla dåre. Tegnell can comment on this new study from, among others, Lund University which shows that his celebrated vaccine can unintentionally change our DNA. What risks he put people through … totally insane. Damn fool.
		Här har du biverkningarna som Pfizer ville dölja i 75 år men som dom blev tvingade att dela med sig av efter domstolsbeslut. Tycker du det verkar vara ett bra vaccin? Varför är det så tyst helt plötsligt? Hitta en sjukdom/biverkning vaccinet INTE ger vore enklare. Here you have the side effects that Pfizer wanted to hide for 75 years but were forced to share after a court order. Do you think it seems like a good vaccine? Why is it so quiet all of a sudden? Finding a disease/side effect that the vaccine does NOT cause would be easier.
		Stor ökning av barn som dött i magen på sina mammor eftersom dessa lyssnat på blodmagipropaganda från healerskor som Agnes Wold. Därtill kommer såklart alla som föds med vaccinskador. Det har inte med någon pandemi att göra utan beror på mRNA-vaccinen Large increase in children who died in their mothers' wombs because these listened to blood magic propaganda from healers such as Agnes Wold. In addition to, of course, everyone who is born with vaccine injuries. This has nothing to do with a pandemic but is due to the mRNA vaccine.
		Normalt dör ca 66/år, nu 649 dödsfall / 16 mån Unga friska idrottsmän drabbas av hjärtstillestånd, hjärtmuskel-, och hjärtsäcksinflammationer och hastig död sedan mRNA genterapi injiceringarna startades. Normally there are about 66 deaths/year, now 649 deaths/16 months. Young healthy sportsmen suffer from cardiac arrest, heart muscle and pericardial inflammations and rapid death since the mRNA gene therapy injections were started.

mRNA vaccine novelty	how well is mRNA tested, why hasn't mRNA been used for any publicly available vaccines before, and what its potential side effects could be; not safe, or possible, to release a mass use vaccine in such a short time frame; the vaccine approved in order to prevent the use of effective medicine; uncertainty about potential long-term side effects that wouldn't be possible to detect in the vaccine's short trial period; doctors warning against mRNA/Joe Rogan-Robert Malone interview	*Vissa covidvaccin innehåller en ny teknik som kallas mrna, genmodifierare, det är första gången man testar denna teknik i stor skala. En studie från Lunds universitetet visar att dessa genmodifierare i vissa fall har hamnat på fel ställen i kroppen efter injicering.* Some covid vaccines contain a new technology called mrna, gene modifier, this is the first time this technology has been tested on a large scale. A study from Lund University shows that these gene modifiers have in some cases ended up in the wrong places in the body after injection. *Det kan inte finnas några argument överhuvudtaget för att injicera ett snabbframtaget otestat genpreparat. #svpolitik* There can be no argument at all for injecting a hastily produced untested gene liquid. #svpolitik *Den som inte har förstått att ett snabbframtaget vaccin (8 månader) som inte är ett vaccin (utan en mRna-injektion) i fas II och som aldrig tidigare har lanserats för människor i stor omfattning är riskabelt är dum i huvudet. Läs artikeln nedan från Lunds Universitet nedan.* Anyone who has not understood that a fast-track vaccine (8 months) that is not a vaccine (but an mRNA injection) in phase II and has never before been used on humans on a large scale is risky is stupid in the head. Read the article from Lund University below. *Det tar 8–12 år att få ett vaccin godkänt, inte några veckor! Så per definition är mRNA-vätskan inte ett vaccin. Det fick ett nödgodkännande och det kan man bara få om det inte finns fungerande läkemedel. Så man förbjöd Ivermektin och Hydroxiklorokin. Varför tror du?* It takes 8–12 years to get a vaccine approved, not a few weeks! So by definition, the mRNA formulation is not a vaccine. It received emergency approval and you can only get that if there are no working drugs. So they banned Ivermectin and Hydroxychloroquine. Why, you think?"

(Continued)

Theme	*Top addressed issues*	*Examples*
		Svininfluensa-vaccinet stoppades. Ändå luras miljoner svenskar 10 år senare att ta ett annat otestat vaccin. Det är svårt att förstå, min tankeverksamhet kollapsar i försöket att förstå. De äldre kan jag förstå. Men alla under 70 – obegripligt. The swine flu vaccine was stopped. Nevertheless, 10 years later, millions of Swedes are deceived into taking another untested vaccine. It's hard to understand, my brain activity collapses in the attempt to understand. I can understand older people. But everyone under 70 – incomprehensible.
		Just därför kanske man ska undvika experimentella – och villkorat godkända mRNA injektioner överhuvudtaget, om man är fullt frisk och stark? Individuell Risk / nytta bedömning och Informerat samtycke kunde ändå vara på sin plats. Men icke när det gäller masskvaxxet! Alla ska med. That's precisely why perhaps one should avoid experimental – and conditionally approved – mRNA injections at all, if one is completely healthy? Individual risk/ benefit assessment and informed consent should still be in place. But not when it comes to the mass quaxxination! Everyone is in/
		Nej, men jag kan läsa och tolka vetenskapliga artiklar och statistik. Jag följer de visselblåsande epidemiologier, läkare och forskare som påtalat farorna med dessa otestade mrna-injektioner som bara i Sverige lett till över 100.000 anmälningar av biverkningar. No, but I can read and interpret scientific articles and statistics. I follow the whistle-blowing epidemiologists, doctors and researchers who have spoken out about the dangers of these untested mrna injections, which have led to over 100,000 side effect reports in Sweden alone.
		När till och med uppfinnaren (Dr Robert Malone) av mrna tekniken varnar så borde man nog tänka efter. Framför allt hävdar han att vacc av barn kan få konsekvenser vi aldrig önskat. When even the inventor (Dr. Robert Malone) of mrna technology warns, one should probably think twice. Most importantly, he claims that vaccination of children can have consequences we never wanted.

mRNA vaccines' (in)effectiveness in protecting against Covid-19	vaccinated people falling ill with Covid-19; Covid-19 not a dangerous illness; correlation between vaccine (in)effectiveness and other measures to prevent the spread; mRNA vaccines more/less effective than other vaccine technologies; lack of clarity about the number of mRNA doses needed	*Trots påståendet fungerar inte mRNA vaccinerna mot vare sig infektion eller spridning. Och i förlängningen förstör dom det naturliga immunförsvaret. Många läkare världen över rapporterar nu att 95% av allvarligt sjuka är dubbelvaccinerade.* Despite claims, the mRNA vaccines do not work against either infection or spread. And by extension, they destroy the natural immunity. Many doctors worldwide now report that 95% of the seriously ill are double-vaccinated.
		Covid är en allvarlig sjukdom ja. Vi vet dock att nuvarande 'vaccin' är oeffektiva mot nuvarande varianter och har inga data över långtidseffekter av att ge barn injektionen. Svininfluensevaccinet var en katastrof, det här kommer sluta ännu värre om vi börjar injicera barn … Covid is a serious disease, yes. However, we know that current "vaccines" are ineffective against current variants and have no data on the long-term effects of giving children the injection. The swine flu vaccine was a disaster, this will end up even worse if we start injecting children …
		Det var en bluff att viruset var en pandemi som skulle vara så farligt att det behövs ett vaccin mot det! Sen är vaccinet en ännu större bluff! Vaccinet skyddar inte dig själv och det fungerar inte heller mot smitspridning! It was a hoax that the virus was a pandemic that would be so dangerous that a vaccine against it was needed! Then the vaccine is an even bigger scam! The vaccine does not protect you and it does not work against the spread of infection either!
		Varför ta ett vaccin som inte skyddar dig ändå … har 4 kollegor som tagit 3 sprutor och 2 hamna på intensiven … de andra 2 blev väldigt sjuka … hela detta vaccin är planerat och ren bluff … allt handlar om kontroll o maktmissbruk mot mänskliga rättigheter. Why would you take a vaccine that doesn't protect you anyway … I have 4 colleagues that have taken 3 injections each, and 2 of them ended up in intensive care … the other 2 got really sick … everything with this vaccine is planned and a clear hoax … everything is about control and abuse of power against human rights.

(*Continued*)

Theme	*Top addressed issues*	*Examples*
		Skräpartikel … märkte inte nån reaktion från media om att många föräldrar vägrade vaccinera sina barn mot farliga barnsjukdomar … vilket borde vara mycket viktigare än vacciner mot covid, då den bevisligen inte skyddar mot sjukdomen, men kan orsaka farliga biverkningar … Junk article … I didn't notice any reaction from the media about many parents refusing to vaccinate their children against dangerous child diseases … which should be much more serious than the Covid-vaccine, which obviously doesn't protect from the disease, but can cause adverse side effects …
		Synd att man fortsätter med de farliga mrna-injektionerna. Tror personligen det varit bättre att undersöka/utveckla Novavax eller liknande traditionella vacciner att rekommendera till gamla och riskgrupper. It's a shame that they continue with the dangerous mrna-injections. Personally I think it would have been better to research/develop Novavax or similar traditional vaccines to recommend to older people and risk groups.
		Hur många sprutor tycker du man ska ta? Har själv haft Covid och tagit två sprutor. Är ett tiotal tillräckligt? How many shots do you think one should take? I have had Covid myself and taken two doses. Are ten enough?
Profits from mRNA vaccines	mRNA technology mass-distributed for profit rather than their effectiveness; allegations of corruption	*Tror man skall vara lite försiktig innan man upphöjer WHO till något slags rättsrådande facit En icke helt transparent organisation Gates foundation skänker stora pengar till WHO – samtidigt som Gates foundation även är tunga investerare i mRNA-tekniken* https://google.com/amp/s/amp.svt.se/nyheter/utrikes/gates-stiftelse-okar-stod-till-who I think one should be a little careful before elevating WHOs decisions to some kind of legal precedent. Not a completely transparent organisation. The Gates foundation donates a lot of money to WHO – at the same time as they also heavily invest in mRNA technology. https://google.com/amp/s/amp.svt.se/nyheter/utrikes/gates-stiftelse-okar-stod-till-who

		Dom visste exakt vad dom gjorde och vilken skada som orsakas. Tänk på att mRNA vaccinens innehåll och grundläggande skaldeförmåga varit under utveckling i många år och att dom till viss del ägs av det amerikanska försvaret – med flera. (DARPA om jag inte minns fel.) They knew exactly what they were doing and what damage was being caused. Keep in mind that the mRNA vaccine's content and basic shielding ability have been under development for many years and that they are to some extent owned by the American defence – and others. (DARPA if I remember correctly.)
		… *Modernas VD intervjuas i TV och erkänner att de haft patent på covid sen 2016 och tjänar miljarder tack vore det under covid bedrägeriet, när allt av det censureras i svensk media* … … Moderna's CEO is interviewed on TV and admits that they had a patent on covid since 2016 and are making billions thanks to it during the covid fraud, when all of it is censored in the Swedish media …
		Och vissa tjänar tydligen massor av pengar för att fortsätta propagera för ett värdelöst och farligt vaccin helt utan verkan! Ni kommer dömas hårt när sanningen kommer fram! And some apparently make a lot of money to continue to promote a useless and dangerous vaccine with no effect! You will be judged harshly when the truth comes out!
mRNA vaccines content/ ingredients	do mRNA vaccines contain dangerous metals; monkeypox; HIV virus; chips/mass control devices	*mRNA-vaccinen innehåller metaller som bildar oorganiska växter" i blodomloppet." #covid19 #vaccin* The mRNA vaccine contains metals that form inorganic plants "in the bloodstream." #covid19 #vaccine
		Alla pfisers vaxx ska enligt uppgift från pfiser innehålla det nya mrna-grafen-pag-skiten från och med i år. Så ta fan inga vaxx om ni vill överleva According to pfizer, all pfizer vaxx will contain the new mrna-graphen-pag crap starting this year. So don't take any vaxx if you want to survive
		Någon som vet om det hör till det normala att stoppa in fragment av HIV (HIV-protein) i vaccin, eller om det är specifikt för just Covid-vaccinet? Tacksam för svar Does anyone know if it is normal to insert fragments of HIV (HIV protein) into vaccines, or if it is specific to the Covid vaccine? Grateful for answers

(*Continued*)

Theme	*Top addressed issues*	*Examples*
		Vilddjurets märke är en realitet. Visste ni att tillverkarna inte behöver avslöja alla ingredienser i ett nödgodkänt vaccin? Anledningen till att de vill TVÅNGS-vaccinera alla är att vaccinerna innehåller ett operativsystem o genmanipulerar folk utan deras vetskap. The mark of the beast is a reality. Did you know that manufacturers do not have to disclose all ingredients in an emergency approved vaccine? The reason they want to FORCIBLY vaccinate everyone is that the vaccines contain an operating system and genetically manipulate people without their knowledge.
		De ska skrämma upp oss igen, undra vad vissa vaccin innehåller … men att det är adenovirus från apor kan vi säkert bortse ifrån. https://www.svd.se/a/V97oq6/fall- They will scare us again, wonder what some vaccines contain … but we can certainly ignore the fact that it is adenovirus from monkeys. https://www.svd.se/a/V97oq6/fall-
mRNA-related conspiracies	chips/mass control devices in vaccines; lab leak; new world order;	*Hela vaccin-och pass-agendan är 100% satanisk. Det är slaveri och de vaccinerade har redan injecerats med ett operativsystem Detta operativsystemkan kopplas till en app men även utan appen kan folk kontrolleras o mindkontrolleras på distans via femG* The entire vaccine and pass agenda is 100% satanic. It is slavery and the vaccinated have already been injected with an operating system This operating system can be connected to an app but even without the app people can be controlled and mind controlled remotely via fiveG
		Mer skräckpropaganda? Ska vi ta och börja med att först redovisa att C19 är isolerat i ett labb, sen studier på "vaxets" långtidseffekt, och vad mRna/nanoteknik gör med människokroppen på cellnivå? Sedan redovisa namnen på ägarna av alla patent på virus och vax. Tack. More horror propaganda? Shall we start by first reporting that C19 is isolated in a lab, then studies on the long-term effect of the "vax", and what mRna/nanotechnology does to the human body at the cellular level? Then report the names of the owners of all patents on viruses and vax. Thanks.

Hej @svenskakyrkan WEF grundare Klaus Schwab skriver i sin bok covid-19: the great reset att han ämnar att förändra människors DNA till att bli en del av AI i smyg, utan att låta människor välja själva, genom injektioner. Vart står ni? Vad skulle Jesus säga om detta?

Hello @svenskakyrkan WEF founder Klaus Schwab writes in his book covid-19: the great reset that he intends to change people's DNA to become part of AI secretly, without letting people choose for themselves, through injections. Where do you stand on that? What would Jesus say about this?

Tidigare Pfizer-konsult: Injektionerna innehåller digitala kontrollplattformar #pfizervaccin #KarenKingston #StewPeters

Former Pfizer consultant: Injections contain digital control platforms #pfizervaccine #KarenKingston #StewPeters

Visst har dom tjänat hundratals miljarder, men det var aldrig målet, Dom som äger dessa bolag "Blackrock" äger redan pengarna, dom äger bankerna! Målet med Plandemin har hela tiden varit Avbefolkning, Genom att lura i så många som möjligt dessa Mrna injectionerna. "De-population"

Of course they have earned hundreds of billions, but that was never the goal, Those who own these companies "Blackrock" already own the money, they own the banks! The goal of the Plandemic has always been depopulation, by cheating these Mrna injections into as many as possible. "De-population"

Notes

1 The Nobel Assembly's decision can be found here: https://www.nobelprize.org/uploads/2023/10/press-medicineprize2023-3.pdf (Accessed on 2023-10-02).
2 https://www.health.gov.au/initiatives-and-programs/covid-19-vaccines/is-it-true/is-it-true-can-covid-19-vaccines-alter-my-dna (Accessed on 2023-05-10).
3 https://www.unicef.org/montenegro/en/stories/covid-19-vaccine-does-not-change-human-dna (Accessed on 2023-05-10).
4 https://www.cdc.gov/coronavirus/2019-ncov/vaccines/facts.html (Accessed on 2023-05-10).
5 https://www.gov.za/covid-19/vaccine/myths (Accessed on 2023-05-10).
6 https://www.who.int/news-room/questions-and-answers/item/coronavirus-disease-(covid-19)-vaccines-safety (Accessed on 2023-05-10).
7 https://doh.wa.gov/emergencies/covid-19/vaccine-information/vaccine-facts (Accessed on 2023-05-10).
8 A score derived from an automated algorithm, representing a weighted count of the amount of attention that a research output has attracted.
9 Out of 21 million research outputs across all sources, this article has done particularly well and is in the 99th percentile, according to Altmetric: https://mdpi.altmetric.com/details/123663306
10 In July 2023, the platform changed its name to X, but as our investigation encompasses material from before this change, we will refer to Twitter instead of X and tweets instead of x's.
11 A report from *Internetstiftelsen* shows the increase of social media use during the pandemic and which platforms the Swedes used the most: https://svenskarnaochinternet.se/rapporter/svenskarna-och-internet-2020/sociala-%20medier/fler-anvander-sociala-medier-under-pandemin/#nio-sociala-medier-i-jamforelse (accessed on 2023-10-03).
12 For the structural topic modelling, we used the R package STM (version 1.3.6).
13 A wealthy family of industrialists and bankers in Sweden.

References

Aldén, Markus, Francisko Olofsson Falla, Daowei Yang, Mohammad Barghouth, Cheng Luan, Magnus Rasmussen & Yang De Marinis. 2022. Intracellular reverse transcription of Pfizer BioNTech COVID-19 mRNA vaccine BNT162b2 in vitro in human liver cell line. *Current Issues in Molecular Biology* 44(3): 1115–1126. https://doi.org/10.3390/cimb44030073

Bartlett, Tom. 2021. The vaccine scientist spreading vaccine misinformation. *The Atlantic*, 12 August 2021.

Bischof, Jonathan & Edoardo Airoldi. 2012. Summarizing topical content with word frequency and exclusivity. *Proceedings of the 29th International Conference on Machine Learning (ICML)*, 9–16. Edinburgh, Scotland, UK.

Blei, David M., Andrew Y. Ng & Michael I. Jordan. 2003. Latent Dirichlet allocation. *Journal of Machine Learning Research* 3: 993–1022.

Blume, Stuart. 2017. *Immunization: How vaccines became controversial.* London: Reaktion Books.

Blume, Stuart & Mariska Zanders. 2006. Vaccine independence, local competences and globalisation: lessons from the history of pertussis vaccines. *Social Science & Medicine*. 63(7): 1825–1835. https://doi.org/10.1016/j.socscimed.2006.04.014

DiFonzo, Nicholas & Prashant Bordia. 2007. *Rumor psychology: Social and organizational approaches*. Washington, DC: American Psychological Association.

Dolgin, Elie. 2021. The tangled history of mRNA vaccines. *Springer Nature* 597: 318–324.

Doona, Joanna. 2024. "Read the room Sweden": Memes, trust and vulnerability in pandemic engagement. In Lars Borin, Mia-Marie Hammarlin, Dimitrios Kokkinakis & Fredrik Miegel (eds.), *Vaccine hesitancy in the Nordic countries: Trust and distrust during the COVID-19 pandemic* (Chapter 5, this volume). London: Routledge.

Eickhoff, Matthias & Runhild Wieneke. 2018. Understanding topic models in context: A mixed methods approach to the meaningful analysis of large document collections. *Proceedings of the 51st Hawaii International Conference on System Sciences*, 903–912. https://doi.org/10.24251/hicss.2018.113

Eklöf, Motzi. 2016. *Variola & vaccinia: Om massvaccination, folkhälsopolitik, vaccinforskning och läkaeretik*. Malmköping: Exempla.

Goldenberg, Maya J. 2021. *Vaccine hesitancy: Public trust, expertise, and the war on science*. Pittsburgh: University of Pittsburgh Press.

Hammarlin, Mia-Marie, Dimitrios Kokkinakis & Lars Borin. 2023. COVID-19 vaccine hesitancy: A mixed methods investigation of matters of life and death. *Journal of Digital Social Research* 5(4): 31–61.

Harrison, Joel A. 2010. Wrong about vaccine safety: A review of Andrew Wakefield's "Callous disregard". *The Open Vaccine Journal* 6: 9–25.

Hausman, Bernice L. 2019. *Anti/Vax: Reframing the vaccination controversy*. Ithaca: ILR Press.

Ivankova, Nataliya V., John W. Creswell & Sheldon L. Stick. 2006. Using mixed-methods sequential explanatory design: From theory to practice. *Field Methods* 18(1): 3–20. https://doi.org/10.1177/1525822X05282260

Knapp, Robert H. 1944. A psychology of rumor. *Public Opinion Quarterly* 8(1): 22–37. https://doi.org/10.1086/265665

Larson, Heidi J. 2020. *Stuck: How vaccine rumors start and why they don't go away*. Oxford University Press.

Larson, Heidi, Leesa Lind & Rob Goble. 2022. Vaccines and the social amplification of risk. *Risk Analysis* 42: 1409–1422. https://doi.org/10.1111/risa.13942

Loomba, Sahil, Alexandre de Figueiredo, Simon J. Piatek, Kristen de Graaf & Heidi J. Larson. 2021. Measuring the impact of COVID-19 vaccine misinformation on vaccination intent in the UK and USA. *Nature Human Behaviour* 5: 337–348.

Lund University. 2022. *Q&A: COVID-19 vaccine study gains attention*, 10 March 2022. https://www.lunduniversity.lu.se/article/qa-covid-19-vaccine-study-gains-attention

MacDonald, Noni E. 2015. Vaccine hesitancy: definition, scope, and determinants. *Vaccine* 33: 4161–4164.

Mimno, David, Hanna M. Wallach, Edmund Talley, Miriam Leenders & Andrew McCallum. 2011. Optimizing semantic coherence in topic models. *Proceedings of the Conference on Empirical Methods in Natural Language Processing*, 262–272. Association for Computational Linguistics.

Pertwee, Ed, Clarissa Simas & Heidi J. Larson. 2022. An epidemic of uncertainty: Rumors, conspiracy theories and vaccine hesitancy. *Nature Medicine* 26: 456–459.

Rao, Sathyanarayana T.S. & Chittaranjan Andrade. 2011. The MMR vaccine and autism: Sensation, refutation, retraction, and fraud. *Indian Journal of Psychiatry* 53(2): 95–96.

Roberts, Margaret E., Brandon M. Stewart & Tingley Dustin. 2019. Stm: An R package for structural topic models. *Journal of Statistical Software* 91(1): 1–40. https://doi.org/10.18637/jss.v091.i02

Rosanvallon, Pierre. 2008. *Counter democracy: Politics in an age of distrust*. Cambridge: Cambridge University Press.

Rosanvallon, Pierre. 2021. *The populist century*. Cambridge: Polity.

Shevell, Michael & Eric Fombonne. 2006. Autism and MMR vaccination or thimerosal exposure: An urban legend? *The Canadian Journal of Neurological Sciences* 33: 339–340.

Sparrow, Betsy & Ljubica Chatman. 2013. Social cognition in the internet age: Same as it ever was? *Psychological Inquiry* 24: 273–292.

Sun, Ling, Yuan Rao, Lianwei Wu, Xiangbo Zhang, Yuqian Lan & Ambreen Nazir. 2023. Fighting false information from propagation process: A survey. *ACM Computing Surveys* 55(10): 1–38. https://doi.org/10.1145/3563388

Vosoughi, Sorous, Deb Roy & Sinan Aral. 2018. The spread of true and false news online. *Science* 359(6380): 1146–1151. https://doi.org/10.1126/science.aap9559

Wallach, Hanna M., Iain Murray, Ruslan Salakhutdinov & David Mimno. 2009. Evaluation methods for topic models. *Proceedings of the 26th Annual International Conference on Machine Learning*, 1105–1112. Montreal.

Watson, Oliver J., Gregory Barnsley, Jaspreet Toor, Alexandra B. Hogan, Peter Winskill & Azra C. Ghani. 2022. Global impact of the first year of COVID-19 vaccination: A mathematical modelling study. *Lancet Infectious Diseases* 22: 1293–1302. https://doi.org/10.1016/S1473-3099(22)00320-6

Zubiaga, Arkaitz & Heng Ji. 2014. Tweet, but verify: Epistemic study of information verification on Twitter. *Social Network Analysis and Mining* 24(1): 1–12. https://doi.org/10.1007/s13278-014-0163-y

11 The COVID-19 vaccine discussion on Twitter

Arguments of sceptics and supporters

Jana Sverdljuk and Bastiaan Bruinsma

Introduction: social polarisation during the COVID-19 pandemic

In many countries, COVID-19 vaccine discussions have been sharply divided across ideological and partisan lines and have exacerbated social polarisation (Mønsted & Lehmann 2022). Algorithm-assisted studies of the COVID-19 vaccine sentiment present on Twitter show that a positive psychological mood around the vaccine has been a prevailing one. Trust and anticipation slightly dominated over neutral and negative sentiments (Greyling & Rossouw 2022). Negative emotions had to do with fear of side effects, rollout plans, lockdowns, and other preventive measures (Lyu et al. 2021). Social tension was especially noticeable in the United States, where adherents of far-right ideologies, gathered around the Twitter (now known as X) account @realDonaldTrump, capitalised on the COVID-19 crisis in their fight against political opponents.

The Nordic countries are known for having a highly developed welfare state model: a system sometimes called "democratic socialism" that combines democratic culture, individual freedom, and comprehensive systems of social security (Koivunen et al. 2021). The region is on top of world rankings for quality of life, individual prosperity, and equality. All these factors result in a prominent level of social trust. At the same time, due to conditions of digitisation, globalisation, and challenges to democracy, signs of social disintegration, political polarisation, and diminished interpersonal and general trust have emerged (Koivunen et al. 2021). During the pandemic, there was a high level of COVID-19 vaccine acceptance. At the same time, studies conducted in Sweden show that vaccine hesitancy was found among rural women and men who vote for Sweden Democrats, a right-wing populist party and the second-largest party in the Riksdag (Swedish Parliament). This group has "little faith in Sweden's democratic system" (Lindvall & Rönnerstrand 2022). Young adults who reside in big cities and who do not consume high-quality media expressed disagreement with the vaccination policy as well (Lindvall & Rönnerstrand 2022). In this context, we need to gain knowledge about the dynamics of social relations in the Nordic countries, and the impact of global media trends on these dynamics. We ask, what were the main discussion topics in the Twitter) vaccine corpus, and how did

DOI: 10.4324/9781003305859-14

those with opposing views argue in favour or against vaccination? How did they treat each other? Did they act within the frameworks of social trust?

Theory: generalised trust and attitudes to special groups

We define trust, after Lucy Gilson, as a relational notion that lies: between people, between people and organisations, between people and events (Gilson 2003: 1454). On an interpersonal level, it can be described as the subjective willingness to become vulnerable to a trustee believing that the latter will act to the subject's benefit (Schilke et al. 2021). Morals and altruism are involved in the relation or feeling of trust (Coulson 1998; Lahno 2001). Solidarity, truthfulness, a belief in fairness, and spontaneous altruism are decisive common principles which underpin this feeling (Ulsaner 2008). When built into the functioning of social institutions and accepted by society, these common principles form a basis for social capital, or generalised trust (Honneth 2007; Rothstein 2005; Rothstein & Stolle 2008; Ulsaner 2008).

Community members who do not share the values and norms of the larger group tend to trust only people with similar mindsets, which can lead them to form subcultures or even criminal gangs, "with goals that are opposed to the broader public interest" (Gilson 2003). These groups can experience negative feelings, and their mistrust of others can lead to conflictual action that, as Gilson (2003: 1459) points out: "clearly brings limited benefits to the wider community and may even initiate a vicious cycle of dis-trust leading people to withdraw from civil life". Another case of conflictual relations might involve groups that have different religious, cultural, and political beliefs. In this context, the question arises of how to treat people who do not share the same values as the rest of the community; e.g., should medical institutions or other members of society stop trusting them? In this context, Gilson points to the problem of healthcare providers demonstrating "different levels of trust towards different groups of patients", showing cases of problematic treatment of members of low-income families or people thought to be using medical services in the wrong way.

To explore the manifestations of trust or mistrust in our research material, study how various groups relate to each other, and especially ask whether the majority acts within the frameworks of social trust and exercises a respectful attitude toward special groups, we deploy ideas about othering and disrespect. The concept of "othering" has been elaborated in philosophy and social sciences. According to Jensen (2011), othering is a discursive process in which powerful groups ascribe problematic and/or inferior characteristics to the subordinate groups to affirm their superiority. Similarly, Honneth (1992) states that disrespectful behaviour is injurious because it impairs the insulted persons in their positive understanding of themselves. In addition, it might be useful to introduce the concept of hate speech, after Brison (1998: 313), here:

> speech that vilifies individuals or groups on the basis of such characteristics as race, sex, ethnicity, religion, and sexual orientation, which (1)

constitutes face-to-face vilification, (2) creates a hostile or intimidating environment, or (3) is a kind of group libel.

The Internet and especially social media have become places where participants do not spare strong words in relation to their interlocutors, allowing themselves expressions from which they would refrain in real life (Gagliardone et al. 2015). As a result, participants have become warier of each other and, in some cases, have stopped respecting those who have different opinions. This situation can produce a negative impact on generalised trust.

Data: Twitter utterances about vaccines

To retrieve the tweets that we needed for our analysis, we deployed the Snscrape library for Python. We then used the search term "vaccin*"[1] and selected only those tweets that were in English. Specifying the algorithm to search among tweets in the period of 1 January 2020 to 1 September 2021 leads to a corpus containing 48,334,908 tweets. Apart from the text of the tweets themselves, we also get information on the hashtags used in them, and about the users who wrote them. For further analysis, we then clean the text of each tweet using the steps suggested by Grimmer et al. (2022). Also, we test for any effects these steps (and their order) might have had on our data by using the preText package by Denny and Spirling (2018). It was necessary to clean our data, given the often-messy nature of Twitter data. As such, we choose to perform the following steps: (a) use of lowercase words, (b) removal of stop words, (c) removal of numbers and punctuation, (d) removal of hashtags and mentions, and (e) application of stemming.[2] While the exact order and choice of steps automatically influence our outcomes (Denny & Spirling 2018), we choose here to follow these steps to both make the data easier to interpret and lighten the work for the algorithm by reducing the total number of terms.

As part of our analysis focuses on the geographical location of the user, and as we study in detail utterances from the Nordic countries, we then sub-set this corpus further based on this. We can do so in two ways. The most obvious is to use the user-defined "location". Yet, while more than 80% of the tweets mention a location, they are often fanciful descriptions (such as "in hell" or "anywhere you like"). As such, we opt to use the geographical location data that Twitter stores if users agree to use this option. While this method does provide us with very precise locations, it comes at the price of reducing our corpus to 1,046,683 tweets, or 2.16% of the full data set. While this is a considerable reduction, a quick comparison between the full and reduced corpora shows that STM creates related topics.

We reduced this number further when we generated a Nordic sub-corpus, which contains 3,401 tweets. It would not be correct to say that the English-language data would be fully representative of the realities in the Nordic countries (since people naturally also write tweets in their native languages – in our case, in Danish, Finnish, Icelandic, Norwegian, and Swedish, as well as in Faroese, Greenlandic, and Sami). Nevertheless, using this data set still makes sense if one perceives voices from the Nordic countries as an inseparable part of the global, or transnational exchange of opinions (and X [formerly Twitter] certainly enables this). These tweets can be statements meant for perception from the outside, reactions to events and agendas of worldwide significance. One may also be aware of the research limitation, that the demographic expressing themselves in English would be different from those posting in the national languages, and that vaccine hesitancy would be more typical for the latter category.

Table 11.1 shows what our reduced corpus looks like, with the frequencies of the tweets arranged per continent. For each continent, we also show the three countries with the highest number of tweets. From this, we see that the

Table 11.1 Frequencies of tweets, per country and continent

Continent	*Country*	*Frequency*
Africa	South Africa	23,894
	Nigeria	8,596
	Kenya	4,696
	Others	11,979
Europe	United Kingdom	158,638
	Ireland	20,370
	Germany	4,091
	Nordic countries	
	Sweden	1,207
	Norway	809
	Denmark	795
	Finland	468
	Iceland	122
	Others	24,357
Latin America	Mexico	2,014
	Brazil	1,766
	Others	7,599
North America	United States	532,340
	Canada	74,121
	Jamaica	3,145
	Bermuda	188
	Others	3
Oceania	Australia	30,398
	New Zealand	3,640
	Fiji	431
	Others	285
South and South-eastern Asia	India	87,155
	Philippines	9,743
	Malaysia	8,293
	Others	18,971
Western Asia	United Arab Emirates	2,750
	Saudi Arabia	1,883
	Israel	1,313
	Others	4,024
Total		**1,046,683**

United States is good for around half of the tweets in our dataset, followed by the United Kingdom (around 15%) and India (around 8%). These numbers are as expected given that we restricted ourselves to English-language tweets. For the Nordic countries, a consequence of this is that their numbers place them behind the United Kingdom, Ireland, and Germany.

Methodology: structural topic modelling and thematic analysis

To process a large corpus of Twitter utterances, and to answer the research questions as to the main topics, arguments, and involved relations of trust/ mistrust, we combined quantitative (structural topic model or STM) and qualitative (thematic analysis) techniques. Doing so allowed us to overcome some of the major drawbacks that tend to plague both types of methods (Jacobs & Tschötschel 2019). That is, while the STM provides the precision that qualitative themes often lack, the qualitative thematic analysis explains the topics' various meanings. Our procedure involves the following steps, alternating between quantitative and qualitative methods.

First, for the quantitative part, to get a general sense of the dominant attitudes regarding the COVID-19 vaccine and the character of social relations (especially the relation of trust) implied in the discussions, we generate a word cloud containing the most frequent words (what we call keywords) that represent the main corpus (see Figure 11.1). Keywords provide insight into what the corpus is all about. This initial knowledge serves as guidance for asking further questions and making more advanced inquiries.

Second, to generate our topics, we use a structural topic model or STM (Roberts et al. 2014). The STM method allows analysts to gain insight into how different texts (in our case, tweets) might talk about the same underlying topic using different word choices. This method provides a structure to our data by dividing it into chunks, which we can identify by looking at the relevant words and the most representative tweets that were characteristic of each of them. Belonging to the wider family of topic models based on latent Dirichlet allocation, or LDA (Blei et al. 2003), STM finds its topics by looking at the relations between the words. The more often words appear together in a text, the more likely it is that they belong to the same topic. As an unsupervised model, STM requires no monitoring apart from the setting of the initial parameters. These initial parameters include the number of topics and any information that can help the algorithm to find the topics. In this study, we provided the date of publication of the tweet as extra information, as we suspected that the topics might vary over time.

As for the number of topics, we followed the advice by Roberts et al. (2019) to run multiple STM models, ranging from 2 to 20 topics. We then used a combination of quantitative and qualitative methods to decide on the final numbers of topics. On the quantitative side, we looked at the *exclusivity* and *semantic coherence* of each of the topic constellations. These measure to what degree topics may contain many overlapping words, and to what degree words

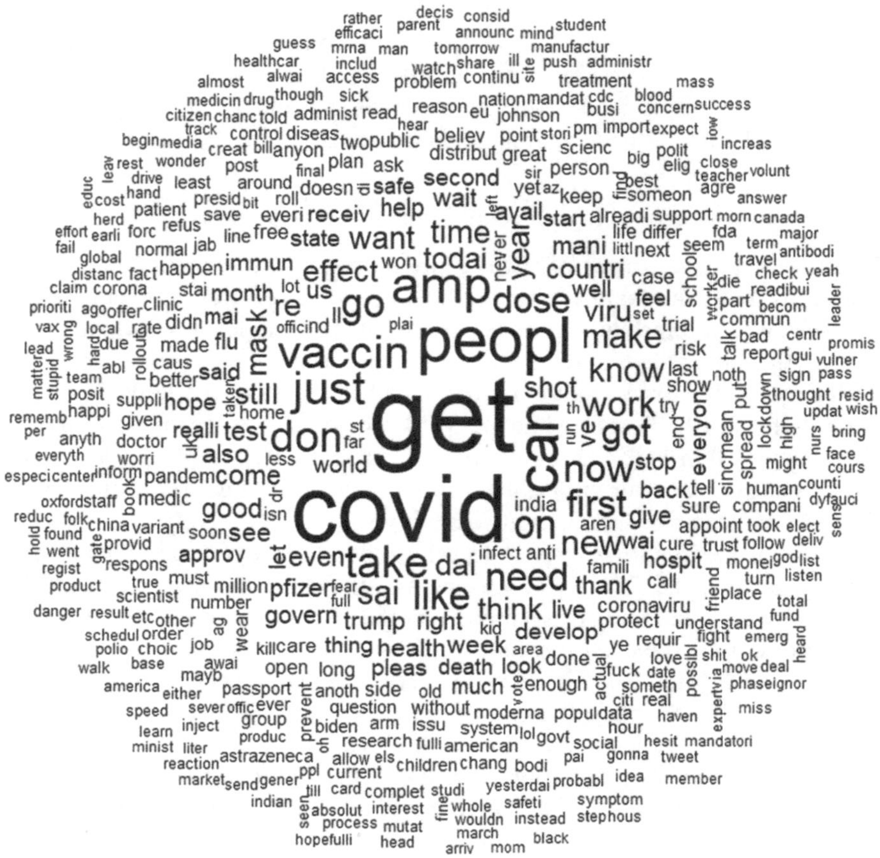

Figure 11.1 Word cloud with the most frequent words in the main corpus.

that occur in the same topic also occur in the same context. Both are good indicators of what human coders would consider valid topics. The result of this is a model containing either six, seven, or eight topics. We then looked at each of these constellations qualitatively to judge the usefulness of each constellation. Based on this, we decided on a model using six topics.

We extracted a list of relevant words for each that have the highest association with that certain topic. For this association, we base ourselves on the FREX (frequency and exclusive) value of each word. This value combines the exclusivity of each word (meaning that a word occurs more often in that topic than in others) while also correcting for its overall frequency (Airoldi & Bischof 2016). To understand our topics better and to label them, we also extracted the 50 most representative tweets for each topic. Doing so for each of the six topics gives us 300 tweets for the main corpus and another 300 tweets for the Nordic sub-corpus. Given the way STM works, each word and each tweet are part of each topic. Unlike clustering methods, in topic models, there is no real "classification" but more of a degree of belonging. Thus, a tweet can belong 99% to Topic 1, but still 0.1% to Topic 2.

At this stage, we defined the common issue that tweets sharing the same topic take up. The algorithm provides a researcher with a transformation of a large corpus, upon which the researcher releases the analysis itself. The researcher's task is to make sense of what the topic model shows when it comes to semantic relations and meaning-making processes in the corpus. The researcher's agency is important to consider while defining the meaning of the topics defined with the help of LDA. While defining the issues central to each topic, one must make a reverse procedure and try to understand why the algorithm united the items under the same topic. According to Jacobs and Tschötschel (2019: 3–4), a piece of text

> can be represented as the outcome of first selecting subjects, then selecting ways of speaking about them, and finally selecting some words associated with that manner of speaking. Topic modelling can be understood as a reversal of this process in which the algorithms use the observed distributions of words across texts in the corpus to infer non-exclusive clusters typically used in common – each representing a mode of speech about a specific subject.

While doing so, we kept the question in mind: "What experiences related to the vaccine did people encounter when writing their tweets?" Taking into consideration that we also related the text to the major events (development, distribution, and the actual vaccination), one can define our methodology as contextualist and characterised by the critical realism theory, which, according to Braun and Clarke (2006: 81), acknowledges "the ways individuals make meaning of their experience, and in turn, the ways the broader social context impinges on those meanings, while retaining focus on the material and other limits of 'reality'". We related the data to concrete events, stories, cases, and actors (politicians, scientists, officials) who might have led the public discussion. In addition, we used elements of applied linguistics, which links linguistic expressions to deliberations, reflections, and actions of the producers of the speech acts, as well as to the social relations in which they are involved (Mills 2004). Thus, the topics in our analysis can be defined as issues, which are common for the utterances placed in the same "basket" by the algorithm and which relate to some aspect of experiences with the general subject of the entire corpus ("vaccines"). Topics in our analysis should not be confused with the themes, as the latter are the results of further qualitative analysis and can go through several topics.

Third, we then studied the behaviour of our topics over time. As we included the day of publication of the tweet in our model, we can plot the prevalence of our topics on each day. This allows us to see if a topic became more prevalent because of certain time-related events.

Fourth, we continued with a qualitative enquiry, choosing a thematic analysis (Braun & Clarke 2006) to present the defined topics (with the help of LDA) as close to the data as possible, while also providing essential background information and identifying the main themes, which go through various LDA-defined topics. The method of thematic analysis presents the data in its richness or broadness, and at the same time allows for simple manipulations, such as coding. While using coding of the most representative tweets within each topic, we separated between various branches of discussions (sub-topics). Further, we divided the items (tweets) between those in favour of and those opposing the COVID-19 vaccine. This latter step was done to establish what topics caused the most controversies or to see which topics contained a large number of utterances against vaccination. This made it possible to analyse the manner of communication of the two groups (proponents and opponents of vaccination), and detect cases of "othering" and hate speech directed towards the "other camp". Finally, we identified common themes, i.e., important persistent concepts and meanings underlying the data set that help answer the main research question (about the implied justifications for vaccine acceptance or scepticism). In the presentation of our analysis, we describe in detail the discussion within the three topics (out of the six LDA-defined topics) by tracing certain variations in the reasoning in favour or against vaccines and paying special attention to the agonistic spirit entailed in various positions. In this way, we concentrate on only a representative fragment of our data, being driven by the theoretical interest, in showing the assumptions behind, and the ways of people's reasoning, rather than by the interest to describe the entirety of the data.

Mistrust between advocates and opponents of vaccination

A qualitative analysis of the selected tweets from the Nordic countries shows that people mostly expressed positive attitudes towards the COVID-19 vaccine and trusted the authorities. The word cloud[3] that represents the main corpus shows that words such as "get" and "covid" appear most frequently. Often, these words are part of utterances about the experiences of getting vaccinated or calls to do so. At the same time, we observed a prominent level of tension in the COVID-19 vaccine discussion, and many of the pro-vaccine statements were built as objections to a real or imaginary opponent. The questions on how to deal with the COVID-19 pandemic, or even whether to acknowledge it as a real health threat, split Twitter users, even though opponents of vaccination represented a clear minority. In their criticism of one another, the pro-vaccine and the anti-vaccine constituencies used sharp tones, mutual accusations of incompetence, ridicule, and obscene language. Often, the pro-vaccine group was appealing to ideals, principles, and established doctrines of left-wing political parties, while the most outspoken opponents of vaccination adhered to right-wing radical views.

A close reading of the phrases with another frequent word – "people" – shows that the use of the word often held negative connotations and denoted various kinds of "others" who appear to be wrong, incompetent, or immoral. For example, those criticising vaccine refusers use such expressions such as: "people I know not getting it [the COVID-19 vaccine] are just scared"; "lots of people have misinformation regarding [the] vaccine". Apart from these kinds of neutral sentences, we also observed harsher expressions, especially when Twitter users sought to punish vaccine refusers, such as: "People who don't want the vaccines should not be treated in a hospital".

Conversely, Twitter users who were vaccine sceptics often took a defensive position trying to protect themselves from all the "people" who allegedly wanted to restrict their freedom. Thus, a Twitter user notes that the majority, that is, those who got vaccinated, treated him dismissively and spoke harshly to him: "people are telling me to die". Others complained about being pressured and angered by society: "people want me to get a vaccine"; "people angrily screaming at people to get vaccinated". Another Twitter user compares COVID-19 vaccine proponents with dictators who deprive others of freedom: "you people are worse than people forcing political thought control" cf. Hammarlin et al. 2024, chapter 10, this volume. Thus, a preliminary analysis of the use of the most frequent words invites a closer look at the general tone and the main pro and con arguments within the vaccine discussion.

Topics retrieved with the help of structural topic modelling

After getting a general sense of the expressed attitudes and social relations involved in the COVID-19 vaccine Twitter discussions, we may want to know what issues or topics caused these disputes. We found six meaningful topics based on our STM analysis of the main corpus. Table 11.2 represents the most relevant words for each of them.[4]

The next step was to define what each topic was about, proceeding from a qualitative reading of the 300 most-representative tweets from the main corpus, and 300 tweets from the Nordic sub-corpus, and paying attention to the relevant words. Overall, these were the topics:

- "Herd immunity": as a way of combating the virus in the absence of a vaccine, or as an outcome of vaccination
- "Approval": official reports about approval and readiness to administer various vaccine types
- "Getting vaccinated": information from vaccination stations about vaccine availability and people's reports about getting first and second doses
- "Reasons": people's reflections around the meaning of getting vaccinated; "Should I – or should I not?"
- "Restrictions": discussions about rules of conduct in public places, such as showing vaccine passports in airports and bars, and on vaccine requirements to attend schools
- "Politicians": reflecting on the roles of various politicians in solving the pandemic crisis

Table 11.2 Top 15 terms most associated with each of the topics, based on their FREX-value

Getting vaccinated	*Politicians*	*Approval*	*Restrictions*	*Reasons*	*Herd immunity*
covid	sai*	covid	go	get	need
dose	trump	new	re*	people	make
first	govern	health	effect	can	viru
got	plan	state	mask	don*	mani*
dai*	world	develop	see	just	wai*
get	country	us	ve*	like	immune
today	medic	amp*	good	on	flu
shot	save	approv	back	know	also
vaccin	try	million	let	work	stop
week	must	coronavirus	test	want	death
thank	noth	trial	thing	vaccin	much
receiv	biden	india	realli*	think	protect
second	trust	country	keep	still	never
next	support	pfizer	long	even	sure
feel	american	uk	side	covid	case

Notes:

1 Note that all the terms are stemmed.

2 The derivations for the stems with an asterisk (*) are explained in note 1.

Table 11.3 Percentages of topic prevalence for the five Nordic countries

	Approval	*Reasons*	*Getting vaccinated*	*Restrictions*	*Politicians*	*Herd immunity*
Denmark	14.5	11.0	21.7	10.8	15.9	17.0
Finland	15.1	10.6	22.0	10.6	15.6	17.5
Iceland	16.6	9.5	17.2	12.3	18.1	17.0
Norway	13.2	11.2	20.6	11.0	16.4	18.6
Sweden	14.5	10.8	18.0	12.0	17.6	17.7

Table 11.3 shows topic prevalence for the Nordic countries. The percentages for each cell represented how prominent that topic was on average over all texts in that country. Thus, in the case of Denmark, a little over a fifth of the tweets concerned themselves with "Getting vaccinated", while for Iceland, only 17% of the tweets were about this topic. Overall, we find that while there were slight variations between the countries, the overall numbers are close to each other, with "Getting vaccinated" being the most popular topic and "Reasons" and "Restrictions" being the least popular. There is no statistical test for the differences, as we wished to focus on an overall idea of the numbers of topics per country and not the differences between countries. When adding the results from the qualitative tweet analysis, we observed that in the Nordic countries, most represented were the topics that involved fewer controversies (such as

"Getting vaccinated"), whereas the topics that contained hot discussions ("Reasons" and "Restrictions") received less attention. This result may indicate a less intense discussion in the Nordic region compared to the rest of the world.

Time graph: Prevalence of topics over time in the Nordic countries

A careful study of the graph (seen in Figure 11.2) showing the prevalence of topics over time confirms our previous conclusions, namely, that herd immunity, experiences of vaccination, as well as, later, the issues related to the COVID-19 vaccine approval and administration, were most frequently occurring throughout the whole studied period. The level of the topic's popularity was tightly knit with the real events, including the approval of the Pfizer-BioNTech COVID-19 vaccine in the UK (and EU) in November 2020, as well as the start of mass vaccination in the summer of 2021 in Europe. Herd immunity as a "natural" way of combating the virus was actively discussed before the vaccine became available. Starting from late autumn and winter 2020 until summer 2021, reports on vaccine approval and administration took off. People described their vaccination experiences even before the COVID-19 vaccine came into play, and since autumn 2020, these reports have been dealing with getting the first and second doses of the COVID-19 vaccine. The role of politicians in solving the COVID-19 crisis was actively discussed during the whole

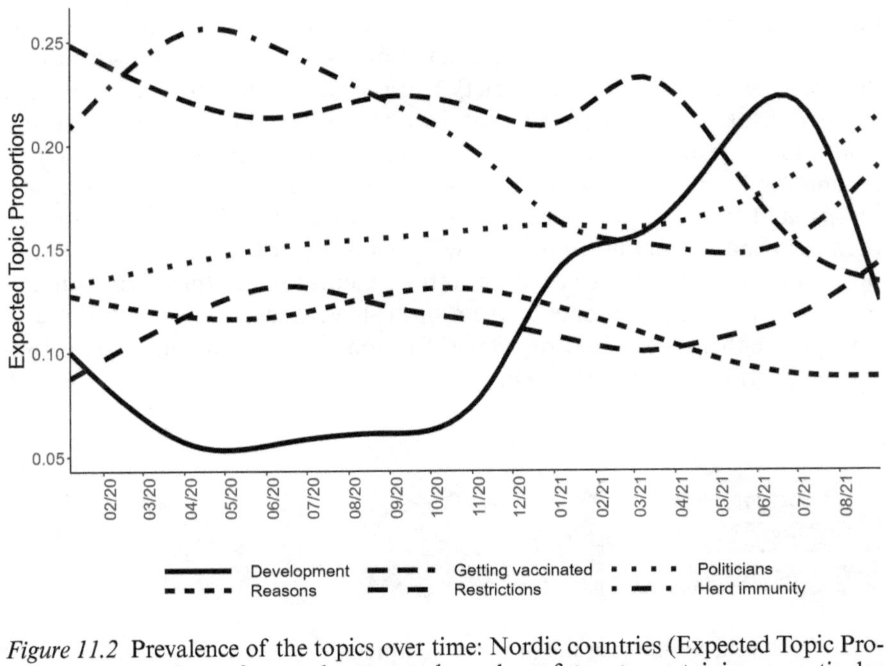

Figure 11.2 Prevalence of the topics over time: Nordic countries (Expected Topic Proportion refers to the expected number of tweets containing a particular topic at any given moment).

period. The same can be said about discussions around reasons for getting vaccinated, and rules of conduct in public places.

Thematic analysis: arguments behind vaccine acceptance or scepticism

A thematic analysis has shown that there was a constant theme of solidarity among the supporters of vaccination, who underlined that it was important to get a vaccine not only to protect oneself but to successfully cope with the virus spread. At the same time, vaccine opponents were most concerned with freedom of choice and associated vaccination with pressure. We show how these arguments were expressed while the users were discussing three controversial topics: herd immunity, official restrictions, and the role of politicians in solving the COVID-19 crisis. First, we show that when it comes to the topic of herd immunity, the free choice argumentation was expressed in the thesis of the least interference in the personal space of citizens. Within the discussion on mandatory vaccination in schools, free choice was associated with the possibility of leading a natural lifestyle and a philosophy of childcare that takes place in harmony with nature. And finally, when speaking of politicians, the users who were concerned with the issue of freedom said that they felt pressure from certain politicians and from members of governments and various organisations. These actors, as they believed, created various structures of control. In other words, often these were adherents of conspiracy theories, such as "big pharma" and "New World Order". Second, while discussing herd immunity, supporters of vaccination put forward a thesis that it can be achieved only if everyone gets vaccinated and shows solidarity with others. Solidarity was interpreted as society's responsibility to end the pandemic. Concerning the issue of mandatory vaccination, solidarity meant ensuring health for all, especially for vulnerable groups, among others, children. When it comes to the discussions on politicians, users emphasised international solidarity and justice and judged various governments and politicians out of their contribution to this. In the following, while describing these several ways of argumentation, we pay attention to the general tone of the discussion and the ways of treating opponents, from both sides. Users' different interpretations of the themes of solidarity versus freedom of choice within various topics are illustrated in the scheme in Figure 11.3.

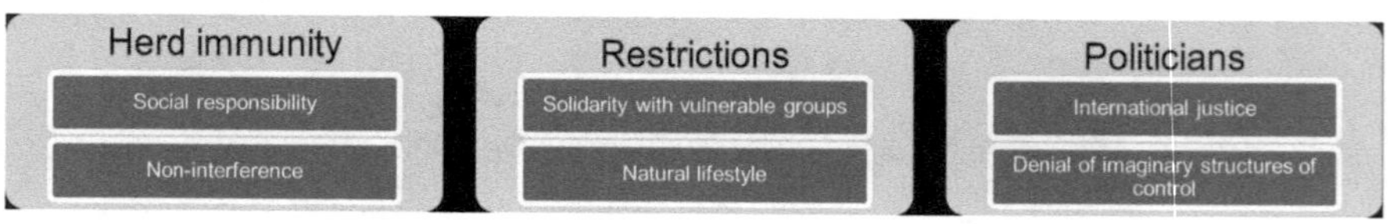

Figure 11.3 Scheme showing the different interpretations of the users regarding solidarity versus freedom of choice.

Herd immunity: passivity and non-interference?

The issue of herd immunity caused heated debates between advocates and opponents of the vaccine. In both the main corpus and in the Nordic sub-corpus, we observed a tendency to assert that herd immunity was the only way to limit the viral spread, especially in the period before the approval of the COVID-19 vaccine, "when vaccines were out of the question". This approach is reminiscent of the point of view that vaccines are not needed at all, and that COVID-19 can be overcome in a natural way: simply by strengthening one's own immunity ("take vitamin C hourly", as one user said), and waiting for part of the population to get sick and recover from the disease. In the United States, former president Donald Trump, one of the greatest influencers on Twitter, believed that herd immunity could be the main strategy to deal with the pandemic. A small group of scientists from a libertarian think tank in the United States published the so-called Great Barrington Declaration in an open letter, in which they argued in favour of stopping lockdowns and the natural herd immunity approach. On a global scale, by 2021, around 50,000 protests had been linked to the pandemic, some of which were violent (Newey et al. 2021). Public health experts preferred to avoid talking about herd immunity as a tool in the absence of vaccines (Aschwanden 2020). In an influential publication in *The Lancet*, herd immunity as a natural strategy for overcoming the pandemic was deemed a "dangerous fallacy unsupported by scientific evidence" (Aschwanden 2020).

Within the Nordic countries, herd immunity discourse was especially popular in Sweden, where there were official policies of maintaining an "open society". Contrary to most of the world, Swedish authorities did not introduce a total lockdown. The country's own unique way of coping with the pandemic was legitimated by the authorities' wish to guarantee fundamental constitutional freedoms (such as freedom of movement) and avoid exerting excessive pressure on citizens. We observed a considerable number of tweets supporting this view in the Nordic sub-corpus. Liberal attitudes to precautionary measures sanctioned by the state might have enforced some people's anti-vaccination stand and caused vaccine hesitancy. Both ways of thinking, about the optionality of lockdown and avoidance of vaccines, presupposes a similar view that the COVID-19 virus is not dangerous, and that it can be fought with natural means, for example through developing "natural herd immunity". Both ways of thinking imply passivity and avoidance of any pressure from the authorities. For example, a user says: "While testing is needed, herd immunity is the only viable long-term option. Remember this is a coronavirus like the common cold, SARS, and MERS. We overcame them without vaccines. We will need to do the same for this one too. We need to forget that there will ever be a vaccine". Coronavirus was equated with the common cold, and herd immunity was seen as the only, natural way out. WHO defines vaccine hesitancy as a "delay in acceptance or refusal of vaccines despite availability of vaccination services" (Shen & Dubey 2019). Vaccine hesitancy implies not a complete denial of, but a slightly negative attitude towards vaccines, and is connected with awareness of own dissimilarity to others and unwillingness to "go with the flow" (Shen & Dubey 2019). It implies a rejection of any pressure from others or authorities. While we do not have any evidence that the Swedish policies of non-interference might have led to more vaccine hesitancy, there are many examples of tweets in which the users who supported authorities and were vaccine sceptics talked about their independence and did not agree to follow the general rules.

At the same time, the Swedish philosophy of non-interference in citizens' behaviour was much criticised as well; Swedish scientists accused the authorities of promoting policies that caused many deaths (Kianzad & Minssen 2020). People criticised the Swedish "special way", saying that keeping bars and restaurants open was very problematic since this policy "helps to spread the virus". One of the main arguments in favour of the vaccine was related to the value of solidarity. For example, a user says:

> A vaccine is not just to protect yourself. The benefit is also that you stop spreading the virus. Vaccinated people do not get sick and do not spread the virus. Everyone should therefore take the vaccine so we can stop the pandemic by herd immunity.

It is worth paying attention to the use of the word "people" in this quote. It applies to the group of those who have been vaccinated. The latter is endowed with all possible positive qualities: they allegedly cannot even get sick or give the virus to another person.

Restrictions during the pandemic: "natural lifestyle" as an alternative?

Another big issue that caused controversies involved restrictions and requirements of conduct in public places such as schools, restaurants, or bars. In the United States, there were especially heated debates connected to the question of whether the COVID-19 vaccines should be mandatory for children in schools, along the lines of other mandated vaccines against rubella, diphtheria, smallpox, polio, and whooping cough. These debates often boiled down to an intense fight between anti-vaxxers and pro-vaccine people. Opponents of vaccines, who have been active since the 1970s in Europe, Asia, Australia, and North America (and who gather around physicians like Gordon Stewart and Andrew Wakefield), promoted the idea that vaccines contain dangerous ingredients that might cause various side effects, autism, and even death. The anti-vaccination movement has its roots in the religious and political movements of 19th-century England. Its adherents proclaimed personal freedom in response to the requirement of the state for mandatory vaccination. Along these lines, during the 1902 smallpox outbreak in the United States, critics came forward stating that compulsory vaccination violates citizens' rights to care for their own bodies as they know best.[5] Parents who decline their children's vaccines claim to stand for the so-called natural lifestyle. The once-fringe movement has intensified during the COVID-19 pandemic. Within the main corpus, but also in the Nordic sub-corpus, we found numerous messages confirming this position.

Proponents of vaccines consider compulsory vaccination programmes to be necessary measures of saving lives and associate them with the values of solidarity and care for others, especially children. At the same time, being a proponent of the value of solidarity is sometimes connected with the strategies of othering and exclusion in relation to the so-called anti-vaxxers. For example, a user objected to a person who believes that vaccines lead to autism, assaulting the latter (calling the person a "bitch") and saying that the latter "wouldn't be able to walk normally" due to polio, would be "coughing because of pertussis" and would have "probably died due to tetanus". In another tweet, a user taunts an anti-vaxxer, sarcastically asking if the latter "enjoyed any polio lately". We noted many other cases of verbal assaults, where anti-vaxxers are called "f*cking idiots", "stupid", and "stubborn", with some Twitter users writing irritated exhortations to vaccinate: "just f*cking do it!" Thus, it is also necessary to take a critical look at the cases of hate speech against vaccine sceptics.

After the vaccine became available, those who were refusing to get vaccinated were accused of being guilty of "potentially prolonging the pandemic" and "contributing to spikes in cases". One user even posted a video response to a tweet that seemed to endorse forced vaccination. In this video, a healthcare worker suddenly attacks a young guy who is sitting calmly in the gym. A masked nurse knocks the young man to the ground and forcibly makes an injection. Although the message is conveyed humorously, audiences can sense the anger being directed towards an irresponsible young person who is being humiliated and treated with disrespect. In this way, solidarity may border with pressure to take the only right collective action. The circle of deviant, irresponsible "others" is defined, and if someone gets into this circle, they can become an object of coercive measures. Even if all this remains at the level of fantasy and a simple joke, statements of this kind can lead to a decrease in the level of trust in society.

Politicians solving the COVID-19 crisis: between conspiracy theories and international justice

The COVID-19 pandemic and vaccines became an excellent occasion for promoting various political ideologies and views. Trump and his Republican followers produced conspiracy theories, including that the COVID-19 virus and the vaccines were secretly invented either by the Chinese or the Democrats (or both) to seize power and establish a "totalitarian world order". Tweets propounding this view were found in the main corpus, and we can see that "Trump" and "Biden" were among the most frequent words in the topic covering politicians. While promoting a panoply of conspiracy theories, among them the emergence of the "New World Order" – a society without nations, borders, or distinct cultures that Democrats allegedly sought to establish through the deployment of secretly toxic COVID-19 vaccines – far-right groups attacked adherents of progressive ideology and their policies, openly proclaiming xenophobia, racism, and sexism. These conservative-leaning members of the Twitterverse embraced what the researcher of the American far-right Camila Liyanage has called “radical traditionalism” (Liyanage 2020: 130). This discourse is characteristic of people who adhered to a popular sort of libertarianism once known as the Tea Party. These people became associated with anti-vaccine movements as the populist Tea Party morphed into pro-Trump libertarian “MAGAs” or “ultra-MAGAs”, finding their voices in criticism of lockdowns and vaccine mandates as assaults on their fundamental freedoms (Butler & Sorell 2022). The “free choice” position began to spread as a response to extensive calls to vaccinate, which these people found to be tiresome, even offensive. From the point of view of those who joined the “free choice” movement, governments put undue pressure on citizens. They perceived themselves as victims of ridicule, social contempt, and even authoritarianism, accusing progressive pro-vax society of being worse than “those who practise political thought control”, thus basically offending and denigrating the authorities and everybody who followed the rules. We find some supporters of the American far-right in both corpora.

However, the prevailing number of tweets were criticising Trump’s anti-vaccine and anti-science stance. In the tweets that came from the Nordic region, people paid a lot of attention to American politics. The majority expressed their sympathies with American Democrats. With the coming to power of Joseph Biden in 2021, whose inauguration took place in the middle of the pandemic, many could sigh with relief welcoming an incoming president who had, as one user put it, “faith in science and knowledge-informed politics and administration”. Another user, welcoming Biden to the White House, writes that the latter “re-joined the WHO” (after Trump had withdrawn the United States from the organisation), rapidly distributed millions of doses of vaccines among the American people, donated to international vaccination efforts, and “brought humanity back into the White House”. Users criticised Republicans for their sceptical attitude towards the COVID-19 vaccine and their refusal to wear masks, perceiving these questions to be a part of the whole “package” of political issues: climate legislation, voters’ rights, democracy, and science-based policies.

Many Twitter users from the Nordic countries in particular criticised Trump for pursuing narrow national interests and expressing little solidarity with other countries. In the tweets, Trump is called a “hypocrite and liar”, the very “definition of evil”, or the one who has a “Nazi-style” of governance. Trump’s practising of what was called “vaccine nationalism” – in which he set orders to hoard vaccines without sharing them with the rest of the world – is seen as “scandalous”. In contrast, people from the Nordic countries promote international images of their states as contributors to the research and development of vaccines and as promoters of global justice. For example, we observed a number of tweets in which their authors point out that Norway has played a key role in building the Coalition for Epidemic Preparedness Innovations

(CEPI), a global coalition founded by Bill and Melinda Gates working to prevent epidemics. Vaccine nationalism and the narrow interests of politicians exist elsewhere, but not in the Nordic region, according to these users. At the same time, we saw tweets offering some constructive criticism as well, when people pointed out that Trump himself may positively influence vaccine sceptics, since many of his supporters do not listen to Democrats or liberal media. Authors of utterances like this demonstrate a certain amount of trust toward Trump supporters and may even inspire them to engage in a dialogue.

Conclusion: better inclusion of special groups

By combining quantitative and qualitative methods, we defined the main discussion topics in global and Nordic Twitter vaccine discussions by paying special attention to the core arguments in favour of and against vaccines and the character of the involved social relations. The issues of herd immunity, mandatory vaccination programmes, as well as separate political figures and their agendas aroused great interest among the Twitter public. Although the majority (including those from the Nordic countries) supported vaccination, the debate resulted in sharp political, philosophical, and values-based divisions between defenders and opponents of vaccination. The main problem, in many cases, was in the manner of communication and the inability to adhere to the basic rules of decency. There were instances of hate speech, disrespect, and othering. Especially problematic was the style of radical groups that practises hate speech in relation to vaccine supporters. Referring to Gilson (2003: 1459), one may conclude that the radical groups stood in opposition to the "broader public interest" and tried to "promote conflictual action". These groups demonstrated mistrust at many levels: towards others, medical institutions, and the whole of society.

At the same time, representatives of the majority, instead of trying to include these groups in a meaningful conversation, made them objects of public ridicule. When using the concept of "othering", it is possible to conclude that those who have more power (and the vaccine sceptics often belong to low-income groups with few resources), made the extremist groups feel even more inferior. Those who become objects of "othering" might experience a lowering of their self-esteem, as well as feelings of social pressure, and, in the end, become unwilling to listen to points of view that differ from their own. Gilson suggests that instead of various kinds of humiliating attitudes and treating groups differently, communities would be better off if they would include such individuals in policy and decision-making and the public deliberation process. This will promote more trustful behaviour on both sides. Further suggestions include creating opportunities for special groups to improve personal self-esteem and raising a sense of moral worth. One suggestion might even be face-to-face meetings to discuss controversial issues, "to confront the mismatches between our own beliefs and those of others, enabling self-reflection and learning" (Gilson 2003: 1461). Promoting inter-group communication and the ability to engage in a constructive debate would be key to establishing a generalised trust.

Notes

1 Note that in the search term, the asterisk (*) represents a wildcard and can stand for any type of character. As such, the term matches not only those tweets with "vaccine", but also those with "vaccination", "vaccinated", and so on.
2 During stemming, inflected and derived words are reduced to their "stem". For example, "says", "said", and "saying" are all reduced to the stem "sai". The idea behind this is twofold: it groups words with a similar meaning together, and reduces the overall number of unique terms, thereby reducing the pressure on the algorithm.
3 The reason the word cloud in Figure 11.1 contains items which are not words comes about as the word cloud was generated *after* cleaning the text. In this process, numbers, digits, spaces, and stop words are removed. In addition, strings are lowercased and stemmed. This means, for example, that "people" and "peoples" are stemmed to "people" – these are the terms that occur in the word cloud. Their interpretation is thus not that of actual words, but of the stems of these words as they occur in the text. Their occurrence is based on the frequency in the text. Also, note that not *all* words occur in the word cloud (for reasons of clarity). A word (or its stem) had to occur *at least* 30 times to be included. This number is not set in stone but was simply that number that led to a readable word cloud at this resolution.
4 The reason the words such as "get", "also", and "much" occur in each of the topics is their overall high frequency. As can be seen in the word cloud in Figure 11.1, these words occur most often in all the texts. While the FREX value tries to correct for this, it can never be perfect. The same would occur if stop words such as *the*, *and*, *our*, etc., would be included. There are various ways to deal with this in topic modelling. Most often, scholars throw them out in order not to let these words "spoil" the topics. As an alternative, one could keep the words and look at the other words in the topic to base their description on them and silently "ignore" those words.

   As for the stemming shown in Table 11.2, "dai" derives from "day" or "days", "sai" derives from "say" or "says", "amp" represents the ampersand (&), which was not taken out during cleaning, "re" and "ve" stem from combinations such as "I've" and "They're", where the apostrophe is removed, and are abbreviations of "have" and "are" respectively, "realli" comes from "really", "don" comes from combinations such as "don't", "mani" and "wai" come from words such as "many", and "way" or "ways". For precise details on the algorithm, see Porter (1980).
5 For more information on this, see College of Physicians of Philadelphia (2022).

References

Airoldi, Edoardo M. & Jonathan M. Bischof. 2016. Improving and evaluating topic models and other models of text. *Journal of the American Statistical Association* 111(516): 1381–1403.

Aschwanden, Christie. 2020. The false promise of herd immunity for COVID-19. *Nature* 587: 26–28.

Blei, David M., Andrew Y. Ng & Michael I. Jordan. 2003. Latent Dirichlet allocation. *Journal of Machine Learning Research* 3: 993–1022.

Braun, Virginia & Victoria Clarke. 2006. Using thematic analysis in psychology. *Qualitative Research in Psychology* 3(2): 77–101.

Brison, Susan J. 1998. The autonomy defense of free speech. *Ethics* 108(2): 312–339.

Butler, Jethro & Tom Sorell. 2022. Does libertarianism provide a justification for vaccine hesitancy? *The Political Quarterly* 93(2): 342–346.

College of Physicians of Philadelphia. 2022. *History of anti-vaccination movements*. https://cpp-hov.netlify.app/vaccines-101/misconceptions-about-vaccines/history-anti-vaccination-movements#Source-1 (Accessed 21 February 2023).

Coulson, Andrew. 1998. Trust: The foundation of public sector management. In Andrew Coulson (ed.), *Trust and contracts: Relationships in local government, health and public services*, 9–34. Bristol: The Policy Press.

Denny, Matthew J. & Arthur Spirling. 2018. Text preprocessing for unsupervised learning: Why it matters, when it misleads, and what to do about it. *Political Analysis* 26(2): 168–189.

Gagliardone, Iginio, Gal Danit, Alves Thiago & Gabriela Martinez. 2015. *Countering online hate speech*. Paris: UNESCO Publishing.

Gilson, Lucy. 2003. Trust and the development of health care as a social institution. *Social Science & Medicine* 56(7): 1453–1468.

Greyling, Talita & Stephanié Rossouw. 2022. Positive attitudes towards COVID-19 vaccines: A cross-country analysis. *PLoS ONE* 17(3): e0264994.

Grimmer, Justin, Margaret E. Roberts & Brandon M. Stewart. 2022. *Text as data*. Princeton: Princeton University Press.

Hammarlin, Mia-Marie, Fredrik Miegel, Dimitrios Kokkinakis & Jullietta Stoencheva. 2024. Fearing mRNA: A mixed methods study of vaccine rumours. In Lars Borin, Mia-Marie Hammarlin, Dimitrios Kokkinakis & Fredrik Miegel (eds.), *Vaccine hesitancy in the Nordic countries: Trust and distrust during the COVID-19 pandemic* (Chapter 10, this volume). London: Routledge.

Honneth, Axel. 1992. Integrity and disrespect: Principles of a conception of morality based on the theory of recognition. *Political Theory* 20(2): 187–201.

Honneth, Axel. 2007. *Disrespect: The normative foundations of critical theory*. Cambridge: Polity Press.

Jacobs, Thomas & Robin Tschötschel. 2019. Topic models meet discourse analysis: A quantitative tool for a qualitative approach. *International Journal of Social Research Methodology* 22(5): 469–485.

Jensen, Sune Qvotrup. 2011. Othering, identity formation and agency. *Qualitative Studies* 2(2): 63–78.

Kianzad, Behrang & Tio Minssen. 2020. Sweden's response to COVID-19: A tale of trust, recommendations, and odorous nudges. https://blog.petrieflom.law.harvard.edu/2020/05/12/sweden-global-responses-covid19/ (Accessed 21 February 2023).

Koivunen, Anu, Jari Ojala & Janne Holmén. 2021. Always in crisis, always a solution? The Nordic model as a political and scholarly concept. In Anu Koivunen, Jari Ojala & Janne Holmén (eds.), *The Nordic economic, social and political model: Challenges in the 21st century*, 1–20. London and New York: Routledge.

Lahno, Bernd. 2001. On the emotional character of trust. *Ethical Theory and Moral Practice* 4(2): 171–189.

Lindvall, Johannes & Björn Rönnerstrand. 2022. Challenges for public-service delivery: The case of COVID-19 vaccine hesitancy. *Journal of European Public Policy* 30: 2601–2622.

Liyanage, Chamila. 2020. Apocalypse now: Conspiracy theories of the radical right. In Tamir Bar-On & Bàrbara Molas (eds.), *Responses to the COVID-19 pandemic by the radical right: Scapegoating, conspiracy theories and new narratives*, 129–131. Stuttgart: ibidem Verlag.

Lyu, Joanne Chen, Eileen Le Han & Garving K. Luli. 2021. COVID-19 vaccine-related discussion on Twitter: Topic modeling and sentiment analysis. *Journal of Medical Internet Research* 23(6): e24435.

Mills, Sara. 2004. *Discourse*. London and New York: Routledge.

Mønsted, Bjarle & Sune Lehmann. 2022. Characterizing polarization in online vaccine discourse: A large-scale study. *PLoS ONE* 17(2): e0263746.

Newey, Sarah, Anne Gulland & Nicola Smith. 2021. Plague and protests: How Covid has sparked a wave of unrest around the world. *The Telegraph*. https://www.telegraph.co.uk/global-health/terror-and-security/plague-protests-pandemic-has-sparked-wave-unrest-around-world/ (Accessed 21 February 2023).

Porter, Martin F. 1980. An algorithm for suffix stripping. *Program: Electronic Library and Information Systems* 14(3): 130–137.

Roberts, Margaret E., Brandon M. Stewart, Dustin Tingley, Christopher Lucas, Jetson Leder-Luis, Shana Kushner Gadarian, Bethany Albertson & David G. Rand. 2014. Structural topic models for open ended survey responses. *American Journal of Political Science* 58(4): 1064–1082.

Roberts, Margaret, Brandon Stewart & Dustin Tingley. 2019. stm: An R package for structural topic models. *Journal of Statistical Software* 91(2): 1–40.

Rothstein, Bo. 2005. *Social traps and the problem of trust*. Cambridge: Cambridge University Press.

Rothstein, Bo & Dietlind Stolle. 2008. The state and social capital: An institutional theory of generalized trust. *Comparative Politics* 40(4): 441–459.

Schilke, Oliver, Martin Reimann & Karen S. Cook. 2021. Trust in Social Relations. *Annual Review of Sociology* 47(1): 239–259.

Shen, Shixin Cindy & Vinita Dubey. 2019. Addressing vaccine hesitancy: Clinical guidance for primary care physicians working with parents. *Canadian Family Physician | Le Médecin de famille canadien* 65(3): 175–181.

Ulsaner, Eric M. 2008. Trust as a moral value. Accessed on February 21, 2023: https://www.researchgate.net/publication/237268768_Trust_as_a_Moral_Value

12 COVID-19, the mark of the beast, and the Last Days

A study on vaccine hesitancy in Norwegian Christian charismatic movements

Tove Ingebjørg Fjell

Introduction

The world has known vaccine hesitancy as long as vaccines have been available: after the introduction of the very first vaccine against smallpox, a certain vaccine hesitancy grew internationally from the 1800s (Baldwin 1999: 274; Moseng 2003: 206; Walsø 2011). In Norway, vaccine hesitancy was communicated from different groups after the smallpox vaccine was made mandatory in 1810: vicars pointed out the extra work caused by vaccine registrations of candidates for confirmation, and doctors were worried about adverse effects like brain infection. Christians were critical towards "tampering with Creation",[1] considering cowpox vaccination meant inoculating pox from cows into human bodies – in other words, deconstructing the line between human and animal (Fjell 2005: 42–43; Schiøtz 2003: 420). In the interwar period, the Norwegian Association for Vivisection criticised the use of cowpox vaccine, claiming it was an act of cruelty to animals (Fjell 2005: 43), and in the 1950s, the Association for Animal Rights and Public Health argued the same (Schiøtz 2003: 420–421). In our time, there have been several vaccine debates, both about the swine-flu vaccine in 2009–2010 (Jansen 2018), and particularly the MMR vaccine. The best-known individual in the MMR debate is Dr Andrew Wakefield, who in 1998 published a study in *The Lancet* on a possible connection between the MMR vaccine and autism (Wakefield et al. 1998). The study was retracted, but it still lives its own life on the internet (Alver et al. 2013; Fjell 2005).[2]

Vaccine hesitancy has historically included religious and medical arguments, as well as arguments based on prevention of cruelty to animals, but these arguments are not necessarily present at the same time in the contemporary debate on corona measures. In a study on vaccine hesitancy, published pre-social media, I found medical arguments only (Fjell 2005). Post-COVID-19, religious arguments have returned to the public vaccine debate, while arguments based on animal cruelty are not found in vaccine hesitancy itself; however, they exist in COVID-19 narratives of origin – presenting the corona virus as having been developed in the endangered species, pangolins, sold in the wet markets in Wuhan (NTB 2020).

DOI: 10.4324/9781003305859-15

Today, all vaccination in Norway is voluntary (cf. Infection Control Act 1994), and the legal protection and free will of the individual is of greater importance than societal considerations. There have been times when, for example smallpox, diphtheria, or tuberculosis vaccination was mandatory (Moseng 2003; Walsø 2011); however, smallpox is now considered eradicated, and other infections are considered controlled through high vaccine coverage.[3] A high vaccine coverage implies a high level of trust in the authorities, and belief in the authorities' corona announcements. In this context, the trust is between individuals and systems, and it "becomes important when there is an implicit imbalance of power due to a high level of information asymmetry"; where "one party accepts a vulnerable position, assuming the best interests and competence of the other, in exchange for a reduction in decision complexity"; and regarding trust in vaccines, there is trust in the vaccine *product*, the *provider* of the vaccine, and in the *policymaker*, which may be government, health system, or researchers (Larson et al. 2018: 1599–1600). However, even with a high level of trust and vaccine coverage, some distrust occurs: with the identification of SARS Coronavirus 2 as the cause of COVID-19, the vaccine hesitancy debate has re-emerged.

Radical measures resulting in conflict – corona measures being an example – have the potential to create counter narratives (cf. Dyrendal & Emberland 2019: 76; Sturm & Albrecht 2020; Bodner et al. 2021): in a previous study on corona hesitancy, I analysed different counter narratives, which to varying degrees express hesitancy towards the authorities' main narratives and offer new truths about COVID-19 (Fjell 2021). I found that hesitancy does not appear from one group in particular, but from different groups. The groups that constitute the corona hesitancy are loosely compounded, with elements of alternatively oriented groups focusing on "natural immunity" and hesitancy towards scientific medicine; anti-globalists, nationalists, neo-Nazis,[4] and political parties on the far right in Norwegian politics,[5] together with Christians, as in Protestant charismatic movements. They come from different positions and find togetherness in a certain hesitancy towards authorities. The diversity is described by Carline Tromp:

> In Norway a group called Red Hats protested frequently in front of Parliament, where people like ex-fitness queen and radical feminist Kari Jaquesson, and previous AKP(m-l) profile Pål Steigan shared the stage with people selling silver water, and Pentecostalists claiming that [prime minister at the time] Erna Solberg was Satan reincarnated.
>
> (Tromp 2020: 300)[6]

This is probably the most sensational consequence of corona hesitancy – and far from a unique Norwegian phenomenon – that very different groups stand side by side in demonstrations and share one another's memes and articles on social media.

In this chapter I will analyse vaccine hesitancy expressed by individuals in Christian charismatic movements. Who are they, in the landscape of Christians in Norway? In 2022, 65% of the population were members of the Church of Norway (Statistics Norway 2022). Torkel Brekke, a historian of religion, explains the lay movements in this landscape (Brekke 2019): there is "a prominent lay movement", where the "main section … tends to be politically moderate", while "offshoots" of the Christian lay movement, literalists in their approach to the Bible, pro-Israel, and anti-socialist, "call for different politics on matters of immigration, same sex marriage, and the place of Christianity in education and in society more broadly" (Brekke 2019: 3). Brekke, who studied this part of the lay movement regarding research on Christian conspiracy theories on a Muslim takeover, refers to them as the New Christian Right. Some of the media expressions that I have studied clearly belongs in the landscape of a New Christian Right, while others are more moderate, regarding the topic of corona measures. They gather followers from, amongst others, Lutheran-evangelical revivalist and Pentecostal movements. For the sake of simplicity, when referring to them, I will use the terms "Christians" and "Christian charismatic movements".

In this chapter, I pose the following research questions: how is vaccine hesitancy expressed in these movements? To what degree are their counter narratives known from other vaccine hesitancy narratives? Why have precisely these groups taken an interest in COVID-19? The aim of the study is to present a nuanced picture of vaccine hesitancy in Christian charismatic movements. Before presenting some answers to the research questions, I will firstly explain the method, research material, and research ethical challenges, and secondly, the relevant background literature.

Method and research material

To answer the research questions, I have studied multifaceted media material. Regarding traditional media, I have searched the database *Atekst* from February 2020 until February 2022, using the search words "COVID-19" and "corona", with words like "Christian", "church", "mission", and "mark of the beast". The data set consists of 60 media items,[7] which include 42 news articles, 5 editorials, and 13 readers' letters. I have carried out a thematic analysis (cf. Braun & Clarke 2006) of media items both where the vaccine is supported, and most importantly identification of different motivations for vaccine hesitancy. Twenty-nine items, or almost half[8] of the data set, are found in the two national Christian newspapers *Vårt Land* and *Dagen*; 11 items[9] are found in local newspapers in the bible belt in the south and west of Norway, and the rest come from national media, in addition to a few regional and local papers in the east and centre of Norway.[10] In the initial coding, I organized the data into two main codes: hesitancy about and support for corona vaccination in Christian movements. After repeated reading, I found three themes: firstly, a disagreement within and between Christian charismatic movements on the question of corona vaccination; secondly, a hesitancy not unlike other corona vaccination hesitancy in society; and thirdly, a hesitancy concerned with Bible passages, in particular Revelation to John. I have further studied a few postings made by pastors on their open Facebook pages, which were referred to in the newspapers, and YouTube videos produced by members of these groups discussing the vaccine in relation to Revelation, and their comment sections.

There are some research ethical challenges: newspapers and public YouTube videos are without access restrictions. The Facebook material included has no access restrictions, and there are large numbers of "friends": "Facebook pages with thousands of members could be regarded as public, despite any technical settings indicating that the group is 'private' or only for 'friends'. The larger the group, the more public the information" (NESH 2022). Comment section participants in traditional and social media may well understand that their statements are public, though not necessarily *made public* (cf. Fjell 2010); e.g., for use in research (NESH 2022). Nevertheless, I cite two online comments, without asking consent, as I consider that no sensitive personal information is presented.

Background literature

Previous studies on international corona resistance and conspiracies, and studies on how this has influenced Christians, have helped me understand this topic.

When authorities' measures are interpreted as radical, counter narratives will be created, which to different degrees distance themselves from authorities' main narrative: such counter narratives are discussed in the study "Covid-1984" (Fjell 2021). Sometimes the distance between counter and main narrative is large and, in these cases, studies on conspiracy theories and *conspiracy talk*, the latter being conspiracies without a theory, rather testing and suggesting connections (Emberland, cited by Tromp 2020: 307; Færseth 2017), are relevant. This study will analyse conspiracy talk rather than actual theories, presented as counter narratives. The interest of individual truths, with little focus on probability, is made possible in a time of post-truth, where a hunch of how things are connected has increased in importance (cf. Larson 2020: xli; McIntyre 2017). Conspiracy talk travels fast on the internet, particularly on social media, and very different groups get inspired from and share each other's statements.

During recent years, several cultural analyses on COVID-19-related topics have been published. One example is "How vaccine rumors start – and why they don't go away" (Larson 2020), where the author discusses the spreading of vaccine rumours, the role of social media as an efficient communicator of the rumours, and the most well-known vaccine rumours that are put into circulation.[11]

American-initiated vaccine rumours, sometimes crossing the line to conspiracy talk, play a role in some of the Christian groups. Why? In an historical study of revivalism in the Norwegian bible belt, it is argued that west and south Norway have been inspired through transatlantic trade, shipping, and emigration, which has had an impact on Christians in these areas (Seland 2020: 135). Furthermore, the previous editor of the Christian newspaper *Vårt Land*, Helge Simonnes, underlines that "[t]he Norwegian relations to Christian movements in the US are extensive" and points to the large amount of American Christian literature translated to Norwegian, the number of Norwegian youth studying in Christian schools, the many American pastors visiting Free Churches, and how religion is being "souped together" with conspiracies (Simonnes 2021: 14). In a book on Trump, God, and the Church, Simonnes points out that common Christian values are thought to be under attack, and considering its severity, it becomes decisive to support politicians who claim they are Christian and work for Christian values (Simonnes 2021: 74–75). Ex-president Donald Trump was considered to have great significance on this matter and received support from Norwegian Christian movements in Norway, who are far more concerned with dissolution of norms in questions regarding, e.g., family, sexuality, and gender than the Church of Norway, or the authorities, or society in general. This points to a distance and a certain marginalization, which must be taken into consideration regarding the Christian movements' degree of trust in communication from authorities.

I do not know of any studies on vaccine hesitancy in Christian charismatic movements in Norway. However, the theologian Carolin Ahlvik-Harju has studied vaccine attitudes among Laestadians in the Pietarsaari region of Finland. She argues that low COVID-19 vaccine coverage in this area may be explained by a certain distrust of authorities, and attention towards alternative medicine, rather than explaining it by the Laestadians' belief (Langh 2021). In the following, however, I will argue that religious belief is an important element in explaining vaccine hesitancy in the Christian charismatic movements that I have studied.

No consensus

There is no consensus regarding corona measures in the Christian movements. After authorities' massive information campaigns on the importance of the vaccine, the media published articles on pastors having recommended vaccination for their members. The pastor in the *Misjonskirken Stavanger* 'Mission Church Stavanger'[12] supported vaccination publicly, and later received text threats, one claiming that he was "the evilest shepherd, and the most necessary idiot that Satan had granted their hometown" (Husebye 2021a). The pastor commented that he was fully aware that some believed the vaccine is part of the Antichrist's game, but that he disagreed. Others have previously been vaccine hesitant but have now changed their minds, one being pastor in the revival centre *Brølende Lam* 'Roaring Lamb'.[13] He toured the west coast in late 2021 and joined prophetic gatherings, with talks, song, and prayers (Dommerud et al. 2022). The pastor, being vaccine hesitant and unvaccinated, got infected, was seriously ill, and ended up in intensive care with respiratory support. After recovering, he publicly thanked the health service.

Some pastors received negative feedback on their vaccine support, while others regretted that they did not get jabbed. The media context is the many articles on Christian movements, which in the early days of the pandemic claimed that there was no coronavirus, and later advised Christians not to get jabbed. One is pastor Hanvold, head of *Visjon Norge* 'Vision Norway',[14] a TV channel of importance for Christians "preoccupied with Israel and the Last Days" (Hoel 2014: 35; Simonnes 2021: 134). Hanvold has moved between two positions: firstly, that he did not believe in the coronavirus; and secondly, to sell "medicine" to treat COVID-19. A few weeks before COVID-19 arrived in Norway, Vision Norway addressed the virus in a live broadcast and asked for donations of 2020 Norwegian kroner. The invited Venezuelan preacher (Simonnes 2021: 147, 153) used these words:

> I challenge you to cover your children with a sacrifice. I will pray for all these prayer-offerings. Every parent who watches. I challenge you, as God's prophet, to call the number on the screen. The Holy Spirit has guided me with 2020 seeds. 2020 *kroner* [NOK 2020].
>
> (Bjerkeseth & Kommandantvold 2020)

According to the national broadcaster NRK, the collection was going to provide three new production buses for live TV productions. Health politicians and parliamentary representatives called the story scandalous, unethical, and quackery. Other Christians called it "anti-Christianity" and "serious abuse of the gospel, and vulnerable people" (Bjerkeseth & Kommandantvold 2020). The pastor later claimed that he did not believe in the coronavirus: he welcomed a guest in his studio four days after lockdown in March 2020, shook hands, and said: "We who don't believe in the corona virus can shake hands" (Walnum et al. 2020). This caught attention and got criticised, but Hanvold explained that it was a joke. Shortly afterwards he was selling "Chaga extract – The Diamond of the Forest – The world's most powerful medical mushroom", presented as an infection- and virus preventative product, "important in these days" (Engebretsen 2020). Even if the word "corona" was not used in the advertisement, the Consumer Authority claimed that it concerned COVID-19, and the sales campaign resulted in a NOK 250,000[15] fine (Gilje 2020). Hanvold also brought up the topic in meetings. Early in the pandemic, he warned that the virus is built upon a lie:

> We have prayed … for this corona virus. We have prayed and prayed and prayed and prayed. Suddenly there was a breakthrough! Amen. We … kind of … hit … the nail … on the head. Amen! And we said: "Lord, *expose the lie*! … regarding corona. In the name of Jesus Christ. Amen!" Then we felt that it became obvious that this virus is built on a lie, it is built on seduction … planted … by powers and authorities. And then … when we started praying … and ffppff [searching for words] … kind of hit the nail on the head in a prayer meeting … It was Wednesday

> morning ... We felt that ... ok ... that we prayed based on a revelation. And then we felt a breakthrough ... in the Holy Spirit. Hallelujah, Thank God and praise the Lord.
>
> (video in Tufan & Engen 2020)

This video was published online and resulted in severe criticism, also from authorities, which referred to it as "suited for creating fear and uncertainty" (Tufan & Engen 2020). Hanvold underlined later that corona was not the lie, but that it was *built on* a lie, which would be revealed by himself and his congregation through prayer. The revelation implies, firstly, that corona is not God's punishment on earth, and secondly, that the virus has been planted by authorities with a certain agenda. The last matter, the virus being planted by authorities, is a well-known counter narrative presented in several other vaccine-hesitant groups.

Two years into the pandemic, there were far fewer statements on the non-existence of the virus than there were early in 2020. In advertising for corona treatments, or praying for a speedy recovery, there is an acknowledgement of the existence of the virus. However, several Christians are critical toward the vaccine, which the authorities claim is important to avoid serious illness.

Jesus fought the virus 2,000 years ago

A Baptist pastor and ambulance driver got into trouble when he, in a contribution to a newspaper, wondered how a Christian can fear a virus that Jesus fought 2,000 years ago. He claimed that it was neither Pfizer nor Moderna that gave protection, but God's son, and that protection against COVID-19 ought not to be vaccines, but "an even more unwavering trust in God's promises of health" (Bjerva 2021; Simonnes 2021: 157).[16] The pastor added that the vaccine was not based on science, a counter narrative known from several other hesitant groups. However, the counter narrative claiming that God protects against COVID-19 is unique for Christian movements, and is not shared by others.

The pastor in World Outreach Mission is also corona vaccine hesitant, but he underlines that he is far from a vaccine resistant. He has been jabbed with traditional vaccines a number of times when going on mission travels, but the mRNA vaccine is different, he says, and points to a known counter narrative, expressed in many vaccine-hesitant groups: the mRNA vaccine has not been through normal approval processes (Husebye 2021b). The preacher Pedersen, founder of *Misjonen Jesus Leger* 'Jesus Heals Ministries',[17] uses harsher words when he claims that the vaccine is poisonous and dangerous: "Don't let the poison damage your children's heart, brain, or lung" (Kåsa 2021; Staurland 2021); that the vaccine results in suffering and death; and that more have died from the vaccine than from COVID-19 (Vadla 2021). He calls the vaccine "a con syringe" (Kåsa 2021), experimental, and poisonous. These are well-known counter narratives. In a Facebook statement, he claims that he knows many who died after having been jabbed: "Women aborted, hundreds of athletes are dead after being jabbed". However, after being jabbed, if the vaccination was not fatal, there is help: "God can heal the sick, and the 'vaccine damaged', he can restart the body, and neutralize the spike protein" (Agderposten 2021). The Norwegian Institute of Public Health (NIPH) refers to Pedersen's statements as "medical false doctrines" (Husebye 2021c), and the editor of the Christian newspaper *Dagen* is quoted as saying that many will interpret these statements as a message from God, and not as "content from questionable antivax websites, read and interpreted by a layman without medical education" (Agderposten 2021). The critique against Pedersen made him later apologize, not for his statements, but for having "created a frontier among Christians" (Gustafsson 2021).

Bible passages and corona measures

Statements about medicine and health, such as healing the "vaccine damaged", or the vaccine being poisonous and therefore best being avoided, are frequent, and well-known outside of Christian charismatic movements. Less frequent, but still appearing, are references to Bible passages. In a weekend gathering, the touring preacher, Terje Johnsen, compared the corona vaccine to the scorpions in Revelation to John. He claimed that the vaccine "has the code number 060606, in other words 666"; that an ingredient is "luciferiers", named after Lucifer or Satan, and that "[i]n a substance in the vaccine is found an artificial and a living organism which stand out and may be compared to the tail of a scorpion" (Hammerstad & Husebye 2021). The preacher referred to Revelation, where locusts, strong as scorpions, were to harm "only those people who did not have the seal of God on their foreheads" (9:4), and "[t]hey had tails with stingers, like scorpions, and in their tails, they had power to torment people for five months" (9:10). He then mentioned that Bill and Melinda Gates are in favour of depopulation, echoing a well-known counter narrative, and pointed to Revelation: "Doesn't it say in Revelation that a fourth of all people are to die? This is serious" (Hammerstad & Husebye 2021). In Revelation to John, we learn about a pale horse, Death, its rider, and Hades behind him: "They were given power over a fourth of the earth, to kill by sword, famine and plague, and by the wild beasts of the earth" (6:8). The preacher paints a severe picture to his audience, and the next preacher enters the stage, addressing the mark of the beast.

Several express that they know someone who sees the vaccine as the mark of the beast, often in contrast to their own view (e.g., Husebye 2021b). The notion of the mark of the beast is taken from Revelation (13:1–18): a beast comes out of the sea, gets power from a dragon, blasphemes God, wages war against God's holy people, and gets authority over everyone. A second beast comes out of the earth, and makes everyone worship the first beast, deceives everyone, and orders them to set up and worship an image of the first beast:

> The second beast was given power to give breath to the image of the first beast, so that the image could speak and cause all who refused to worship the image to be killed. It also forced all people, great and small, rich and

> poor, free and slave, to receive a mark on their right hands or on their foreheads, so that they could not buy or sell unless they had the mark, which is the name of the beast or the number of its name.
>
> (Revelation 13:15–17)

This is not the first time during the last decades that the mark of the beast has been discussed in media. Previously, it has been connected to the introduction of the Visa card, bar codes, and the internet, and is now reintroduced in connection with the corona pandemic.

Some claim that the mark is a chip in the vaccine, that is being entered into the body in the jab process. Some believe that the mark is the corona passport, or the *Smittestopp* app.[18,19,20] Others are critical to the reintroduction of the mark of the beast. A pastor in Stavanger Mission Church says: "When they place the vaccine in a spiritual world, and say it is a sign of Antichrist's coming and dominance, I throw in the towel" (Vaarland 2021). A member of the Christian think tank *Skaperkraft* 'Creative Power' claims that the reintroduction is the result of Christians with the apocalyptic notion that the vaccine is part of the establishment of a totalitarian state (Vaarland 2021). Others connect the mark of the beast to the corona passport: pastor Reite got a vaccination appointment, but on the day of the appointment, he felt "a severe unrest", and cancelled. He thinks, along with other sceptics, that the vaccine is not well examined, and that the vaccine itself may create mutations. He continues:

> And then there is the corona passport! What on earth is that? We see already that if one cannot prove vaccinations on a mobile app, one is not allowed to travel, go to concerts etc. This is coercion! Will we sometime soon not be allowed in the supermarket without a corona passport? There are so many odd and scary things going on at the moment. And the corona passport may have a connection with the mark of the beast 666, as it says in Revelation. Nobody can buy or sell unless they have the mark of the beast.
>
> (Nordal 2021)

The pastor does not imply that the corona passport *is* the mark of the beast, but that there may be a connection. The mark of the beast is of a certain interest, and pastor Røysland in the Moria[21] congregation has published two YouTube videos addressing the topic. In the first video, titled "COVID-19 and the Mark of the Beast" (Røysland 2020),[22] published one week after lockdown in 2020, the pastor opens the talk by underlining that we live in highly prophetic times, in joyous expectation of the Last Days. The pandemic is not to be feared, it is just a warm-up round before the coming of the Last Days. Now it is important not to worship the mark of the beast, and the pastor shows on his screen what will happen to those who do:

> A third angel followed them and said in a loud voice: "If anyone worships the beast and its image and receives its mark on their forehead or on their hand, they, too, will drink the wine of God's fury, which has

> been poured full strength into the cup of his wrath. They will be tormented with burning sulfur in the presence of the holy angels and of the Lamb. And the smoke of their torment will rise for ever and ever. There will be no rest day or night for those who worship the beast and its image".
>
> (Revelation 14:9–11)

Those who worship will be lost, but not those who deny to worship, says the pastor, and shows this verse on his screen:

> I saw thrones on which were seated those who had been given authority to judge. And I saw the souls of those who had been beheaded because of their testimony about Jesus and because of the word of God. They had not worshipped the beast or its image and had not received its mark on their foreheads or their hands. They came to life and reigned with Christ a thousand years.
>
> (Revelation 20:4)

When the Antichrist arrives, he will use a system built on the number 666, and according to the pastor, this system is operative, and ready for use. The mark started off with an apparently innocent chip in the Visa card, now a chip in the mobile phone, and possibly a chip inside one's hand: older people in the United States are chipped, and so are some Swedes, he claims.

The coronavirus creates fear, which is far more dangerous than the virus, according to the pastor. Fear results in authorities setting aside rights, and thus the virus may be seen as a catalyst for launching of the mark of the beast. In critical times, like ours, humankind is pushed "a quantum leap closer to the mark of the beast", he claims.

A year later, a new video was published, titled "The Vaccine and the Mark of the Beast" (Røysland 2021).[23] The pastor received several requests after the first video, motivating him to publish a second. In the new video, smilingly, he says that the vaccine is not connected to the mark of the beast. He points to his own yellow fever passport, used on mission travels, to document that he is not a potential carrier. The pastor received several positive responses in the comment section; however, a few are not content with his video presentation. One writes: "Hello … this vaccine is not a normal vaccine!!!!! – don't you know that?" Another addresses the pastor:

> Why are you so convinced? I believe it's scary that you go all in for this. What if it is [dangerous], even if you interpret it differently!? One is that you don't believe it is [dangerous], but the truth is, that you don't know!

The comment section does not hold much in the way of resistance towards the pastor's message on the vaccine being a catalyst, and not the actual mark of the beast. But there is no consensus among Christian movements regarding this topic. Preacher Pedersen of "Jesus Heals Ministries" posts on social media:

> Soon the mark of the beast will be upon us, where nobody can buy or sell without a chip in the right hand, or forehead. But spiritually blind pastors in their "safe congregations" don't understand this. Yea-sayer preachers stay on as friends with the authorities' syringe politics.

The Moria pastor publishing the videos may be interpreted as a yea-sayer by Pedersen, as the former in 2021 does not clearly disapprove of the corona vaccine. There is no consensus either on the authorities' corona policy, on the content of the vaccine, when the Last Days are to happen, or how believers are supposed to act in the Last Days.

Conclusion

The aim of this chapter has been to grasp the nuances of Christian movements' vaccine hesitancy. The vaccine hesitant in the charismatic movements are few, but through social media, with high-speed posting and sharing on several platforms, the hesitancy becomes quite visible. The Christian counter narratives receive extra attention in traditional media and also in Christian newspapers, where the message is found to be provocative, by exposing "vulnerable" congregation members to illness, even death, by advising them to not get jabbed (cf. Bjerkeseth & Kommandantvold 2020).

There are both corona vaccine supporters and hesitants among the Christians, often in an outspoken disagreement inside and between the charismatic movements, and regarding the hesitancy, there is a wide spectrum of counter narratives performed. Some are strongly inspired by other hesitant groups, and distrust in authorities is found in counter narratives on the non-existence of the virus: that it is a lie planted by authorities, in the development of a totalitarian state; that the vaccine is experimental; that it changes DNA; that it lacks scientific basis or final approval; that one is getting chipped by the vaccine; etc. However, another type of distrust is communicated, presented in counter narratives with Bible references. An insider explains that it is easier for Christians to accept conspiracy theories, because "one lives in a cosmology, where the Last Days are central, with strong and conflicting powers. Then it's not just a question of whether to get jabbed or not, but a spiritual fight against Satan's clever plans" (Finsveen 2021). It is a question of believing and therefore trusting the Bible, rather than believing and trusting some health advice presented by authorities.

Apart from the Christian charismatic movements' obvious interest in Bible narratives, how can these movements' recognition and attention of corona measures, and distrust, be explained? Researchers point out that religious minorities, a label that fits these Christian movements in Norway, have lower trust in health care systems: "This distrust can be traced back to historical mistreatment and systematic neglect or abuse of these populations by health and governmental systems" (Larson et al. 2018: 1600). It is not fair to say however, that the Christian charismatic movements in question are either neglected or abused in Norway today. But they do find themselves in a marginalized position, with a certain distrust of, and disagreement with, liberal values and authorities' scientific medical know-how, and decades of unwanted financial attention. Together with sound knowledge of Bible narratives, and a strong belief in God's help by praying for recovery, which sometimes may contradict the authorities' health advisory, this may be a potential explanation for the great attention that these groups have paid to the coronavirus.

Notes

1 All direct quotes from research literature and sources, originally in Norwegian, are translated.
2 This presentation was published in 2005, in a study I did on vaccine support and hesitancy (Fjell 2005).
3 Norway has since the end of the 1940s a child vaccination programme, starting at 6 weeks and ending at 15 years of age (NIPH 2022a). The programme is voluntary and one of the most important individual preventative measures (Elvbakken et al. 1994). The vaccine coverage is high also regarding the COVID-19 vaccine. Per June 2022, 90.9% of over 18s have been jabbed twice with a COVID-19 vaccine (NIPH 2022b).
4 In a Swiss magazine the term "Nippies" is used, merging the words "Nazi" and "Hippie" (Stahl 2022).
5 The political parties in question are without much influence: *Alliansen* 'The Alliance', *Demokratene* 'The Democrats', and *Liberalistene* 'The Liberals'. An example of a party on the political right that appeals to some Christians, and where certain members are openly hesitant towards corona measures on social media, is *Partiet De Kristne* 'The Christians' party', which during 2022 changed their name to *Konservativt* 'Conservative'.
6 AKP(m-l) is the former Norwegian Workers' Communist Party, and part of the Marxist-Leninist movement in Norway.
7 The data corpus consists of 84 media items in total, of which 24 items regard vaccine hesitancy without mentioning Christians, or corona vaccine hesitancy among Christians outside of Norway. The 24 items are not part of my analysis, which leaves the data set with 60 media items.
8 The 29 media items, or 48%, are found in *Vårt Land* (13 news articles and 5 readers' letters) and *Dagen* (6 news articles, 4 readers' letters, and 1 editorial).
9 The 11 media pieces are 6 news articles, 4 editorials, and 1 reader's letter, found in *Agderposten*, *Lyngdals Avis*, and *Vennesla Tidende*.
10 The rest contain 20 media items, of which 17 are news articles (8 of those are published by the national broadcaster NRK), and 3 are readers' letters.
11 Some studies have analysed violent actions towards authorities, in connection with corona measures (Jolley & Paterson 2020; Sturm & Albrecht 2020). In Norway such criminal acts are primarily death threats and other threats against authorities, and secondarily some attempted break-ins at vaccine stations, and attempts to interrupt ongoing vaccination (Dagsavisen 2022; Grimstad et al. 2022).
12 Mission Church Stavanger is a member of Mission Covenant Church of Norway, which holds 91 congregations and has 10,000 members (Langhelle 2022).
13 I have not been able to find the revival centre's number of members.

14 Vision Norway is a satellite channel launched in 2003, airs 24/7, has 60 paid employees, in addition to volunteers, and partners with, amongst others, TV Vision Sweden (Vision Norway 2022). They are financed through donations.
15 NOK 250,000 is equivalent to 21,000 British pounds.
16 After massive critique, the pastor apologised. He explained that he is not antivaccination, and that he meant to say that one does not have to fear.
17 Jesus Heals Ministries was founded in 1990 by Svein Magne Pedersen, and has since 2003 sold for 230,000,000 Norwegian kroner, which is equivalent to 19,090,000 British pounds (Birkeland & Elle 2021). In 2022 Jesus Heals Ministries was on a warning list on the Norwegian Control Committee for Fundraising (Norwegian Control Committee for Fundraising 2022).
18 The *Smittestopp* app, introduced by NIPH, had to be downloaded on mobile phones. The intention was to prevent the spreading of COVID-19, by sending a message to an individual who has been in contact with an infected person for more than 15 minutes, who also had downloaded the *Smittestopp* app. The app was discontinued in August 2022.
19 See also Dag Hoel (2014: 17, 58) on political Christianity on what else may be considered as the mark of the beast.
20 Norwegians may use corona passports when travelling abroad. There have been debates on whether to introduce corona passports for use at concerts, bars, etc., but so far it has not been introduced.
21 Moria was founded in 2019, and had 70 members in 2020 (Moria Norge 2022). Moria broadcasts through *Kanal 10* 'Channel 10', which has been on the warning list of the Norwegian Control Committee for Fundraising (Birkeland & Elle 2021).
22 The 54-minute-long video was published on 20 March 2020. Viewing numbers per June 2022 were 55,505, the number of likes was 552, and there were 155 comments. The channel has over 3,000 subscribers.
23 The 45-minute-long video was published 16 April 2021 by Moria Norge. Per June 2022, the viewing number was 21,317, the number of likes was 217, and there were 135 comments.

References

Agderposten. 2021. Når vaksinemotstanden kommer fra en helbredelsespredikant er den ekstra farlig. [When vaccination resistance comes from a healing preacher, it is more dangerous.] Editor. 23 August 2021.

Åleskjær, David. 2021. Åpent brev til Svein Magne Pedersen. [Open letter to Svein Magne Pedersen.] *Dagen*. 20 August 2021.

Alver, Bente Gullveig, Tove Ingebjørg Fjell & Teemu Ryymin. 2013. *Vitenskap og varme hender: Den medisinske markedsplassen i Norge fra 1800 til i dag*. [Science and warm hands: The medical marketplace in Norway from 1800 to today.] Oslo: Scandinavian Academic Press.

Baldwin, Peter. 1999. *Contagion and the state in Europe, 1830–1930*. Cambridge: Cambridge University Press.

Birkeland, Camilla & Ingrid Elle. 2021. Kristen-TV på verstingliste. [Christian TV on the worst-of list.] *Kapital*. 28 May. https://kapital.no/reportasjer/naeringsliv/2021/05/28/7675709/kristen-tv-pa-verstingliste (27 June, 2022).

Bjerkeseth, Anders Wam & Maria Kommandantvold. 2020. Ba om penger til Visjon Norge for å bli beskyttet mot koronaviruset. [Asked for money for Vision Norway in order to be protected against the corona virus.] NRK.no. 28 February. https://www.nrk.no/osloogviken/ba-om-penger-til-visjon-norge-for-a-bli-beskyttet-mot-koronaviruset-1.14922251 (2 April, 2022)

Bjerva, Hans Petter. 2021. Bråk etter vaksineinnlegg. Risørpastor Bjørn Kristiansen i hardt vær. [Trouble after vaccination comments. Risør pastor Bjørn Kristiansen in stormy weather.] *Aust Agder Blad*. 14 January 2021.

Bodner, John, Wendy Welch, Ian Brodie, Anna Muldon, Donald Leech & Ashley Marshall. 2021. *Covid-19 conspiracy theories: Qanon, 5G, the New World Order and other viral ideas*. Jefferson: McFarland & Co.

Braun, Virginia & Victoria Clarke. 2006. Using thematic analysis in psychology. *Qualitative Research in Psychology* 3: 77–101.

Brekke, Torkel. 2019. Christianity betrayed: Conspiracy theory about a Leftist-Muslim plot against Christianity in Norway. *Journal of Religion and Society* 21: 1–15.

Dagsavisen. 2022. Vaksinemotstander anmeldt etter hærverk på teststasjon i Bergen. [Vaccine opposer reported after vandalism at test station in Bergen.] 6 January 2022.

Dommerud, Tine, Arnfinn Mauren & Tomm W. Christiansen. 2022. Pastoren havnet i koma: -Som tidligere vaksineskeptiker har jeg nå fått et annet syn. [Pastor ended up in a coma: -As a former vaccine sceptic, I now have a different view.] *Aftenposten*. 24 January 2022.

Dyrendal, Asbjørn & Terje Emberland. 2019. *Hva er konspirasjonsteorier?* [What are conspiracy theories?] Oslo: Universitetsforlaget.

Elvbakken, Kari Tove, Svanaug Fjær & Thor Øyvind Jensen. 1994. *Mellom påbud og påvirkning: Tradisjoner, institusjoner og politikk i forebyggende helsearbeid*. [Between injunction and influence: Traditions, institutions, and politics in preventative health work.] Oslo: Ad Notam.

Engebretsen, Laila Nguyen. 2020. Ville selge "virushemmende" kosttilskudd – kan få 250.000 kroner i bot. [Wanted to sell "virus-inhibiting" nutritional supplements – could be fined NOK 250,000.] NRK.no. 26 March 2020. https://www.nrk.no/osloogviken/visjon-norge-butikk-ville-selge-_virushemmende_-kosttilskudd-_-kan-fa-250.000-kroner-i-bot-1.14960636 (2 April, 2022).

Færseth, John. 2017. *KonspiraNorge*. [ConspiraNorway.] Oslo: Humanist forlag.

Finsveen, Jesper Nordahl. 2021. Kaller vaksiner 'gift': -Setter folk i livsfare. [Calls vaccines 'poison': -Puts people's lives in danger.] *Dagbladet*. 19 August, 2021.

Fjell, Tove Ingebjørg. 2005. Fri tvang eller tvingende frihet – eller begge deler? Om vaksineringspraksiser i samtids-Norge. [Free coercion or coercive freedom – or both? About vaccination practices in contemporary Norway.] *Tidsskrift for kulturforskning* 4: 41–54.

Fjell, Tove Ingebjørg. 2010. Offentliggjort, men inte offentligt? Några tankar om bruket av Internetkällor. [Published, but not public? Some thoughts on the use of Internet sources.] *Nätverket* 17: 77–82.

Fjell, Tove Ingebjørg. 2021. Covid-1984. En studie av motnarrativ om koronatiltak. [Covid-1984. A study of counter narratives about corona measures.] *Tidsskrift for kulturforskning* 1: 61–81.

Gilje, Caroline Teinum. 2020. Forbrukertilsynet gir Visjon-Norge bot på 250.000 kroner. [The Norwegian Consumer Protection Agency fines Vision Norway NOK 250,000.] *Vårt Land*. 24 April 2020.

Grimstad, Tonje, Svein Vestrum Olssonm Intisaar Ali, Fouad Acharki & Torgeir Knutsen. 2022. Vaksinemotstandere tok seg inn på vaksinesenter – målet var å stjele vaksiner. [Vaccine opponents broke into vaccine centres. The aim was to steal vaccines.] Nrk.no. 27 January 2022. https://www.nrk.no/osloogviken/vaksinemotstandere-tok-seg-inn-pa-vaksinesenter-1.15830653 (2 April 2022)

Gustafsson, Klaus. 2021. Predikant beklager 'harde ord og vendinger' i vaksinedebatt. [Preacher apologizes for 'harsh words and phrases' in vaccine debate.] *Dagen*. 24 August 2021.

Hammerstad, Bjørn Olav & Johanna Magdalena Husebye. 2021. Her advarer predikanten mot koronavaksine. [Preacher warns against the corona vaccine.] *Dagen*. 14 December 2021.

Hoel, Dag. 2014. *Armageddon Halleluja! Møter med politisk kristendom*. [Armageddon Halleluja! Encounters with political Christianity.] Oslo: Spartacus.

Husebye, Johanna Magdalena. 2021a. Fikk truende SMS da han støttet koronavaksinen. [Received threatening text message when he supported the corona vaccine.] *Dagen*. 23 July 2021.

Husebye, Johanna Magdalena. 2021b. Pastor Terje er skeptisk til koronavaksinen. [Pastor Terje is skeptical about the corona vaccine.] *Dagen*. 26 July 2021.

Husebye, Johanna Magdalena. 2021c. Forkynner vil 'rense' folk fra koronavaksinen. [Preacher will 'cleanse' people from the corona vaccine.] *Dagen*. 16 December 2021.

Infection control act. 1994. [Smittevernsloven] https://lovdata.no/dokument/NL/lov/1994-08-05-55 (9 April 2022).

Jansen, Karine Aasgaard. 2018. Å bli vaksinert, eller ikke å bli vaksinert, er det (det eneste) spørsmålet? Norske holdninger til vaksinasjon og svineinfluensapandemien i 2009 til 2010. [To be vaccinated, or not to be vaccinated, is that the (only) question? Norwegian attitudes to vaccination and the swine flu pandemic in 2009 to 2010.] *Tidsskrift for kulturforskning* 1: 73–88.

Jolley, Daniel & Jenny L. Paterson. 2020. Pylons ablaze. Examining the role of 5G COVID-19 conspiracy beliefs and support for violence. *British Journal of Social Psychology* 59: 628–640.

Kåsa, Jon Berntsen. 2021. Reagerer kraftig på FB-skriverier til predikant. [Reacts strongly to Facebook posts from preacher.] *Vennesla Tidende*. 24 August 2021.

Langh, Sara. 2021. Tidningen Läraren: Vaccinationsfrågan är mycket känslig i Larsmo. [The vaccination issue is very sensitive in Larsmo.] *Svenska Yle*. 25 September 2021. https://svenska.yle.fi/a/7-10006481 (30 June 2022)

Langhelle, Svein Ivar. 2022. Misjonskirken i Norge. [Mission Church in Norway.] Store norske leksikon. https://snl.no/Misjonskirken_i_Norge (27 June 2022).

Larson, Heidi J. 2020. *Stuck. How vaccine rumors start – and why they don`t go away*. New York: Oxford University Press.

Larson, Heidi J., Richard M. Clarke, Caitlin Jarrett, Elisabeth Eckersberger, Zachary Levine, Will S. Schultz & Pauline Paterson. 2018. Measuring trust in vaccination: A systematic review. *Human Vaccines & Immunotherapeutics* 14(2): 1599–1609.

McIntyre, Lee. 2017. *Post-truth*. London: MIT Press.

Moria Norge. 2022. About us. https://www.morianorge.no/om-oss (27 June 2022).

Moseng, Ole Georg. 2003. *Det offentlige helsevesen i Norge 1603–2003*. Bind 1 [The public health service in Norway, 1603–2003. Vol. 1]. Oslo: Universitetsforlaget.

NESH. 2022. The Norwegian national research ethics committees: A guide to internet research ethics. https://www.forskningsetikk.no/en/guidelines/social-sciences-humanities-law-and-theology/a-guide-to-internet-research-ethics/ (1 April 2022)

NIPH. 2022a. Norwegian Institute of Public Health: Childhood Immunisation Programme. https://www.fhi.no/en/id/vaccines/childhood-immunisation-programme/ (1 April 2022)

NIPH. 2022b. Norwegian Institute of Public Health: Coronavirus vaccination – statistics. https://www.fhi.no/en/id/vaccines/coronavirus-immunisation-programme/coronavirus-vaccination---statistic/#norway-number-vaccinated (27 February 2022).

Nordal, Svein. 2021. Nei til vaksine. [No to vaccine.] *Møre-Nytt*. 24 August 2021.

Norwegian Control Committee for Fundraising [Innsamlingskontrollen] 2022. About us. https://www.innsamlingskontrollen.no/about-us/ (27 June 2022).

NTB. 2020. Kinesiske forskere hevder skjelldyr kan ha spredt Wuhan-viruset. [Chinese scientists claim shellfish may have spread the Wuhan virus.] 8 February 2020. https://www.vg.no/nyheter/i/JogPO8/kinesiske-forskere-hevder-skjelldyr-kan-ha-spredt-wuhan-viruset (2 April 2022).

Røysland, Inge. 2020. Covid-19 og Dyrets Merke. [Covid-19 and the Mark of the Beast.] YouTube. 20 March 2020. https://www.youtube.com/watch?v=NFN89vwTBxI&t=33s (2 January 2022)

Røysland, Inge. 2021. Vaksinen og Dyrets Merke. [The vaccine and the Mark of the Beast.] YouTube. 16 April 2021. https://www.youtube.com/watch?v=U_hjLxFDa9w&t=1869s (2 January 2022).

Schiøtz, Aina. 2003. *Det offentlige helsevesen i Norge 1603–2003*. Bind 2 [The public health service in Norway, 1603–2003. Vol. 2]. Oslo: Universitetsforlaget.

Seland, Bjørg. 2020. The Norwegian bible belt: Geographical and cultural historical perspectives. *Historisk tidsskrift* 2: 128–143.

Simonnes, Helge. 2021. *Trump, Gud og kirken*. [Trump, God, and the church.] Oslo: Verbum.

Stahl, Antje. 2022. Darf Kunst mit den Waffen der neuen Rechten kämpfen? *Republik*. 9 March 2022.

Statistics Norway. 2022. Church of Norway. https://www.ssb.no/en/kultur-og-fritid/religion-og-livssyn/statistikk/den-norske-kirke (27 June 2022)

Staurland, Geir Magne. 2021. Går ut mot predikants vaksinemotstand. [Speaks out against preacher's vaccine opposition.] *Vårt Land*. 23 August 2021.

Sturm, Tristan & Tom Albrecht. 2020. Constituent Covid-19 apocalypses: Contagious conspiracism, 5G, and viral vaccinations. *Anthropology & Medicine* 28(1): 122–139.

Tromp, Carline. 2020. *Kulturkrig: Det nye ytre høyre og normaliseringen av det ekstreme*. [Culture war: The new far right and the normalization of the extreme.] Oslo: Cappelen.

Tufan, Øzgur & Astrid Engen. 2020. Kontroversiell TV-pastor sa at koronaviruset bygget på en løgn. [Controversial TV pastor said the corona virus was based on a lie.] NRK.no. 22 March 2020. https://www.nrk.no/norge/kontroversiell-tv-pastor-sa-at-koronaviruset-bygget-pa-en-logn-1.14956164 (2 April 2022).

Vaarland, Mattis C. O. 2021. Peker på kristne som tror at vaksinen er 'dyrets merke'. [Points to Christians who believe the vaccine is 'the mark of the beast'.] *Vårt Land*. 25 January 2021.

Vadla, Amalie. 2021. FHI: Ikke bekymret for vaksinemotstand. [NIPH: Not worried about vaccine opposition.] *Vårt Land*. 3 August 2021.

Vision Norway. 2022. About Vision Norway. https://www.visjonnorge.com/eng/about-us (27 June 2022).

Wakefield, Andrew J., S. H. Murch, A. Anthony, J. Linnell, D. M. Casson, M. Malik, M. Berelowitz, A. P. Dhillon, M. A. Thompson, P. Harvey, A. Valentine, S. E. Davies & J. A. Walker-Smith. 1998. Ileal-lymphoid-nodular hyperplasia, non-specific colitis, and pervasive developmental disorder in children. *Lancet* (RETRACTED) 358: 637–641.

Walnum, Amanda Nordhagen, Madeleine Liereng & Steinar Solås Suvatne. 2020. Beklager håndtrykk-spøk. [Sorry for the handshake joke.] *Dagbladet*. 17 March 2020.

Walsø, Vilde Christoffersen. 2011. *Fra plikt til rettighet: Tvang og frivillighet i norsk vaksinasjonslovgivning fra 1947 til 1994*. [From duty to rights: Coercion and voluntariness in Norwegian vaccination legislation from 1947 to 1994.] Master thesis. University of Bergen.

13 "Infections without properties"

Trust and cultural difference in the Norwegian public debate about minorities and COVID-19 before the vaccination

John Ødemark, Vetle Hove, Trine Krigsvoll Haagensen, and Tony Sandset

Introduction: framing COVID and culture before vaccination

In an article on COVID-19 and "ground-zero empiricism", Lorraine Daston asserted that "[t]here was no settled script for how to go about knowing" the virus and its effects and compared this situation to that of early modern science (Daston 2020). The lack of an epistemological script for studying the virus had a socio-cultural counterpart; in the liminal period before mass vaccination reinstated a kind of normalcy, there was no script for regulating social behaviour, and many old and worn cultural scripts for framing difference and danger were reemployed.

In this chapter, we examine how concepts of "culture" were used and were related to "trust" to frame the situation in Norway before the vaccination. We study this through an examination of the news coverage of COVID-19 and minority groups, and how these were presented in a selected sample of mainstream newspapers from the first lockdown in March 2020 to the beginning of the public vaccination programme in December 2020. The point of departure is an observation of what we (influenced by the strong programme in the sociology of science) will call an asymmetrical use of "culture" in the debate; i.e., "culture" is what "others" (like ethnic minorities) have. Members of the majority were mostly held individually responsible for complying with rules for social distancing. A further observation is that both the right wing and the liberal position implicitly concurred in the asymmetrical talk about culture, although the assessment of the role of culture in the spread of the disease varied widely.

The COVID-19 pandemic entailed close surveillance of infection rates, frequent updates on the epidemic situation, as well as advice and regulations from national health authorities to the populace at large. Even if everybody was affected, it is also well documented that the pandemic affected different groups in different ways. Research on health disparities have demonstrated that the pandemic hit some communities more than others (Bowleg 2020;

DOI: 10.4324/9781003305859-16

Horton 2020). A case in point would be how BAME (Black, Asian, and minority ethnic) communities in England had higher risk of COVID-19 infection and higher risk of severe disease outcome (Cheshmehzangi 2022; Sandset 2021). Similarly, in the United States, African Americans and other racialised communities were hit disproportionally at the start of the pandemic (Garcia et al. 2021; Tai et al. 2021). Linked to this has been the emergent realisation that many of the frontline workers in the healthcare sector, many of them belonging to BAME communities, were at increased risk of contracting COVID-19:

> A disproportionate number of ethnic minority NHS staff members from various socio-economic backgrounds, including hospital consultants, nurses and healthcare assistants, have died as a result of COVID-19.
>
> (Manderson et al. 2021: 115)

Thus, many of the frontline workers who died fighting COVID-19 belonged to the same groups that were blamed for spreading the virus (Bonilla-Silva 2022). The framing of COVID-19 as the "China Virus" or "Wuhan Virus" was a staple in these racist and discriminatory discourses (Hahm et al. 2021). Moreover, other discriminatory and racist tropes have also been levied at racialised and ethnic minority communities during the pandemic (Dalingwater et al. 2022; Kaur-Gill 2020), and against Muslims in Britain (Poole & Williamson 2023).

In Norway, people born in Somalia, Pakistan, Iraq, Afghanistan, and Turkey seemingly had the highest risk of infection (Indseth et al. 2021: 4). This led to a public debate about cultural factors in the spread of the virus. A leading Norwegian centre-right newspaper, *Aftenposten*, first coined the term *innvandrersmitte* 'immigrant infection' to address what the newspaper construed as an emerging problem, but rapidly retracted when they saw the commotion created by this coinage (Journalisten 2020). The term was contested both internally in the newspaper, and by interest groups, like *Unge antirasister* (*Young Anti-racists*), who challenged both health authorities and media, and observed that:

> The media has rolled out numbers and statistics. They have made lists of which districts in Oslo are "best" and "worst" and they have thrown out words such as "immigrant infection".
>
> (*Young Anti-racists*, op-ed, VG 2020a)[1]

While it was repeatedly claimed that the Norwegian success in disease control was due to a high level of trust in the authorities, the spread of COVID-19 in migrant and minority communities was often interpreted as a lack of collective, social responsibility on the part of immigrants by anti-immigration politicians (who regularly expressed distrust in social authorities themselves). In line with a much-deployed pattern of alt-right rhetoric, it was also asserted that mainstream media and establishment politicians closed their eyes to the dangers and contagions represented by immigrants (Nettavisen 2021a).

To be sure, liberal voices contested this interpretation and pointed to what we can call social and economic factors behind the spread of COVID-19 among migrants and minorities (e.g., economic factors like overcrowded housing and occupations where social distancing was impossible). This socio-economic framing was, however, challenged when *Folkehelseinstituttet* (The Norwegian Institute of Public Health, hereinafter FHI) – a Norwegian government agency dedicated to producing evidence-based health policy – in April 2021 published a report titled *COVID-19 among Persons Born Outside Norway*. The report stated that:

> Foreign-born persons as a group are significantly overrepresented among those with confirmed infection and among those admitted with COVID-19. The overrepresentation in confirmed infections and hospitalizations decreases somewhat when we adjust for age, sex, and municipality of residence, but still remains high. The overrepresentation in both confirmed infections and hospitalizations changes only to a small degree after we in addition adjust for socio-economic conditions such as income, education and overcrowding. Nor does the adjustment for medical risk between different groups affect the overrepresentation to any great degree. When we adjust for all these factors together, it has a certain effect, but the overrepresentation among foreign-born is still significant. The reasons for the overrepresentation among different parts of the immigrant population *can thus not be explained with the data we have had available in this report*. It is important to gain more knowledge about the potential causes of the overrepresentation, including any associations with lack of or delayed access to health services (including testing and contact tracing) and undetected infection in some groups.
>
> (Indseth et al. 2021: 10; our emphasis)

Thus, FHI concluded that neither socio-economic nor genetic factors explained what was called a "significant overrepresentation". We observe that the authors of the report add that the data available to them do not indicate why the socio-economic and genetic explanations fail to account for the overrepresentation. While this surely may be the case, accounting for the statistical overrepresentation can be a question not only of available data, but also of how to construe and frame the data. It is a truism in the history and philosophy of science that data are theory-laden and hence inevitably construed through preconceptions (e.g., Gilje 2019: 162–164). Therefore, the question of how to construct, frame, and interpret the data – for instance, in relation to categories such as economy, society, biology, or culture – becomes essential.

In this chapter, then, we study the use of one such framing category in the public debate. More precisely, we aim to examine how concepts of "culture" were used and were related to "trust" in the public debate about COVID-19 and ethnic minorities in Norway, i.e., in the public debate to which the report was partially a response, and into which it was "reinserted" after publication.

Our aim is both analytical and theoretical; we will examine the use of "culture" in the Norwegian public debate and rethink the conceptual aspect of relating "culture" to COVID-19 and epidemiology. Our approach is based upon an articulation of a key notion in the history and sociology of knowledge with perspectives from the political and historical critique of the culture concept in anthropology and cultural studies. We will reemploy the principle of symmetry from the so-called strong programme in the sociology of knowledge (e.g., Bloor 2001). This principle asserts that true and false beliefs – winners and losers of scientific polemics – should be dealt with using the same kind of sociological explanation. Thus, David Bloor claims that we should not

> study one side of a scientific dispute while leaving the other side unexamined because it seems right or obvious. "Symmetry" means that this equally distributed curiosity should issue in the same general kinds of sociological explanation regardless of how the knowledge is evaluated. All beliefs confront the same problems of credibility and depend on the same contingencies. True beliefs have no more intrinsic credibility than false ones.
>
> (Bloor 2001: 59)

We will investigate talk of culture and COVID-19 in Norway with reference to notions of symmetry and asymmetry. Our point of departure is an observation of the largely asymmetrical use of "culture" in the context of the pandemic. On the one hand, members of the majority were mostly held individually responsible for not complying with rules for social distancing. This then was mostly seen as a lapse of reasoning or as a moral failure. On the other hand, the perceived risk behaviour of ethnic minorities was often related to "culture", seen as a shared system of meaning and collective practice. "Culture" thus construed is what "others", like ethnic minorities, have, and as such it is opposed to the true beliefs produced by science. Used in such an epistemological sense, "culture" is a fundamental asset for making claims and beliefs epistemologically asymmetrical. An illustrating case in point is a quote from a chief physician at FHI, who, early in the pandemic, contrasted culture with science to discredit the use of masks:

> It is a cultural thing in parts of Asia that you use a lot of masks when there are various viruses such as the flu. But there is no good evidence that it has any effect.
>
> (Hanna Haug Røset, news article, VG 2020b)[2]

To be sure, there are discourses about Norwegian (majority) culture, and contexts where national culture is called upon as a cherished cultural heritage. However, customs that in other contexts and discourses are important in claims about Norwegian cultural identity and heritage, such as Christmas celebrations and Easter holidays, were rarely framed as a particularly "cultural" and collective danger for public health. The news reporting on the most likely point of entry for COVID-19 into Norway illustrates this. The virus most likely came to Norway with majority Norwegians who had been on vacations in Ischgl, a popular Austrian ski resort. FHI concluded that around 695 cases of COVID-19 could be traced back to this event, which coincides with the Norwegian Easter holiday, when Norwegians customarily go on ski holidays. Yet, this event was never framed as a part of a particular Norwegian custom and cultural tradition.

In the next section, we will present our sources and methodological approach. Next, we will turn to the analyses of the material, and what this can tell about culture and trust during the first phase of the pandemic in Norway.

Sources and methodological approaches

Sources

We have examined Norwegian news coverage of COVID-19 and minority groups, and how these groups were presented in a selected sample of mainstream newspapers. We limited the search to the period between 12 March and 27 December 2020; that is, from the start of the lockdown to the beginning of the vaccination. The lockdown and the accompanying regulation of social life were described by the government as "the strongest and most invasive measures we have had in Norway in peacetime" (regjeringen.no 2020).[3] The vaccination began on 27 December, with the vaccination of the older and vulnerable people as a kind of national media event, foreshadowing a long-awaited closure.[4] Our periodisation is thus particularly apt for this study, as the media in this liminal period with few settled scripts (cf. Daston) focused on the dangers of the virus, discussed the national and local regulations, and worried about people disregarding rules, non-compliance that could potentially harm everybody.

While debates about the pandemic played out on all media platforms, including social media, we limited our search to mainstream printed press and online newspapers with national or regional impact. In times of crisis, established mainstream media plays an important role in orchestrating and setting the agenda as well as managing the societal responsibility of the press. The Norwegian Media Authority demonstrated that COVID-19 influenced media use. According to their annual report, editor-controlled journalistic media became more important as news sources during the shutdown, an observation that indicates that people considered these outlets their main source of news in our period (The Norwegian Media Authority 2021: 65).

As our concern is the coverage of COVID-19, minority groups, culture, and trust, we selected several search terms relevant for our topic. We searched in *Retriever Atekst*, a digital database and archive which gives access to Norwegian newspapers. We selected sources from different newspapers from different parts of the country using several different search terms (including "Korona", "Innvandr*", "Etnisitet", "trangbodd", "kultur*", "tillit" ['Covid', 'Immigrant *', 'Ethnicity', 'over crowed housing', 'culture *', 'trust')].[5] The thematic criterion of relevance was that the texts discussed causal relations between infection, ethnic minorities, and culture. From the first search results, most articles were discarded due to low relevance with reference to this criterion. The discarded results also included texts containing few of the search terms, or few occurrences of the terms in the article. In addition, we aimed to gather sources from a range of newspapers, regions, and genres. Based on these criteria, we constructed a small corpus of texts which were relevant for our investigation and our analytical strategies (20 in total; see Appendix A). Of the 20 selected articles, 14 deal with non-ethnic Norwegians or migrant workers. The remaining six primarily deal with ethnic Norwegians and/or do not specify ethnicity at all. This gives what we will refer to as a surveyable presentation of the public debate (cf. Savickey 2014).

Our examination of the news coverage of COVID-19 and minority groups is a qualitative study. Our interest is in how the notion of culture was used in the public debate about minorities, culture, and COVID-19. Consequently, we take a pragmatic approach, i.e., the focus is upon the usage in our sources. It follows that the aim is not to contest usage in individual cases, but to read for a pattern in usage by relating individual statements to our overarching analytical grid; the question of cultural symmetry and/or asymmetry in majority-minority relations. To get an even better understanding of the construction of this discursive pattern, we add, in a few cases, other newspaper sources found to be particularly eloquent examples of the discussions of culture and COVID-19. In sum, it must be underscored, that our objective is to hermeneutically construct a clear depiction of a pervasive discursive pattern with implications for how we deal with culture and health, rather than a statistically adequate representation of all newspaper talk about COVID-19 in the period.[6] We do not claim that our survey is statistically representative (let's say of the frequency with which "culture" collocated with "immigrant" in relation to COVID-19 in the period). We contend, however, that the sample is representative in the sense that they demonstrate assertions that were repeatedly uttered during the pre-vaccination phase of the pandemic in Norway. Accordingly, this newspaper discourse and the public debate it expresses also forms a part of the intellectual contexts in which FHI – and others – struggled to find categories to frame and interpret their data about demography and overrepresentation.

Approach: symmetry, science studies and the critique of "culture"

Our interpretative approach is based upon a fusion of a key notion in the history and sociology of knowledge and science with the historical critique of the culture concept, and the political implications of objectifying groups of people, practices, and knowledges as culture/s. As observed, the principle of symmetry contends that all kinds of knowledge, true and false, required the same kind of sociological explanation. This is easily relatable to how different notions of "culture" distribute knowledge and practices into a universal and a local pole. On the one hand, "culture" thematises freedom and the human ability to raise above one's original circumstances, and the local culture, customs, and traditions one was born into. On the other hand, "culture" also references the structures that regulate individual behaviour and as such functions as "a handmaiden of social order" (Bauman 1999: xvi). Being "cultured" is being cosmopolitical and free to enjoy the world and its arts and sciences, while having a "culture" refer to being determined by a local pattern of thought and action, being a prisoner of custom and tradition (Bauman 1999; Rosaldo 1988).

The deployment of "culture" in the media discourse in our sources follows an asymmetrical epistemology of what culture is and how it is related to the risk of COVID-19. When "culture" collocates with terms like "immigrant" or "ethnic minority" – that is, is used as an anthropological or sociological concept, as referencing a particular form of life (not "high culture" and "being cultivated") – it also collocates with "risk" for infections, and "wild dissemination". Hence, a clear pattern of collocations is established: "culture" is used in the collective, anthropological sense and is further associated with risks for infecting majority society (cf. Baker 2011: 51–91 on collocations). Conversely, when "culture" and COVID collocate in the majority context, this generally relates not to infections but to the economy of the culture sector (the arts) during the pandemic.[7] Hence, another conceptualisation of the term "culture" (art, high culture) is in play.

In our material, "culture" thus emerges as an explanatory, accounting for why ethnic minorities have disproportionally higher rates of COVID-19 infections than ethnic Norwegians. In line with the citation of the chief physician of FHI on masking (cited earlier), "culture" here predominantly designates the opposite of true, scientifically warranted knowledge. Such a polar distribution of true knowledge and cultural belief is reminiscent of B. Latour's construal of the asymmetrical grounding of "scientific modernity", where the nature-culture distinction translates into a distinction between cultures; or rather between "scientific moderns" with access to real nature through the natural sciences and all other cultures with mere symbolic access to nature.[8] The "great Divide between Us and Them", then, is really the transposition of the asymmetrical relation between "humans and nonhumans", culture and nature, to the relation between cultures: "we have objective nature and hence true knowledge, they don't" (cf. Ødemark 2017).[9]

In the post-colonial critique of the culture concept, the relation between race and culture is also crucial. With reference to the principle of symmetry, we could say that the uses of "culture" in our material turn certain beliefs and practices into phenomena in need of a particular kind of explanation, and that the necessity of such a supplementary explanation often involves ethnic minority communities. In the context of the pandemic, this is also because certain beliefs and practices were seen as constituting risks for society. The threatened majority was construed as what D. Lloyd has called the "subject without properties" (Lloyd 1991). Lloyd sees the anthropological concept of culture as historically developed from the notion of high culture in aesthetic philosophy, and a concomitant programme for creating "disinterest" by disciplining the human body. Eighteenth-century aesthetic philosophy, Lloyd asserts, has contributed to the creation of a "subject without properties" inextricably linked to a normative construal of human development. At the highest level of both the formation of the individual and the development of humanity, only the formal representation of the physical object is relevant; aesthetic judgements are "disinterested" – and, hence, presuppose the ability of the cultivated subject to free itself from all corporal and local determinations, e.g., from local, culture.[10] The subject without properties thus constitutes a yardstick against which others have been construed as culturally different and is itself not marked by any particularistic traits such as gender, race, dialect – or by local culture (Lloyd 1991).

Culture and COVID – asymmetry and symmetry

Trust – and the culture of the majority

The lack of symmetry in talk about culture and COVID in the Norwegian public discourse often implied "black boxing" culture, making it into a "complex" and "closed" whole – where the cracks "culture" always contains, as well as the entanglements between culture and other aspects of human experience, were disregarded. As C. R. Janes shows, in the context of epidemiology and Ebola, such explanatory use of the concept amounts to "seeing culture as a thing in and of itself arising sui generis to govern social life" (Janes 2006: 261). Moreover, "culture" in this construal is "autonomous" and "explainable only via reference to the 'working out of its own internal and particularistic logic'" (Janes 2006: 261; Singer et al. 1988 cited by Janes 2006). Thus, "culture" is a form of particularity reserved for ethnic others, while "foreign" practices become hyper visible in relation to real or assumed risks of COVID-19 infections. Referencing Lloyd's idea of the "subject without properties", we can say that in the case of ethnic-majority Norwegians, their risk of infection was mostly framed as a pure medical risk disconnected from local, cultural properties, even in cases such as Ischgl, or in relation to customs otherwise strongly associated with cultural identity and heritage, like Christmas celebrations and Easter holidays. Whereas Lloyd talks about the "subject without properties", a subject that is "universal where all others are particular, partial, this Subject is the perfect, disinterested judge formed for and by the public sphere" (1991: 70), we could say that risk of COVID-19 infection when it collocates with ethnic-majority Norwegians is mostly construed as "universal" and pure biomedical risk, a risk that confronts bodies as biological entities, not as cultured and social beings. For the majority, then, culture plays no role in COVID-19 infections. Rather, their infections are "infections without properties" and thus also framed as "naturally occurring".

One cultural characteristic, however, was often applied to the majority in our corpus. Many articles reiterate the idea that the Norwegian success in disease control was due to a high level of popular trust in the authorities (Bergens

Tidende 2020; Nidaros 2020). Here, then, we have a specific cultural property associated with the majority. On this topic, the majority subject itself turns out to be a subject with properties. "Trust" is pinpointed as a social and cultural characteristic of the Norwegian, and even broader Nordic, model. When the Norwegian Academy of Sciences and Letters published a book comprising lectures held (digitally) during the first phase of the pandemic, this was entitled *Tillit i koronanes tid* [*Trust in the Time of Corona*] (Graver et al. 2020). It turns out that in the preface, the editors wished to call attention to the situation where fear erodes trust and breaks down the normal civil liberties in a liberal society. To avert this, *opplysning* 'enlightenment' and *kunnskap* 'knowledge' are enrolled to combat the (apparently irrational, populist?) fear that makes people trade their civil liberties for protection from the government (Graver et al. 2020: 8).

The preface to *Trust in the Time of Corona* makes it eminently clear the authors and editors fully identify as an elite responsible – through the propagation of reason and science – of harnessing both the populace and political authorities so that social trust and the common good can be preserved even in the liminal period of the pandemic. Trust, it is often said, is rooted in the experience of the general reliability of the authorities. In this discourse, then, we can imply that trust has to do with the singular way hierarchy is said both to manifest itself *and* abolish itself – when authorities act in a *disinterested* manner, in accordance with the procedural rules of society, and in the interest of the social whole. Since equality is another socio-cultural property regularly used to compare Norway and other Nordic countries (favourably) with other nations, it is interesting that the function of trust as an identity feature has everything to do with social hierarchy, i.e., with the hierarchical relation between those who govern and those who are governed: "We trust our elites because we're equal!"

While the academy seemed to distrust both the people and the government, our sources show the idea that the Norwegian success in disease control was due to a high level of popular trust in the authorities. Listen, for instance, to the physician Marit Dypdal Kverkild,

> The head of infection control [Kverkild] has one answer to why we Norwegians are so obedient when the State interferes with the Christmas celebration: Trust. – Without trust, people do not listen to us.[11]
>
> (N.N., interview with Marit Dypdal Kverkild, Nidaros 2020)

Hence, trust makes people willing to comply with rules of social distancing. We note that Christmas here is treated not as a cause of infection, but as part of a (normal) way of life that needs to be protected. In relation to Lloyd's idea about the "subject without properties", moreover, it is also important to note that this talk of "trust" is made in a context where – explicitly or implicitly – a relation to other societies, less characterised by trust, is involved. Consequently, these statements are mostly made in a mode of comparison, where the identity of the Norwegian culture is constructed in contrast to others:

> Norway managed what Germans, Danes, British and French have not achieved. This is how Norway stopped the virus in August.
>
> (Per Anders Johansen, news article, Stavanger Aftenblad 2020)[12]

This comparison also works inside the Nordic contexts. Turning back to Kverkild, the head of infection control cited earlier, she adds that,

> Sweden has had faith in the specialists. In Norway, we have seen this from both a health perspective and a societal perspective, i.e., both professionally, administratively and politically. We have understood that this is not only a health crisis but also a societal crisis.
>
> (N.N., interview with Marit Dypdal Kverkild, Nidaros 2020)[13]

Here, then, the notions of democracy and equality make an amicable crack in the construction of a common Nordic culture of trust, and through this foreground Norwegian equality and social solidarity.

Trust and cultural difference

While it was regularly claimed that the Norwegian success in disease control was due to a high level of popular trust in the authorities, the spread of COVID-19 in migrant and minority communities was in some cases interpreted as a lack of social responsibility, i.e., as a break of trust with the majority (Varden 2020). In contrast, members of the majority were generally held *individually* responsible for complying with, for instance, rules for social distancing. Majority Norwegians were more likely to be allowed to speak for themselves, as individuals (not as representing ethnic groups); and they were more likely to be judged as individually according to moral standards. Of the six articles dealing with infections and ethnic Norwegians, individuals identified with proper names were interviewed in two of them. This includes the article "70.000 i bøter for én fest: —De angrer" (Bergensavisen 2020).[14] People fined for violating COVID regulations are cited as repentant, and the transgressions are construed as instances of individual moral failure. In another article, students are interviewed about the high infection rates. Here, the singularised interviewees make it clear that "most young people [take] the crisis seriously" (NRK 2020a).

In contrast, individuals are allowed to speak for themselves, not for "their group", and be cited in direct speech in only 4 of the 12 articles on non-ethnic Norwegians and immigrants. In the articles where non-ethnic Norwegians and immigrants are cited directly, the position of enunciation is also mostly given to politicians or other public figures who represent minority groups. Hence, speech here goes through an instance of meditation, a spokesperson that represents a group and a certain "worldview" linked to the group to the majority culture and the political establishment (cf. Spivak 1988). A case in point is "Koronasmitte på somalsk" ["Corona infection in Somali"] where Amira Ibrahim, a Norwegian Somali, and the project manager in *Likestilling, Inkludering og Nettverk* (Equality, Inclusion and Network) addresses stereotypes about Norwegian Somalis. Ibrahim also contests the FHI report *COVID-19 among Persons Born Outside Norway*, and claims that the "official" discourse lacks a class perspective:

> The public conversation and the authorities lack focus on how socio-economic conditions and class perspectives affect the spread and effect of measures against coronary heart disease. FHI's, the government's and the public discourse's focus on country background is a derailment that overshadows these perspectives.
>
> (Amira Ibrahim, op-ed, Vårt Land, 2020)[15]

Abdi Said, a Norwegian-Somali politician representing the Socialist Left Party (SV), is also cited as a representative of a particular group on the high level of infection among Norwegian Somalis:

> Said believes that Norwegian-Somalis' culture of being social makes them particularly vulnerable to the coronavirus. – We Somalis are social, we talk, and live close together and this is not good now that one has a virus that spreads as fast as the coronavirus now does, he says.
>
> (Hans Ivar Moss Kolseth et al, news article, NRK 2020b)[16]

If we turn from the issue of linguistic representation to the question of "culture", we note a difference between Abdi Said and Amira Ibrahim. In contrast to Ibrahim, Said maintains that something that can be called culture plays a role in the uneven demography of the pandemic. Interestingly, Said's reflection on the role of culture in the pandemic involves both caring for the form of life involved ("[w]e Somalis are social, we talk, and live close together"), and despairing over the lack of "fit" between this "culture of being social" and the epidemic situation ("this is not good now that one has a virus that spreads as fast as the coronavirus"). Abdi Said thus used culture in a way that could easily and effectively have been made symmetrical. Norwegian customs connected to Christmas are also characterised by "living close together" – at least temporarily.

Purifying biocultural phenomena

In contrast to the possible symmetry found earlier, people both on the right and the left concurred in asymmetrical talk about culture, although the assessment of the role of culture in the spread of the disease varied. Particularly from the right, lacking integration was seen as a cause behind the high degree of infections in minority demographics (e.g., Aftenposten 2021a). In contrast to this, others expressed something resembling anthropology's "salvation intent"[17] to shield minorities from claimed associations between specific "cultures" and COVID-19. They did this by pinpointing:

i socio-economic factors that are culturally "neutral"; in the sense that overcrowding is universally connected to low income and inequality, not a cultural preference of certain groups, or
ii genetics and biology, which turned the infection rate into a biomedical fact.

In line with Amira Ibrahim (cited earlier), several articles see immigrants and ethnic minorities as scapegoats. At least two articles use antisemitism and the accusation of Jews for causing the plague during the Middle Ages as an analogy from history (cf. Aftenposten 2021b; VG 2020a).

Both the right and the left tended to purify phenomena, seeing them as pure nature or pure culture, not the hybrid biological and cultural phenomenon an epidemic or pandemic necessarily is. In some cases, the ethnic distribution of incidences of COVID-19 was articulated with right-wing rhetoric, and – reminiscent of Donald Trump's "China virus" – framed the pandemic as a new episode in an old cultural and civilisational war, where others are blamed for the disease that afflicts "us".[18] Negating all association between particular groups and overrepresentation (as the FHI report claimed for certain minorities) by referencing the deep cultural history of the scapegoat is, obviously, an inversion politically, but it still this remain inside the cultural domain. Both these strategies turn what we will call a hybrid bio-cultural fact (cf. Kristeva et al. 2018) into a pure social or cultural phenomenon based upon a polar logic (us vs. them), which also underplays the biological and epidemiological nature of the disease.[19] Like other infectious diseases, however, COVID-19 spreads even among social insiders and friends, on the inside of socio-cultural boundaries. Hence, epidemics also obey rules other than the social ones that regulate the traffic between insiders and outsiders, the ascriptions of identity and self-identifications that, according to F. Barth, are operative in the construction and crossing of ethnic groups and boundaries (Barth 1969; cf. Gerd Baumann 1999). Epidemiology will consequently need to consider, and translate across, both socio-cultural and biological domains, because virus transmission does not conform to a strict separation of nature/biology and culture/society.

Culture and risk

In the public discourse on ethnic minorities and the role of culture, we have identified several examples where the word "culture" is explicitly used to name an epidemiological risk factor. Take the following citation from the chief infectious disease physician in Oslo, where cultural perspectives on communal and human intimacy is seen as a factor complicating compliance with rules for social distancing:

> In Somali culture, people are much closer to each other and the messaging on social distancing can be harder to understand in the Somali group, says the chief infectious disease physician in Oslo.
>
> (Hans Ivar Moss Kolseth et al, news article, NRK 2020b)[20]

Likewise, Lars Gule, a philosopher, social scientist, and well-known media commentator, published an op-ed that singled out the cultural aspects of the spread of the coronavirus. In line with the city chief physician and Abdi Said (the Norwegian-Somali socialist politician cited earlier), Gule pinpointed that social distancing has a cultural dimension (Lars Gule, op-ed, Nettavisen 2021b).[21] Moreover, Gule also tried to distinguish between economic and cultural aspects of the phenomena:

> Overcrowding is not just about economics, but also about cultural and religious ideals associated with large families. This means that there is, so to speak, one cultural factor that to some extent predisposes to the spread of infection – or at least makes it difficult to control the spread of infection.
>
> (Lars Gule, op-ed, Nettavisen 2021b)[22]

Referencing the FHI in *COVID-19 among Persons Born Outside Norway*, he adds that

> If these findings are correct, and can be reproduced in other studies, it requires in-depth explanations. Then we must go into the cultural difference to look at what may be relevant *differences between immigrants and the rest of the Norwegian population*.
>
> (Lars Gule, op-ed, Nettavisen 2021b; our emphasis)[23]

Thus, the FHI report *COVID-19 among Persons Born Outside Norway* entered the news cycle as the point of departure for new polemics about the issue of culture and COVID. Gule's insistence on the presence of "cultural factor that to some extent predisposes to the spread of infection" does not necessarily involve singling out immigrants. In fact, he – symmetrically, we could say – points to other minority groups inside the ethnic Norwegian majority, like free churches, and to orthodox Jews in Israel as sharing the belief in a religiously ordained destiny with Muslims (Lars Gule, op-ed, Nettavisen 2021b). If such a religious idea and practices associated with it crisscross the opposition between insider and outsider, majority and minority, religions and cultures, there would be no need to associate generalised cultural properties, practices, ideologies, and attitudes with ethnonyms (Norwegian, Somali etc.). Nevertheless, the inherent power of the discourse to structure collocations in frequent patterns of association between terms appears to construct a distinction inside the Norwegian nation between immigrants and all others (cf. "relevant differences between immigrants and the rest of the Norwegian population" in the previous quotation).

A group of researchers and medical doctors led by Bushra Ishaq also challenged the focus on culture and ethnicity in the discourse on the pandemic (including in the FHI report [Aftenposten 2021c]) in an op-ed in *Aftenposten*:

> However, we call for a focus on factors other than ethnicity, culture and religion as causes of high infections among immigrants. These factors are part of what the World Health Organization defines as social health determinants, i.e., the conditions we live under in adolescence, working life and old age. They include factors such as education, occupation, income, neighbourhood and physical environment, employment and social support networks, as well as access to health services.[24]
>
> (Bushra Ishaq et al., op-ed, Aftenposten 2021b)

Ishaq and her co-authors both wanted to turn attention away from "culture" and "ethnicity" and opened for the possibility of more nuanced uses of "culture" and "religion" to understand pandemic demographics.[25] Interestingly, they also asked for a more symmetrical perspective upon culture and religion; religious phenomena should be examined across cultural and religious boundaries:

> Mosques in Oslo have been closed for a long time, without the police in Oslo reporting any violations. … Christian congregations have also been criticized for meetings with an increased risk of infection … So what is it about religion that is the explanatory variable? If there is a need for more research on covid-19 infection related to religious acts, it should be carried out across religions.[26]
>
> (Bushra Ishaq et al, op-ed, Aftenposten 2021b)

"Culture", then, should be seen not as a bounded and closed whole, a totality with borders wrapped up around social groups, but as a comparative space. If you inquire about the role of mosques, that same enquiry must also be made of the role of churches.

Concluding remarks

We have demonstrated that the use of "culture" in the media discourse in our sources generally follows an asymmetrical usage. When "culture" collocates with terms like "immigrant" or "ethnic minority", it also collocates with "risk" for infections, and "wild dissemination". Thus, a pattern of fixed collocations is established. Analytically, such marking of culture produces a subject position (immigrant) wherein culture is causally connected to COVID-19 infection, whereas for ethnic-majority Norwegians, culture is rarely used to explain infections, leaving ethnic-majority Norwegians unmarked by culture, as it were. Consequently, ethnic-majority Norwegians and their "culture" is never marked as a particular risk factor. In this matrix of culture, risk, and COVID-19, ethnic-majority Norwegians and their infections are left constructed as part of the biomedical universal risk narrative, whereas "immigrants" are marked as particularly at risk through their particular cultural practices. This creates an asymmetrical framing of culture where only "immigrants" and their culture are operationalised as a risk factor, while cultural practices of the ethnic-majority population are left unmarked.

In this discourse, immigrants and their risk of COVID-19 infection are not only framed as a marked by culture and cultural "properties", but are also discursively marked through what they lack. This is an interesting supplement to the ways in which "immigrant" culture is marked as a particular form of "having" culture, i.e., possessing a particular collective culture that puts "immigrants" at risk for infections. Discourses of lack in the material often focus on lack of language skills, lack of health literacy, and lack of trust. We should, however, note that the lack of these are noted as factors that lead to health inequities. Language barriers, low health literacy, and low levels of trust are all well-documented barriers to health care and can be seen as determinants of health. However, what is particular in our case is how "lack" is regularly framed asymmetrically as something that only immigrants have.

In contrast to this, we argue for the necessity of taking cultural factors of health and epidemiology seriously by treating culture in a symmetrical way. We cited Abdi Said's reflection on the role of culture in the pandemic involving caring for a form of life ("[w]e Somalis are social, we talk, and live close together"), and despairing over the lack of "fit" between the culture and the epidemic situation ("this is not good now that one has a virus that spreads as fast as the coronavirus"). This usage – and care for aspects of a particular form of life – could easily be made symmetrical, without reducing culture to economy or class relations, or denying the entanglements between different aspects of our life worlds.

Text corpus

Date	*Newspaper*	*Article*
2020-04-16	*Aftenposten*	Kraftig smitteøkning blant innvandrere
2020-07-19	*Avisa Nordland*	Nær én av to smittede i Norge er født i utlandet
2020-02-10	*Avisen Agder*	Skivebom av Avisen Agder
2020-11-19	*Bergensavisen*	70.000 i bøter for én fest: - de angrer
2020-12-17	*Dagsavisen*	Covid-forløp og dødelighet basert på fødeland
2020-03-17	*Fremover*	Tilliten til Erna Solberg var elendig, men etter de tørre tiltakene er tilliten på vei opp
2020-04-10	*Gjengangeren*	Koronasmitte og etnisitet – en tilslørende sammenknytning

(*Continued*)

Date	*Newspaper*	*Article*
2020-11-13	*Journalisten*	Aftenposten endret tittel om «innvandrersmitte» etter interne og eksterne reaksjoner
2020-12-26	*Khrono*	Hvem bør stå først i vaksinekøen?
2020-12-20	*Nidaros*	Festbremsen Marit: - Hadde aldri trodd det skulle gå an å bestemme så mye over folks liv
2020-04-11	*Nordlys*	Tegn på at koronasituasjonen ikke tas på alvor av alle i bransjen: - Dette er ingen selskapslek!
2020-04-01	*NRK*	Abid Said (SV) om koronasmitte blant norsk-somaliarar: - Eg synest det er trist
2020-09-11	*NRK*	Halvparten av norske unge: Burde vere forbod mot heimefestar inntil vidare
2020-11-15	*NRK*	FHI bekymret for skjult smitte blant innvandrere
2020-08-21	*Stavanger Aftenblad*	Norge klarte det tyskere, dansker, briter og franskmenn ikke har fått til. Slik stoppet Norge viruset i august
2020-03-28	*Utrop*	Norsk-somaliere tar opp kampen mot korona
2020-12-10	*Varden*	Smitten blant utenlandskfødte er alarmerende høy
2020-12-08	*VG*	Oslo-smitten nær halvert: Raymond Johansen takker Oslo-folk
2020-12-16	*VG*	"25 under 25": Smittetallene er ikke minoritetens feil
2020-04-15	*Vårt Land*	Koronasmitte på somalisk

Notes

1 The Norwegian original version of passages quoted in the text will be provided in square brackets directly in the text or in notes, as here: [Mediene har rullet ut tall og statistikk. De har laget lister over hvilke bydeler i Oslo som er 'best' og 'verst' og de har kastet fra seg ord som 'innvandrersmitte'.]

2 [Det er en kulturell greie i deler av Asia at man bruker mye munnbind når det går ulike virus som influensa. Men det er ingen gode holdepunkter for at det har noe for seg.]

3 [de sterkeste og mest inngripende tiltakene vi har hatt i Norge i fredstid]

4 The term "media event" was coined by Daniel Dayan and Elihu Katz in 1992 to describe pre-planned, scripted, and conciliatory television live broadcasted events that constitute history.

5 The sources gathered through *Retriever Atekst* include *Aftenposten*, *Avisa Nordland*, *Bergensavisen*, *Dagsavisen*, *Gjengangeren*, *Khrono*, *Nordlys*, *NRK*, *Stavanger Aftenblad*, *Utrop*, *Varden*, *VG*, *Vårt land*, *Nidaros*, *Avisen Agder*, *Fremover*, and *Journalisten*. The full list of search terms is: "korona", "covid", smitte" 'infection', "innvandrersmitte" 'migrant infection', "innvandr*" 'immigrant', "etnisitet" 'ethnicity', "minoritet" 'minority', "etnis*" 'etni*', "utenlandsfødte" 'foreignborn', "Norge" 'Norway', "norsk*" 'Norwegian*', 'nordm*" 'Norwe*', "trangbodd" 'overcrowded housing', "trang*" 'overcrowded', "kultur*" "culture", "sosial*" 'social', "Grorud" and "Bærum" and "tillit" 'trust'.

6 Cf. Greenhalgh et al. (2018) on narrative and hermeneutic reviews as supplements to the systematic review. See also Agamben (2009) on paradigms and exemplarity as methodological instruments in the humanities.

7 See for instance: https://www.presset.no/kultur/tag/korona
8 Cf. "[Latour] argues that it was not scientific thinking per se that fueled modernity but rather the construction of cultural domains of 'society' and 'science' as separate and autonomous. One the one hand, science was deemed to be not a social product but to be derived from a sphere of nature that existed apart from humans; Enlightenment thinkers viewed society, on the other hand, as constructed by humans" (Bauman & Briggs 2003: 4).
9 Cf. "In order to understand the Great Divide between Us and Them, we have to go back to that other Great Divide, between humans and nonhumans … In effect, *the first is the exportation of the second.* We Westerners cannot be one culture among others, since we also mobilize Nature. We do not mobilize an image or symbolic representation of Nature, the way other societies do, but Nature as it is, or at least as it is known to the sciences" (Latour 1993: 97; italics in the original).
10 In Kant's *Kritik der Urteilskraft*. The primitive is written at the beginning of this story, and at the bottom of the human evolutionary hierarchy, because his interest is in the lower body and sensory regions. The Iroquois and the Caribbean are attracted to strong colours they can use to paint their own bodies, Kant can tell; they are not concerned with formal reflection on the object. According to Lloyd, it is this normative narrative of human Bildung that lies behind the ideological applicability of the concept of aesthetic culture, for this thematises a liberation from sensory and bodily determination, as well as the local determination of the individual (Lloyd 1991; Ødemark 2017).
11 [Smittevernsjefen har ett svar på hvorfor vi nordmenn er så lydige når Staten legger seg borti julefeiringa: Tillitt. -Uten tillit hører ikke folk på oss.]
12 [Norge klarte det tyskere, dansker, briter og franskmenn ikke har fått til. Slik stoppet Norge viruset i august.]
13 [Sverige har hatt tro på spesialistene. I Norge har vi sett dette fra både et helseperspektiv og et samfunnsperspektiv, altså både faglig, forvaltningsmessig og politisk. Vi har tatt inn over oss at dette ikke bare er en helsekrise men også en samfunnskrise. Vi må vurdere pandemien på en helhetlig måte, sier Marit.]
14 [70,000 in fines for one party: -They regret].
15 [Den offentlige samtalen og myndighetene mangler fokus på hvordan sosioøkonomiske forhold og klasseperspektiver påvirker spredningen og effekten av tiltak mot koronasmitte. FHIs, regjeringens og den offentlige samtalens fokus på landbakgrunn er en avsporing som overskygger disse perspektivene.]
16 [Said meiner norsk-somaliarar sin kultur for å vere sosiale gjer dei særleg utsette for koronaviruset. -Vi somaliarar er sosiale, vi snakkar, og bur tett saman og det er ikkje gunstig no som ein har eit virus som spreier seg så fort som det koronaviruset no gjer, seier han.]
17 V. Argyrou asserts that anthropology is based on what he calls a wish to save "others" from cultural inferiority by postulating that what apparently is different in the final anthropological instance is the "same". "From its early stirrings in the writings of the Spanish missionaries and theologians in the sixteenth century to its inception as an academic discipline in the nineteenth to the present day, ethnological thought and practice has been deeply marked by a salvation intent. … This aim is none other than the redemption of Otherness in the eyes of its Western observers and critics. Anthropology takes it upon itself to save Others from the calumny of inferiority – whatever this presumed inferiority's historical manifestations – by striving to demonstrate that they are ultimately the same as the Self … It does not so much seek to discover the truth about them as to demonstrate what it already knows and posits as the truth" (Argyrou 2002: 28).
18 E.g. Calling COVID-19 the "Wuhan Virus" or "China Virus" is inaccurate and xenophobic (Yale School of Medicine); for Norway, e.g., Alkoholforbud hindrer ikke norske muslimer i å bruke håndsprit. Faktisk.

19 Cf. Latour (1993) on such purification processes. Characteristic of "modernity" are a sharp separation of the ontological domains of "nature" and "culture", but also the continuous processes of translation and meditation that link nature with culture/society, and thus reconnect the domains. But these translations are balanced by processes of "purification" that reestablish the borders. Together these interacting processes create "hybrids" of nature and culture that make modernity work (Latour 1993: 10–12; cf. Bauman & Briggs 2003: 4).

20 [-I somalisk kultur er folk mykje nær kvarandre og bodskapen med sosial distansering kan derfor ha vore vanskelegare å forstå I den somaliske gruppa, seier smittevernoverlegen i Oslo.]

21 Cf. "Different forms of social interaction can be important — with far greater emphasis on frequent contacts with relatives and friends. … Failure to visit relatives and friends or to reject such visits is considered unheard of, simply something one does not do. If you are socialized into such a cultural practice, this can be something that can be very difficult to change. Even when visiting relatives involves crossing national borders. And it is especially difficult to opt-out of participation in social events such as weddings and funerals" [Det å unnlate å besøke slekt og venner eller å avvise slike besøk anses for uhørt, rett og slett noe man ikke gjør. Er man sosialisert inn i en slik kulturell praksis, er det noe som kan være veldig vanskelig å endre. Selv når besøk hos slektninger innebærer å krysse landegrenser. Og spesielt vanskelig er det å unnlate deltakelse i sosiale begivenheter som bryllup og gravferder]. (Lars Gule, op-ed, Nettavisen 2021b).

22 [Trangboddhet handler ikke bare om økonomi, men også om kulturelle og religiøse idealer knyttet til store familier. Det innebærer at det så å si foreligger en kulturfaktor som i noen grad predisponerer for smittespredning – eller som i alle fall vanskeliggjør å kontrollere smittespredning.]

23 [Dersom disse funnene er riktige, og lar seg reprodusere i andre studier, krever det utdypende forklaringer. Da må vi gå inn i kulturforskjellen for å se på hva som kan være relevante *forskjeller mellom innvandrere og resten av den norske befolkningen*]

24 [Vi etterlyser imidlertid fokus på andre faktorer enn etnisitet, kultur og religion som årsaker til høy innvandrersmitte. Disse faktorene inngår i det Verdens helseorganisasjon definerer som sosiale helsedeterminanter, det vil si forholdene vi lever under i oppveksten, arbeidslivet og alderdommen. De inkluderer faktorer som utdanning, yrke, inntekt, nabolag og fysisk miljø, sysselsetting og sosiale støttenettverk, samt tilgang til helsetjenester.]

25 Cf. "In the article, we maintain, for example, culture and religion as possible additional factors in the explanation of immigrant infection. As of today, however, there is no research-based evidence showing that culture and religion are the cause of the immigrant infection." [I kronikken angir vi for eksempel kultur og religion som mulige tilleggsfaktorer i forklaringen av innvandrersmitte. Pr. i dag finnes imidlertid ingen forskningsbasert evidens for at kultur og religion er årsaken til innvandrersmitten] (Aftenposten 2021b).

26 [Moskeer i Oslo har vært stengt i lang tid, uten at politiet i Oslo har rapportert om brudd. … Også kristne forsamlinger har fått kritikk for møter med økt smitterisiko … Så hva er det med religion som er den forklarende variabel? Dersom det er behov for mer forskning på covid-19-smitte relatert til religiøse handlinger, bør det utføres på tvers av religioner.]

References

Aftenposten. 2021a. Ni ganger så høy smitte blant pakistanere. Hvorfor? 2021-04-22. https://www.aftenposten.no/meninger/kommentar/i/dlEjrz/ni-ganger-saa-hoey-smitte-blant-pakistanere-hvorfor

Aftenposten. 2021b. Hvorfor er koronasmitten så høy blant minoriteter? Vi trenger grundige analyser. 2021-04-19. https://www.aftenposten.no/meninger/kronikk/i/9Owo1W/hvorfor-er-koronasmitten-saa-hoey-blant-minoriteter-vi-trenger-grundige-analyser

Aftenposten. 2021c. Det finnes ingen forskningsbaserte beviser for at kultur og religion er årsak til smitte. 2021-05-09. https://www.aftenposten.no/meninger/debatt/i/pAz9BE/smitte-blant-innvandrere-vi-forholder-oss-i-aller-hoeyeste-grad-til-eksisterende-forskning

Agamben, Giorgio. 2009. *The signature of all things: On method*. New York: Zone Books.

Argyrou, Vassos. 2002. *Anthropology and the will to meaning. A postcolonial critique*. London: Pluto Press.

Baker, Mona. 2011. *In other words: A coursebook on translation*. 2nd edition. Abingdon: Routledge.

Barth, Fredrik. 1969. Introduction. In Fredrik Barth (ed.), *Ethnic groups and boundaries: The social organization of culture difference*, 9–38. Bergen and Oslo: Universitetsforlaget.

Bauman, Richard, & Charles L. Briggs. 2003. *Voices of modernity: Language ideologies and the politics of inequality*. Cambridge: Cambridge University Press.

Bauman, Zygmunt. 1999. *Culture as praxis*. London: Sage.

Baumann, Gerd. 1999. *The multicultural riddle: Rethinking national, ethnic, and religious identities*. New York: Routledge.

Bergensavisen. 2020. 70.000 i bøter for én fest: – De angrer. 2020-11-19. https://www.ba.no/5-8-1484125

Bloor, David. 2001. Strong program, in sociology of scientific knowledge. *International Encyclopedia of the Social & Behavioral Sciences* 15208–15210. https://doi.org/10.1016/B0-08-043076-7/03155-7

Bonilla-Silva, Eduardo. 2022. Color-blind racism in pandemic times. *Sociology of Race and Ethnicity* 8(3): 343–354. https://doi.org/10.1177/2332649220941024

Bowleg, Lisa. 2020. We're not all in this together: On COVID-19, intersectionality, and structural inequality. *American Journal of Public Health* 110(7): 917. https://doi.org/10.2105/AJPH.2020.305766

Cheshmehzangi, Ali. 2022. Vulnerability of the UK's BAME communities during COVID-19: The review of public health and socio-economic inequalities. *Journal of Human Behavior in the Social Environment* 32(2): 172–188. https://doi.org/10.1080/10911359.2021.1875949

Dalingwater, Louise, Elisabeth Mangrio, Michael Strange & Slobodan Zdravkovic. 2022. Policies on marginalized migrant communities during Covid-19: Migration management prioritized over population health. *Critical Policy Studies* July: 1–21. https://doi.org/10.1080/19460171.2022.2102046

Daston, Lorraine. 2020. Ground-zero empiricism. *Critical Inquiry* 47(52). https://doi.org/10.1086/711436

Garcia, Marc A., Patricia A. Homan, Catherine Garcia & Tyson H. Brown. 2021. The color of COVID-19: Structural racism and the disproportionate impact of the pandemic on older Black and Latinx adults. *The Journals of Gerontology. Series B, Psychological Sciences and Social Sciences* 76(3): E75–80. https://doi.org/10.1093/geronb/gbaa114

Gilje, Nils. 2019. *Hermeneutikk som metode: Ein historisk introduksjon*. Oslo: Samlaget.

Graver, Hans Petter, Øystein Hov & Tone Tønjum. 2020. *Tillit i koronaens tid*. Dreyer perspektiv 16. Oslo: Dreyers forlag.

Greenhalgh, Trisha, Sally Thorne & Kirsti Malterud. 2018. Time to challenge the spurious hierarchy of systematic over narrative reviews? *European Journal of Clinical Investigation* 48(6): e12931. https://doi.org/10.1111/eci.12931

Hahm, Hyeouk Chris, Casey D. Xavier Hall, Kana Tsurudome Garcia, Anna Cavallino, Yoonsook Ha, Yvette C. Cozier & Cindy Liu. 2021. Experiences of COVID-19-related anti-Asian discrimination and affective reactions in a multiple race sample of US young adults. *BMC Public Health* 21(1): 1563. https://doi.org/10.1186/s12889-021-11559-1

Horton, Richard. 2020. Offline: COVID-19 is not a pandemic. *The Lancet (British Edition)* 396(10255): 874. https://doi.org/10.1016/S0140-6736(20)32000-6

Indseth, Thor, Ingeborg Hess Elgersma, Bjørn Heine Strand, Kjetil Telle, Angela S. Labberton, Trude Arnesen, Karin Maria Nygård & Anna Godøy. 2021. Covid-19 among persons born outside Norway, adjusted for occupation, household crowding, medical risk group, education and income. FHI. https://www.fhi.no/en/publ/2021/Covid-19-among-persons-born-outside-Norway-adjusted/

Janes, Craig R. 2006. Commentary: "culture", cultural explanations and causality. *International Journal of Epidemiology* 35(2): 261–263. https://doi.org/10.1093/ije/dyi238

Journalisten. 2020. Aftenposten endret tittel om 'innvandrersmitte' etter interne og eksterne reaksjoner. 2020. 2020-11-13. https://journalisten.no/aftenposten-innvandring-korona/aftenposten-endret-tittel-om-innvandrersmitte-etter-interne-og-eksterne-reaksjoner/435963

Kaur-Gill, Satveer. 2020. The COVID-19 pandemic and outbreak inequality: Mainstream reporting of Singapore's migrant workers in the margins. *Frontiers in Communication* 5. https://doi.org/10.3389/fcomm.2020.00065

Kristeva, Julia, Marie Rose Moro, John Ødemark & Eivind Engebretsen. 2018. Cultural crossings of care: An appeal to the medical humanities. *Medical Humanities* 44(1): 55–58. https://doi.org/10.1136/medhum-2017-011263

Latour, Bruno. 1993. *We have never been modern*. Cambridge: Harvard University Press.

Lloyd, David. 1991. Race under representation. *Oxford Literary Review* 13(1): 62–94. https://doi.org/10.3366/olr.1991.004

Manderson, Lenore, Nancy Jean Burke & Ayo Wahlberg. 2021. *Viral loads: Anthropologies of urgency in the time of COVID-19*. Embodying inequalities: Perspectives from medical anthropology. London: UCL Press.

Nettavisen. 2021a. Jon Helgheim om koronasmitte blant innvandrere: – Har vært berøringsangst. *Nettavisen*. 2021-04-27. https://www.nettavisen.no/12-95-3424119889

Nettavisen. 2021b. Smitte i innvandrermiljøer: Religiøse og kulturelle faktorer må belyses – og kritiseres. 2021. *Nettavisen*. 21-04-2021. https://www.nettavisen.no/5-95-220431

Nidaros. 2020. Festbremsen Marit: – Hadde aldri trodd det skulle gå an å bestemme så mye over folks liv. 2020-12-20. https://www.nidaros.no/5-113-149008

NRK. 2020a. Halvparten av norske unge: Burde vere forbod mot heimefestar inntil vidare.2020-09-10.https://www.nrk.no/kultur/stor-nrk-undersoking-viser-at-ungdomen-har-koronafestvett-1.15144849

NRK. 2020b. Smittevernoverlege i Oslo: – Meir ny smitte i bydelar med mange innvandrarar. 2020-04-01. https://www.nrk.no/norge/smittevernoverlege-i-oslo_-_-meir-ny-smitte-i-bydelar-med-mange-innvandrarar-1.14968771

Ødemark, John. 2017. Interkulturell og global idéhistorie. In Ellen Krefting, Espen Schaanning & Reidar Aasgaard (eds.), *Grep om fortiden: Perspektiver og metoder i idéhistorie*, 185–206. Oslo: Cappelen Damm akademisk.

Poole, Elizabeth & Milly Williamson. 2023. Disrupting or reconfiguring racist narratives about Muslims? The representation of British Muslims during the Covid crisis". *Journalism* 24(2): 262–279. https://doi.org/10.1177/14648849211030129

Regjeringen.no. 2020. Omfattende tiltak for å bekjempe koronaviruset. *Regjeringens historiske arkiv*. (2022-12-15). https://www.regjeringen.no/no/dokuxmentarkiv/regjeringen-solberg/aktuelt-regjeringen-solberg/smk/pressemeldinger/2020/nye-tiltak/id2693327/

Rosaldo, Renato. 1988. Ideology, place, and people without culture. *Cultural Anthropology*, 3(1): 77–87.

Sandset, Tony. 2021. The necropolitics of COVID-19: Race, class and slow death in an ongoing pandemic. *Global Public Health* 16(8–9): 1411–1423. https://doi.org/10.1080/17441692.2021.1906927

Savickey, Beth. 2014. Wittgenstein and Hacker: Übersichtliche Darstellung. *Nordic Wittgenstein Review* 3(2): 99–123. https://www.nordicwittgensteinreview.com/article/view/2300

Singer, Merrill, Lani Davison & Gina Gerdes. 1988. Culture, critical theory, and reproductive illness behavior in Haiti. *Medical Anthropology Quarterly* 2(4): 370–385. https://doi.org/10.1525/maq.1988.2.4.02a00060

Spivak, Gayatri Chakravorty. 1988. Can the subaltern speak? In Cary Nelson & Lawrence Grossberg (eds.), *Marxism and the interpretation of culture*, 271–313. Urbana: University of Illinois Press.

Stavanger Aftenblad. 2020. Hun hadde ferie og sto i hagen da utbruddet kom. Slik stoppet kommunelegene 32 smitteutbrudd i august. 2020-08-31. https://www.aftenbladet.no/innenriks/i/0ne716/norge-klarte-det-tyskere-dansker-briter-og-franskmenn-ikke-har-faatt-til-slik-stoppet-vi-viruset-i-august

Tai, Don Bambino Geno, Aditya Shah, Chyke A. Doubeni, Irene G. Sia & Mark L. Wieland. 2021. The disproportionate impact of COVID-19 on racial and ethnic minorities in the United States. *Clinical Infectious Diseases* 72(4): 703–706. https://doi.org/10.1093/cid/ciaa815

The Norwegian Media Authority. 2021. *Mediemangfoldsregnskapet 2020*. Annual report. (06-12-2022). https://www.medietilsynet.no/globalassets/publikasjoner/mediemangfoldsregnskap/210129-mediemangfold_bruksperspektiv_2021.pdf

Bergens Tidende. 2020. Hun fikk Norges største utbrudd i august i fanget. 2020-08-31. https://www.bt.no/nyheter/innenriks/i/e824p9/norge-klarte-det-tyskere-dansker-briter-og-franskmenn-ikke-har-faatt-til-slik-stoppet-norge-viruset-i-august

Varden. 2020. Smitten blant utenlandskfødte er alarmerende høy. (2020-12-10). https://www.varden.no/meninger/smitten-blant-utenlandskfodte-er-alarmerende-hoy/

Vårt Land. 2020. Amira Ibrahim: 'Koronasmitte blant norsk-somaliere handler om sosiale helseforskjeller'. (2020-04-14). https://www.vl.no/meninger/verdidebatt/2020/04/14/koronasmitte-pa-somalisk/

VG. 2020a. Debatt: '25 under 25': Smittetallene er ikke minoritetenes feil. (2020-12-16). https://www.vg.no/nyheter/meninger/i/WOm54a/25-under-25-smittetallene-er-ikke-minoritetenes-feil

VG. 2020b. Mener munnbind ikke fungerer mot virus: – En kulturell greie. (2020-01-30). https://www.vg.no/i/g7O1KB

Index

Pages followed by "n" refer to notes.

MIX
Papier | Fördert gute Waldnutzung
FSC® C083411

Kolibri 360 GmbH
Ferdinand-Jühlke-Straße 7
99095 Erfurt, Deutschland
produktsicherheit@kolibri360.de